Bioethics in Search of Virtue

Bioethics in Search of Virtue

A Character-Based Approach

First Edition

Edited By James H. Joiner, Ph.D.

Northern Arizona University

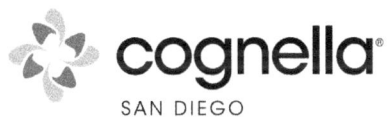

cognella®

SAN DIEGO

Bassim Hamadeh, CEO and Publisher
Craig Lincoln, Project Editor
Abbey Hastings, Senior Production Editor
Emely Villavicenio, Senior Graphic Designer
Laura Duncan, Licensing Coordinator
Natalie Piccotti, Director of Marketing
Kassie Graves, Senior Vice President, Editorial
Alia Bales, Director, Project Editorial and Production

Cover image: Copyright © 2019 iStockphoto LP/Sinhyu.

ISBN: 9781793530127

Contents

Unit III   Moral Issues   121

Unit I

Moral Theory

Consequentialism

Charles Cadwell

According to an old saying, "the road to hell is paved with good intentions." This presumes that the *consequences* of our actions are what really count in moral assessment. It doesn't matter what your intentions or motives are, the outcome is everything. If you save a drowning person, you have done the morally right thing whether you did it seeking some personal reward—a moment of fame, perhaps—or because you felt some unexplained obligation to do so, or even if you simply reacted without thinking. This is, at any rate, the consequentialist take on the matter.

Any theory that evaluates the morality of an action based solely upon outcomes is called **consequentialist**. At least three competing notions of the good give rise to consequentialist ethics.

Ethical Egoism

How does one live a good life? Look out for number one! That's the ethical egoist's answer: when you pursue your own self-interest, you maximize your chances of attaining a good life.

One motivation for subscribing to ethical egoism has been the acceptance of psychological egoism. **Psychological egoism** is a descriptive theory alleging that persons do in fact always act in their own self-interest, at least as they perceive it to be.

Without "as they perceive it to be," psychological egoism would be pretty implausible.

People often act in ways that (as any competent outsider can clearly see) are not in the actor's best interest—not even for the short run. And, of course, there are human vices, the (often habitual) actions that provide immediate pleasure or satisfaction but have adverse long-term consequences. Such actions do not promote one's true best interests. To allow for these facts, the psychological egoist must assume that persons do, upon occasion, misconceive or misunderstand what is in their best interests.

Such misconceptions create a need for ethicists to serve in, shall we say, a **therapeutic role**. If psychological egoism held true, the ethicist's appropriate job would be to help persons understand what is and is not (or would and would not be) in their best interests. Socrates and Plato seemed to have accepted psychological egoism and took exactly this tack towards ethics.

But does psychological egoism correctly describe human behavior?

Once upon a time (it is said), Abe Lincoln, riding in a carriage along a country road shortly after a heavy rain, spotted a mother pig in distress. Her piglets were unable to escape from the bottom of a roadside drainage ditch. The mud-covered banks were so slippery that the piglets tumbled to the bottom every time they tried to climb out. Lincoln ordered the carriage driver to stop, then threw his great coat on the slope, and the muddy piglets quickly scrambled up it, out of the ditch, to their mother. The carriage driver praised Lincoln for his remarkable altruism, but Lincoln would have none of it. He claimed that he had rescued the piglets purely from self-interest. Had he not done so, he said, he would have gone to bed with the images of the distressed mother and her trapped piglets in his mind and would have been unable to get a good night's sleep. As he self-interestedly desired a good night's sleep, he determined to help the piglets.

Any satisfactory descriptive theory must be **falsifiable**. That is, there must be some test by which a theoretical claim might be shown to be mistaken. The Lincoln story suggests that psychological egoism may not be falsifiable: if one wished to be dogmatic about it, one could always claim that any action whatsoever is or was done out of self-perceived self-interest, and no one could disprove this claim. Psychological egoism won't pass muster as a scientific theory.

But even without backing from a scientific theory, ethical egoism has some plausibility. **Ethical egoism** holds that one *should* act in one's self-interest. In short, the good is seen as self-interest, understood as **long-term self-interest**. Short-term or immediate self-interest too often leads to unfortunate outcomes: Overeating may satisfy my immediate interest in being nourished, but when persistently done, overeating results in obesity and cardiovascular disease. Disease is not characteristic of a good life. Self-interest, then, must be understood with a long-term perspective.

At first, the whole idea that looking out for number one will produce highly moral behavior might strike one as thoroughly implausible. Wouldn't a world full of egoists be a horrible place filled with really nasty, self-centered people? Definitely not, claim the ethical egoists. To determine what actions are in your best interests, you must consider how other persons, also looking out for themselves, will respond. If I scratch your back, you will scratch mine. If I poke you in the eye, you will poke back. Clearly, it will normally be in my long-term self-interest to treat other persons honestly and with respect. In short, ethical egoists have a direct response to the objection that their theory does not do the basic things (like resolve moral conflicts) that an ethical theory should do. They note simply that it is in their long-term self-interest to find amicable solutions to moral conflicts. Indeed, say its advocates, if you really work out the details, you will find that ethical egoism yields exactly the basic moral rules that we learn on our momma's knee.

The catch to all this is that ethical egoism tells us to follow these rules *only when it is to our long-term advantage to do so*. We should, however, break the rules whenever we can get away with it, provided only that breaking the rules would then be to our long-term advantage. This catch strikes most persons as a serious flaw in the theory. Somehow, an ethical theory that advocates breaking its own moral rules seems almost oxymoronic.

Radical Altruism

Ethical egoism is sometimes contrasted with a radical form of altruism—the unselfish concern for the welfare of others.[1] Instead of looking out for number one, radical altruism has us totally ignoring our own needs and looking out solely for the long-term best interests of others—that is, the good would be the long-term best interests of everyone *except* the actor.

Some of the moral teachings of Jesus seem to come very close to a radical altruism; I suspect, however, that there are very few if any genuine, radical altruists. For one thing, by totally ignoring their own needs, they would not long survive. A touch of altruism almost surely shows up in every viable ethical theory; radical altruism, however, takes altruism too far.

Moral Standing

When we first examined the roots of normative predicates, we observed that morality can be understood as the expression of our strongest, most precious values … the ones we are least willing to give up or change … the ones we believe apply universally among creatures having moral standing. Such universality means that two entities may receive morally different treatment only if there is a morally relevant difference between them.

There is some confusion among ethical egoists as to whether the self-interest principle is universal or not. Should each person act in his or her own long-term self-interest, or does the egoistic principle apply solely to you or to me? Would the ideal be for me to be a radical egoist and everyone else to be a radical altruist?

This last question gives a clue to what may be the most serious objection to both ethical egoism and radical altruism: both theories make a moral distinction when there is no morally relevant difference, and thus both violate universality. For any moral theory, the good *defines* the **morally relevant dimension(s)**. All creatures who are alike in this dimension thereby have like moral standing. Thus, for example, if the good is *action in accord with practical reason*, any creature capable of acting in accord with practical reason has moral standing. Universality requires that all creatures of like moral standing in like circumstances must receive like treatment. If the good is *action in accord with long-term self-interest*, then any creature with the capacity to so act based on its judgments of its long-term self-interest must be accorded the same moral standing as any other like creature. Ultimately, ethical egoism and radical altruism fail because they assign

---

1. This contrast, like that between *richest* and *poorest*, is one of extremes and is not intended to suggest that there could be nothing in between.

different moral standing to those who are selected on the basis of some criterion other than the one given by the good. Thus, ethical egoism and radical altruism divide all creatures who can act in accord with long-term self-interest into two groups: me and everybody else (or you and everybody else, if you prefer). But this is a distinction without a morally relevant difference, and so it is illegitimate.

The same point can be made about **racism** and **sexism**, for example. Unless race or gender is explicitly a moral dimension flowing from the good—whatever that good may be—different moral treatment based on differences in race or gender is illegitimate because it makes a moral distinction without a morally relevant difference.

Utilitarianism

Ethical theory remains a work in progress. As such, every theory comes in several variations, differing in detail but sharing certain common core ideas. (The common core is what makes it legitimate to apply a common name to the differing versions.) As we shall see, utilitarianism exhibits so much variation that it might better be thought of not as a single theory but rather as a family of theories bound together by agreement on the principle that *those acts are moral which produce the greatest good for the greatest number.*[2] This is called the "**principle of utility**."

To get a sense how the principle of utility works, consider this: In 1912, after having reached the South Pole (only to discover that Amundsen had beaten them by a month), Captain R. M. Scott's expedition set out on a hasty return to the safety of the coast. Unfortunately, one of Scott's explorers was injured and could travel only by being carried on a stretcher. Although knowing it would slow them dangerously, Scott decided not to abandon the man. As a result, all perished.

A utilitarian would, without hesitation, claim that Scott acted immorally. The lives of the many outweigh the life of one: Scott should have abandoned the injured man so that the rest of the expeditionary force could have survived.

Utilitarian theories tend to be ruthless in allowing absolutely no differences in treatment based upon anything other than differences that derive directly from the good. (Some regard this as utilitarianism's greatest virtue; others see it as the wellspring of its greatest flaw.) Typically, utilitarian theories are strongly universal and starkly democratic—no one counts for more or less than anyone else, but the many count for more than the one. Indeed, utilitarianism has provided a strong theoretical moral underpinning for democratic governance and for free-market economics ... and has been dominant in the formation of much public policy, most obviously policy relating to public health.

2. The clause, "for the greatest number," traces back at least to Francis Hutcheson in his *Inquiry into the Original of our Ideas of Beauty and Virtue* (1725, Treatise II, Section 3). It was repeated by Beccaria, Bentham, J. S. Mill, and a host of others up to and including the present day. Even so, many contemporary philosophers would not include it when stating the principle of utility.

Internal Problems with Utilitarianism

Utilitarians agree that the principle of utility is central to ethics, but they disagree on just about everything else. These disagreements can be grouped into four main internal problems with utilitarianism.

(1) Proponents cannot agree on what is to count as the good [3]

The most influential utilitarian theorists have probably been Jeremy Bentham (1748–1832) and John Stuart Mill (1806–1873). They advocated what is sometimes called "hedonistic" utilitarianism. The ancient hedonists contended that the only intrinsic good is stress-free pleasure. Bentham and Mill held that the ultimate motivation for all human action is the seeking of happiness—remember Aristotle?—and they identified happiness with pleasure and the avoidance of pain; hence, the good amounts to pleasure *minus* pain. Mill supported this view with a very simple, empirical argument: The only way to know that something is visible is to recognize that it is seen. Similarly, the only way to know that something is desirable is to recognize that it is desired. As all persons desire to experience pleasure and to avoid pain, pleasure without pain is desirable!

But just as different views of the good can yield wholly different theories, different views of the good within the context of the principle of utility can yield significant differences within the utilitarian family itself. Not all utilitarians accept a hedonistic hypothesis. Some contend that happiness comes only with a plurality of goods including, for example, education, the experience of beauty, freedom, health, knowledge, peace, and power. This view is an element of so-called "pluralistic" utilitarianism. Exactly which of these goods are to be included in ethical evaluations and exactly how said goods are to be balanced out has never been settled.

Some recent utilitarians, apparently sympathetic with the pluralists (but very democratically not wanting to impose any particular set of goods on anyone), have found in the economic theory of preference rankings a happy solution. Economists have shown that it is possible to rank and compare individual preferences in a quantitative way, without any necessity for consideration of the grounds for these preferences. Thus, in a sense, for these so-called "preference" utilitarians, the good is whatever is in fact most highly preferred.

Because preference can be quantitatively ranked, preference utilitarians feel they have solved the second internal problem with utilitarianism, namely,

(2) Proponents cannot agree on how to measure utility, that is, to quantify measures of goods so that the greatest good for the greatest number can be comparatively determined.

Bentham tried to produce a "calculus of pleasure" that evaluated actions as to probability of success in producing pleasure, how many would be affected, intensity of any resulting pleasure, its duration, and its fruitfulness. (Fruitfulness has to do with creating or enhancing future pleasures: if I see a movie, I might gain additional pleasure by having read the book upon which the movie is based.)

Bentham's critics, reprising the ancient hedonists' critics, charged that, pigs being as capable of pleasure as humans, utilitarianism is an ethical theory best fit for pigs. In response to this criticism, J. S. Mill

---

3. One might contend that Utilitarians do in fact agree that the good is simply to *produce the greatest good for the greatest number*. However, this won't work because utilitarians don't agree about which good is to be maximized. That lack of agreement makes the proposed statement hopelessly vague.

tried to differentiate pleasures by quality as well as by quantity. Mill contended that "a beast's pleasures do not satisfy a human being's conceptions of happiness." Mill supported this contention with a straightforward observation:

> Few human creatures would consent to be changed into any of the lower animals for the promise of the fullest allowance of a beast's pleasures; no intelligent human being would consent to be a fool, no instructed person would be an ignoramus, no person of feeling and conscience would be selfish and base, even though they should be persuaded that the fool, the dunce, or the rascal is better satisfied with his lot than they with theirs.

In short, Mill concluded in a now-famous passage, "It is better to be a human being dissatisfied than a pig satisfied; better to be Socrates dissatisfied than a fool satisfied. And if the fool, or the pig, are of a different opinion, it is because they only know one side of the question. The other party to the comparison knows both sides" (*Utilitarianism*, Chapter 2, London, 1863).

In making this move, Mill credits some persons with expertise unavailable to others and so undermines the radical-equality characteristic of Bentham's utilitarianism. No longer can we regard each and every person as an equally important judge of utility. After all, the judge might be a fool, a dunce, or a rascal.

The move also undermines the strong moral underpinning for democratic government and replaces it with a foundation for bureaucratocracy—government by bureaucrats who presumably have special expertise in deciding what is best for the people. (Mill surely did not see this consequence and would definitely not have been pleased with it.)

There is a philosophical moral here: a seemingly minor change in a theory can have major consequences. But I have gotten ahead of myself. All that needs to be concluded here is that measuring utility is no small task and remains unsolved (except perhaps, as we said, if utility is taken to be identical with preference as the economist measures it).

We can now turn to the third internal problem with utilitarianism.

(3) Proponents cannot agree on what the maxim "greatest good for the greatest number" actually means.

To explain the problem, assume we have solved the problem of assigning total happiness points not only to each person, but (by adding) to the world itself. Now consider a population of five persons, each of whom we will identify by using the letters A–E. These persons are to inhabit one of two tiny alternative worlds, with differing amounts of happiness points in each world. The happiness distribution of both worlds is recorded in the table below. The question before us is "which of these two worlds is to be preferred according to utilitarian theory?"

Happiness Distribution in Alternative Worlds I and II

Person	World I	World II
A	3	8
B	2	1
C	2	1

D	2	1
E	2	1
	==	==
total:	11	12

Notice that World II has the greater total happiness and the greater average happiness. Notice also, however, that four persons have greater happiness in World I than they would have in World II. By contrast, only one person would have greater happiness in World II than in World I. The phrase "greater [greatest] happiness for the greater [greatest] number" is ambiguous. Depending upon whether you emphasize the "greater happiness" or the "greater number," each alternative world seems to qualify as the one with the greater happiness for the greater number.

So, does the maxim require that total good be maximized? Does it require that average good be maximized? Does it require that a greater distribution of goods goes to the greatest number (even if that means lesser total good)? Or does it require something else? Utilitarians don't agree.

This brings us to a final internal problem with utilitarianism:

(4) Proponents cannot agree whether the principle of utility governs at the level of individual acts, of rules, or of codes.

Act utilitarians say that we must evaluate each act individually, comparing it with each viable alternative in order to determine which will produce the greatest good for the greatest number. Thus, for example, if I am quite sure in one specific case that telling my friend the truth about something will cause great pain, that a well chosen lie will produce joy, and that I will not be found out, I should lie. Of course, I shouldn't always lie. Sometimes I should tell the truth. It depends on the particular case. There is no strict rule on the matter of truth-telling and lies: I should do whatever will yield the greatest good for the greatest number under the specific circumstances at hand. This is act utilitarianism.

Rule utilitarians, by contrast, see morality as inherently tied to rules. (Mill himself characterized morality as "the rules and precepts for human conduct.") Rule utilitarians are appalled at some of what act utilitarianism allows. For example, a "reality" TV series where two people fight to the death would presumably be allowed by act utilitarianism because such a series would bring great pleasure to millions of viewers, the total pleasure far exceeding the pain of the participants. Rule utilitarians see act utilitarianism as producing too many cases that come out contrary to their gut instincts, and indeed, contrary to the general rules, which, when consistently followed and in comparison to alternative rules, produce, on the whole, the greatest good for the greatest number. Such rules are, according to the rule utilitarian, the standard for judging morality. (What are these rules? They are, in general, just the commonsense ethical rules that have been worked out over the centuries and that our mothers teach us when we are children.)

Act utilitarians remain unswayed by the rule utilitarians and their concerns. Act utilitarians note that blind adherence to rules can also produce horrific outcomes. In such cases, they observe, we either override the rule, basing our exception on act-utilitarian analysis, or else we modify the rule according to the details of the specific case and act-utilitarian analysis. Since act-utilitarian analysis trumps the rule, the rule itself is superfluous; only the act-utilitarian analysis matters.

Code utilitarians, also recognizing that rules have problems, are not happy with having rules selected individually, even though on utilitarian grounds. Unlike the act utilitarians, however, they suggest that the solution lies in moving "up," not "down." We must, they contend, compare entire moral codes and choose the alternative that itself, if followed uniformly, would yield the greatest good for the greatest number. Whether this can be done well enough to test, however, has yet to be seen.

Act, rule, or code? Each perspective seems to have problems that are "solved" at another level; no perspective solves all problems, and so utilitarians can't agree which perspective is best.

Sidebar: Five Cases

All of this has been pretty abstract, so let's get concrete. Here are five cases to consider. In each case, consult your intuition as to the correct moral decision. Then, work out what the various utilitarians would advise (and why). [...]

1. You are a switchman for a railroad. The switch you control directs the train either through a two-mile long, very narrow tunnel or across a trestle spanning a deep canyon with a river at the bottom. As no train is scheduled to go through the tunnel and some minor repair work needs to be done in the middle of the tunnel, a crew of ten has walked a mile inside the mountain and is working on repairs. You have switched the track to send trains across the trestle. Suddenly, you receive a panic call from the engineer of a train one mile away. The throttle is stuck and the train, with fifty souls on board, is barreling along at 60 mph. Two seconds after you receive this message, a barge hits the trestle's foundation and the trestle crashes to the bottom of the canyon. You have a choice: leave the switch as it is and send the fifty on the train plunging to their deaths in the canyon or switch the train to the tunnel, saving the fifty on the train while simultaneously causing the ten workers in the tunnel to be killed by the train. Which should you do and why?

2. Five patients with the same tissue type need organ transplants to live. One needs a heart, two need kidneys, one needs lungs, and one needs a liver. A homeless person who has no living family comes into a clinic for a free checkup. This person is healthy and has the same tissue type as those who need organs. You have a choice: harvest the healthy organs from the one and save the five or send the healthy person on her way and allow the five to die. Which should you do and why?

Consider: In both cases above, one life would be sacrificed in order to save five lives. What, if any, morally relevant differences distinguish the two cases?

3. You have befriended a certified genius who is working on a cure for cancer. She is convinced that she lacks only one piece of the puzzle—and she is correct about this. One day you bring your father to meet her. As you enter her lab, she is doing an experiment. She welcomes you but says she is right in the middle of her experiment and can't stop what she is doing. She is excited, however, because she has just realized what that missing piece is. She now has the cure! As soon as she finishes the experiment, she will write it down, and then you can talk. Your dad stands just behind her to get a better view of the experiment. Suddenly, things go horribly wrong. There is an explosion, knocking the cancer doc backwards so that she bumps heads with your dad. Both lie unconscious on the floor. Fortunately, the blow is not so severe that the doctor will forget that piece that she has just figured out. Unfortunately, there are flames everywhere and they are spreading fast. You have three options: Grab the doctor and get out of there. Grab your dad and get out of there. Just get out of there. (Once you are out, the flames will not allow you to reenter and anyone left behind will be killed in the fire.) Which should you do and why?

4. You are a night watchman at a freight transfer warehouse. The warehouse is unheated and it is the middle of winter. Leonardo da Vinci's priceless painting the *Mona Lisa* is being stored overnight pending shipment. The building has been "swept" and locked. On your 3:00 a.m. rounds, you smell smoke. You unlock the warehouse door and are horrified to see an obviously homeless person who has somehow managed to elude the sweep. He has passed out from drinking too much wine. He had built a little fire to keep warm, but once he passed out, the fire spread wildly. There are flames everywhere. You have three options: Grab the crate holding the *Mona Lisa* and get out of there. Grab the homeless fellow and get out of there. Just get out of there. (Once you are out, the flames will not allow you to reenter and the fire will destroy whatever remains.) Which should you do and why?

5. There has been a rash of technology theft on campus. Monitors, computers, DVD players, projectors, and other items are going missing. Campus security has no idea who is actually doing the thievery. However, the head cop has figured out how he can make it look like you are the thief. He presents his case to the administration officials, and they decide to build stocks in the middle of the quad. Above the stocks there is a big sign saying, "This is what happens to technology thieves at our school!" Campus security grabs you and puts you in the stocks. While you are there, the real thief wanders by and, seeing you in the stocks, decides to commit no further larceny. All technology theft stops. The head cop gets a pay raise and everyone—except you!—is happy. What does morality tell us regarding these events?

External Problems with Utilitarianism

In addition to problems raised by its advocates, utilitarianism has been subjected to "outside" criticisms from those who find utilitarian theories less than promising. We have already mentioned the objection that hedonistic utilitarianism, at least, lowers morality to the level of the beasts.

The most troublesome outside objections hit act utilitarianism the hardest, and have been one motivating force behind those who advocate rule or code utilitarianism. Of the objections raised, I will mention only three:

(1) Utilitarianism undervalues rights and justice as central moral considerations. In Case 5, for example, the person in the stocks is *innocent*, but that fact does not directly affect the utilitarian calculation.

(2) Utilitarianism undervalues obligations that arise from actions (such as promising) and from relationships (such as those with family and friends). In Case 3, for example, the utilitarian would not condone giving any preference to your father if that preference arose just because he is your father.

And an objection raised notably by Kant, not only to utilitarianism but to all consequentialist theories:

(3) We can be held morally responsible *only* for what is in our control; we can predict outcomes, but we cannot control them, hence we cannot be held morally responsible for them.[4] If, for example, I let a friend stay in my house while I am on vacation, and while he is asleep a giant sink-hole swallows up the house with my friend in it, I am surely not responsible for his death.

Whether you find these objections telling or not will largely determine whether you find utilitarianism as promising as its advocates do. After we outline the steps a utilitarian follows in analyzing a situation, we will turn to utilitarianism's main competitor, deontology. As we do, compare the strengths and weaknesses of each theory, and decide for yourself which seems most promising.

Putting Utilitarianism to Work

Confusion and objections notwithstanding, utilitarianism is widely subscribed to as the most promising approach towards finding an objective ethics. And confusions and objections notwithstanding, utilitarianism is quite intuitive in its application to real world cases. We may not have a way to assign numbers to overall good, but we can usually predict the likely outcome of two alternative actions sufficiently well so as to compare the resultant overall good. The act utilitarian response to the rule utilitarian suggests that utilitarian analysis is most interesting and fundamental at the act utilitarian level. The **steps of analysis** are roughly as follows:

> 1. Determine the relevant facts of the situation, the alternative actions (including inaction) that are possible, and identify everyone who will be in some way affected (either directly or indirectly).

---

4. This external objection generates yet another internal issue: Shall we count *actual outcomes* in moral evaluation or do we count (reasonably) *expected outcomes*? A strict consequentialist would be committed to the former, but some utilitarians argue for the latter. Purists then may charge the "expectationists" with abandoning genuine utilitarianism in favor of some unusual sort of deontology.

2. Make the best determination you can as to what outcome each action will most likely produce.

3. Evaluate these outcomes intuitively, taking into consideration everyone affected, considering intensity, duration, immediacy (or remoteness), fruitfulness, quality, and the relative importance of each of these dimensions.

4. Choose the action that most likely produces the greatest net good for the greatest number (where net good weighs bad consequences against good).

These steps may look deceptively simple: to do them well takes serious effort and considerable practice. And even after mastery, we must be ever mindful that consequentialists can never know whether they have in fact chosen rightly or wrongly until *after* the action plays itself out. The sort of utilitarian analysis sketched above gets one no more than a "best bet."

Deontology

Charles Cadwell

The word "deontology" traces back to Greek words meaning "the study of duty." Deontologists totally reject the consequentialist idea that the outcome of an act determines its morality. Deontologists contend that morality turns wholly on acts and motives, and that consequences are at best peripheral to the matter. Morality, they argue (as we shall see), is fundamentally tied to **duty**. As to exactly where duty comes from and how we find out what our duties are, there is less agreement.

Varieties

Intuitionist deontologists claim that duties—the most basic ones, at least—are self-evident or directly perceived, much as logical truths are self-evident or colors and sounds are directly perceived. The United States Declaration of Independence, which opens with an intuitionist statement regarding rights, reminds us how plausible intuitionism is. Even so, intuitionism is often challenged on the grounds that in any given situation, different persons may "perceive" different duties—duties that may conflict with or even contradict each other. Resolving such conflicts by use of intuition seems problematic, since intuition looks to be the very source of conflict. In response, intuitionists contend that the issues are in fact identical with ones regarding such things as color: persons correctly perceive color only when certain conditions are met. Disagreements about any kind of perception may arise when one or more perceivers fail to meet the relevant conditions. The real challenge is to identify the necessary conditions for accurate perception, and that is just as much a challenge for colors as for values or duties.

Contractarian deontologists contend that duty arises with agreements—sometimes formal, sometimes merely implied—and the relationships that these agreements support. One's duties to one's child, for example, are different than one's duties to a neighbor's child. In order to live in a civilized society, every member must implicitly agree to accept certain duties (and grant the corresponding rights) to others. For contractarians, the real challenge of ethical study is to discover the conditions necessary for the legitimacy of a contract, to discover the content of actual implied contracts, and to explicate any duties that they yield.

To discover the conditions necessary for legitimacy of contracts, it should be evident, one cannot turn to contractarianism itself. One must find some independent ground. Some[1] find this ground in the mathematical theory of games.[2] Most contemporary contractarians, however, find this independent ground in formalism.

Formalism

Indeed, the most generally influential deontological approach is formalist. A formalist holds that *form* is the fundamental basis of classification. In ethics, this means that the form of moral claims will determine moral right and moral wrong.

In one way, the ethical formalist is like the logical formalist. Rules of inference like *modus ponens*[3] or *modus tollens* are themselves purely formal: they have no content. But when content is introduced, the form guarantees that truth will be preserved. Ethical formalism is similar: the most basic rules of ethics have no content, but when content is introduced, the rules guarantee conformity with morality. Immanuel Kant (1724–1804) has been the most influential formalist in ethics.

Kant's Approach

Kant developed his ethical theory in three works: *Foundations of the Metaphysics of Morals* (sometimes called *Grounding for the Metaphysics of Morals*), *Critique of Practical Reason*, and *Metaphysics of Morals*. The first two lay out the theoretical foundations; the third examines problems of practical judgment in concrete situations.

In his *Foundations of the Metaphysics of Morals*, Kant contends that he has not discovered anything fundamentally new about ethics, but is merely clarifying what everyone already knows. He opens by praising what he calls "the good will."

All other faculties, Kant points out, are valuable for what they can accomplish. All other faculties can

---

1. Notably, Canadian-American philosopher David Gauthier.
2. Game theory investigates strategies by which competing "players" can optimize outcomes in accord with their own differing interests.

be used for good or evil. Only the good will can be wholly valued for itself and itself alone. Without a good will, no one would ever *deserve* happiness.

What is the will? Today, we sometimes marvel at persons whose determination and perseverance enable them to accomplish some seemingly impossible task. We say they did it "through the sheer power of their will" or "through sheer will power." That idea of will is what Kant has in mind. More precisely, Kant identifies the **will** with practical reason and explains that it is "a faculty of determining oneself to action in accordance with conception of certain laws."

The expression "determining oneself to action" somewhat awkwardly expresses the idea of autonomy (i.e., self-governance). The "certain laws," Kant tells us, are ones that can be assigned by reason alone, independent of "anthropology." Thus, in praising the good will, Kant is simply praising autonomy of the sort that can be found only among rational beings. In short, for Kant, the good is **rational autonomy**. Rational autonomy is itself intrinsically valuable, is the defining characteristic of persons, and thus is the quality that gives persons their intrinsic value.

Kant rejects the "serpent windings" of consequentialism on the grounds that one cannot be held responsible for what one cannot control. We can predict outcomes, but we cannot control them. Sometimes our most noble efforts backfire and produce only harm; sometimes our most sinister efforts backfire and benefit the target. This inability to control consequences, Kant says, means that morality cannot be tied to them. Rather, morality must be tied to what we can control, namely: motives and actions.

How, exactly, is morality tied to motives? Kant observes that acts done out of prudence or for self-gain do not seem worthy of *moral* praise. The only acts obviously deserving such praise are those that in fact go against one's own interests but are *required by duty*. To have moral worth, Kant concludes, an act must be done not only in accord with duty, but *from* duty.

Suppose an act is done from duty. It then has moral worth. But what actuates that moral worth? To understand Kant's answer, we must understand what a maxim is. A **maxim** is a (subjective) principle of action, a practical guide for volition (often expressed in a pithy form): For example, "If you want to make big money, you should go into sales," or "If you owe someone money, you must pay them back," or "Thou shalt not commit murder." For Kant, only maxims that give the motivation for our actions count as morally significant. These maxims will generally comprise some variation of the following form: "In order to achieve [specific end] in [circumstance], I will do [action]." Kantian maxims thus include purpose, but purpose differs from duty. Action, Kant contends, "derives its moral worth not from the purpose which is to be obtained by it, but from the maxim by which it is determined."

The idea is actually quite straightforward: certain principles will yield immoral actions; other principles will yield moral actions; still others will yield actions that are neither moral nor immoral. The principle of action determines the moral worth of the act it specifies.

Kant also reminds us that "duty is the necessity of acting from respect for the law." Hobbes made the same point. The only difference is that Hobbes was writing of civil duty and civil law, whereas Kant addresses moral duty and moral law.

Considering these points, Kant asks what sort of law could, while totally disregarding any of its effects, determine an unqualifiedly good will. Once all effects of the law are excluded from consideration, all that remains is universal conformity to the guiding principle of law in general. Such conformity is exemplified in a single principle: ***Act only in such a way that you could willthe maxim of your action to be a universal law.***

Kant calls this principle **the Categorical Imperative**. An imperative, as any English teacher will tell you, is a command. "Categorical" simply means without qualification—no ifs, ands, or buts. A categorical imperative may be contrasted with a hypothetical imperative, or one that poses a condition to be satisfied before the command takes effect: "If you are in the library and must speak, speak very softly," for example. Unless the condition being-in-the-library-and-finding-it-necessary-to-speak obtains, the speak-very-softly command does not apply. A categorical imperative has no such condition to satisfy.

Rational Autonomy

This very sketchy outline of Kant's introduction of the Categorical Imperative raises questions as to how one might use this principle for moral guidance. We shall turn to this matter shortly. First, however, let us more thoroughly consider the idea of rational autonomy. We can look at rational autonomy from at least two distinct perspectives. We can look at it in the abstract, and we can look at its concrete embodiment in a class of beings.

In the abstract, rational autonomy simply means governing oneself in accord with reason. To govern oneself is to create laws and act in accordance with them. To be rational, these self-created laws must conform to the dictates of reason (rather than to the dictates of emotion or prudence, for example).

A basic concept of civil law is that it shall apply universally to all who have standing as citizens. By extension, moral law must apply universally to all who have standing as moral beings. Kant's idea is really quite simple, then: All rationally autonomous beings have moral standing. Each makes self-governing laws, but each such law, if it is a *moral* law, must be such that every rationally autonomous being would willingly self-impose that same law and submit to it. It follows that an act will be moral if and only if the subjective motivating principle that governs it—that is, the maxim of the action—can rationally be generalized into an intersubjectively acceptable universal law-like statement. More particularly, if I wish to determine whether an act is moral, I must identify the maxim governing it, generalize that maxim to apply to all beings with moral status, and determine that I, as a rational person, would be willing for that generalization to be a law that I (and everyone else) must obey. Such a law will be properly understood as objective—that is, intersubjectively verifiable—because every rational autonomous being would accept it.

From the concrete perspective, we recognize that the embodiment of rational autonomy is what gives persons their great intrinsic worth: all are infinitely valuable ends in themselves. Accordingly, we can put the Categorical Imperative in a second form: ***Always treat persons, including yourself, as ends in themselves, never as a means toan end only.*** The "including yourself" emphasizes the universal character of the Categorical Imperative; the "only" emphasizes that others can become a means to our ends, but do so in accord with their own ends, and hence are not *used* in the pejorative sense of that word.

Since each form of the Categorical Imperative simply expresses rational autonomy as seen from a particular perspective, both forms really say the same thing and both can be expected to yield the same results when applied to real-world problems.

Putting Content into the Categorical Imperative

The Categorical Imperative (when viewed from either an abstract or a concrete perspective) gives us a morals-conforming pattern which itself lacks "anthropological" content. That content comes from the situations to which we apply the form as we engage in moral evaluation.

Kant observes that duties may be to ourselves or to others. He also notes that some duties are "perfect"—that is, allowing no exceptions—whereas others are "imperfect." (The meaning of "imperfect" should become clearer, shortly.) In short, there are four kinds of duties that must be considered, and we can, of course, consider each as seen from either the abstract or the concrete embodiment of the Categorical Imperative.

Let's start with the abstract perspective. Here, the Categorical Imperative tells us that we shall act only in such a way that we can will the maxim of our action to be a universal law. In short, we start with the maxim, generalize it, and then decide whether it could be willed to be law.

If it can be so generalized, any action in accord with that law is in accord with morality, that is, is morally permissible. (But remember, for Kant, action in accord with morality has moral worth only if it is *actually motivated* by the law itself.)

In applying the Categorical Imperative, it is sometimes more revealing to see what turns out to be prohibited. Consider, for example, a person who needs money. One way to get money is to borrow it. But suppose the prospective debtor knows full well that s/he will not be able to repay any loan. May s/he nevertheless borrow? To find out, we consider what maxim—what subjective motivation—could bring one to do so. I presume the maxim would be something like: "When I need money and also know that I cannot pay back any loan, I should nevertheless borrow it." Now, we must generalize this to a proposed law: Whoever needs money and knows that they cannot pay back any loan shall nevertheless borrow money.

Could a rational person will this law? Clearly not, for what would happen? Very soon, no one would lend anybody any money, and at that point it would be impossible to do as the law demands. The law would be self-contradictory in the sense that it would lead to its own destruction. Self-contradictory laws are irrational.

When a maxim leads to a self-contradictory law, action based on that maxim is forbidden and the directly opposite law presents a perfect obligation. Borrowing money only when you can pay it back (and then actually paying it back) is, therefore, a perfect obligation to others.

Here is another case: Suppose a person has some talents, but s/he is in comfortable circumstances and decides not to devote any effort to developing any of them. Is this morally acceptable? Again, we consider the motivation expressed in the form of a maxim: When I'm comfortable, I won't develop my talents. Now we generalize: No one who is in comfortable circumstances shall develop their talents. Could a rational person will such a law? This case differs notably from the one just above in that the proposed law does not in any way lead to a contradiction, so it is not irrational because it is logically flawed. Nevertheless, no rational person could will such a law.

When a maxim does not lead to its own destruction but nevertheless cannot be rationally generalized to a universal law, its direct opposite presents an imperfect obligation. Each of us has an imperfect obligation to ourselves to develop our talents. Intuitively, the obligation is imperfect, because it would be impossible to develop all our talents to the fullest. There isn't enough time. We must choose some over others.

Let's now consider a couple of cases that apply the Categorical Imperative in the form arising from the concrete embodiment of rational autonomy: *Treat persons, including yourself, always as ends in themselves and never as a means only.*

Suppose a person is depressed and contemplating suicide. Is suicide permissible? It is not. No rational person destroys that which is an end-in-itself, that which has infinite intrinsic worth. Suicide destroys the person. It is an act that uses the person as a means only (to end suffering). It is, therefore, forbidden. One has a perfect duty to oneself to live one's life. (How could you confirm that this is a perfect duty?)

Or you encounter a person who is down and out on his or her luck. Should you assist him or her? Even though down and out, the person is nevertheless a person and therefore an entity of infinite worth. And so it is indeed a duty to help others when they are in need, provided one rationally can do so. (As it would be impossible for any one person to help everyone who needs help every time help is needed, the duty to help is an imperfect one.)

Objections to Kant's Formalism

There are a number of objections commonly raised against Kant's moral theory. It is claimed, for example, that the theory

(1) is abstract and difficult to apply,

(2) excludes too many acts from the moral domain,

(3) denies moral standing to small children (and animals)—but they are people too!

(4) ignores outcomes, and

(5) provides no way of choosing among incompatible acts, each of which may conform with the Categorical Imperative.

How serious are these objections?

Let us grant that the theory is abstract and difficult to apply. So what? In physics, quantum mechanics is abstract and difficult to apply. But this fact is irrelevant to what really matters, namely, whether the theory is correct.

And what about the alleged "exclusionary" character of the theory? What is excluded? No matter what act you want to consider, the Categorical Imperative will tell you whether or not that act is in accord with what is morally permissible. Thus, it does not seem to exclude anything from the moral domain that we would expect to be included. Of course, the Categorical Imperative doesn't tell us what is in the heart of the actor. Is the actor motivated by the desire to conform to moral law? Or is the motivation prudence? The real issue is perhaps whether one buys Kant's contention that whether any particular act has moral worth depends upon what is in the actor's heart. If Kant is correct, very few ordinary acts count as *moral* acts, even though fully in accord with morality, simply because the motivation has not specifically been to fulfill a duty. Surely, however, one could choose to take a more inclusive stance and evaluate all acts simply by whether they are in accord with morality, leaving out the issue of motive.

To say that children or animals lack moral standing is only to say that they are either not at all capable of governing themselves by reason or that they have a very limited capability to do so. There is nothing surprising here: we do not hold animals in any way responsible for their actions, and we hold children responsible only to the degree that they are rational and in self-control. This limitation does not mean that we may mistreat or abuse children or animals, it only means that the reasons for not doing so must come by way of philosophical argument deriving from the Categorical Imperative rather than from the intrinsic worth of children or animals.

As for ignoring outcomes, some knowledge of outcomes clearly plays a role in the practical reasoning one uses when analyzing a proposed universal law. (Think of what you must consider to recognize that a law advocating borrowing when there is no ability to repay a debt is self-destructive.) But the real issue is probably whether we accept Kant's argument regarding what he calls the "serpent windings" of consequentialism.

The fifth objection is a serious one. If deontology in general and Kant in particular provide no way of choosing among sets of incompatible duties, each justified by the theory, deontology fails to satisfy an important theoretical desideratum. I am inclined to say that this objection can be largely answered by recognizing that the most widely known of Kant's examples tend to be simplistic ones and thereby somewhat misleading. Take the anti-suicide analysis, for example. As Kant presents the case, suicide can never be justified. But Kant also argued that capital punishment was the appropriate punishment for certain crimes and indeed was the only way to respect the rational autonomy of the person who was to be executed for having committed some heinous crime. How the maxim is cast thus turns out to be of utmost relevance. It seems to me that it would be perfectly rational to generalize the maxim that a person for whom natural death is very near, for whom there is no prospect of anything more than a delay of death, and who will suffer excruciating, unbelievable pain until freed by death, may terminate his or her life at will. You may disagree, but Kant held that the way to work this disagreement out is by philosophical argument. The question as to whether deontology can decide "hard" cases remains an open one.

Putting Deontology to Work

As with utilitarianism, deontology remains a work in progress with the sort of confusions and objections that that status implies. And as with utilitarianism, objections notwithstanding, deontology is widely regarded as the most promising approach towards finding an objective ethics. Indeed, as a practical matter, utilitarianism and deontology are the only two horses still in the race.

Taking all of the points raised above into consideration, we can suggest steps for a duty-based analysis, one with Kantian elements but differing from Kant in identifying the morally *permissible*, *obligatory*, or *forbidden* without requiring *respect for the idea of law* as *motivation*. Because deontology comes as a work in progress, we must do as we did with utilitarianism and apply the steps intuitively rather than with the strictness that a fully polished theory would allow. That being understood, here are the **steps of analysis**:

1. Determine the relevant facts of the situation, the alternative actions (including inaction) that are possible, who will be affected (either directly or indirectly) by each, and which, if any, generally recognized duty (or duties) is (or are) directly applicable.
    a. If there is no conflict among duties and no universalizable exception, these duties settle the matter.
    b. If no generally recognized duty applies, if there may be a conflict among applicable duties, or if there may be some universalizable exception to an applicable duty, continue with Step 2.
2. Determine whether the action treats persons as ends in themselves, never as a means only.
    a. If so, the action is morally permissible;[3] continue with Step 3.
    b. If not, the action is morally forbidden.
    c. If the matter of respect for persons seems not to apply, the action may fall outside of the moral domain; continue with Step 3.
3. Determine whether all persons could rationally will the maxim of the action to be a universal law.
    a. If so, the action is at least morally permissible; continue with Step 4.
    b. If not, the action is either morally forbidden or falls outside the moral domain; continue with Step 4.
4. Generalize an opposing maxim, one that leads to an opposing action.
    a. If the generalized opposing maxim yields a self-destroying practice, the morally permissible action comprises a perfect duty.
    b. If the generalized opposing maxim does not yield destruction of the practice, but still could *not* itself be willed as law, the permissible action comprises an imperfect duty.
    c. If the generalized opposing maxim could also be rationally enacted (though, perhaps, not willed) as a universal law,[4] the issue is not one of morality.

As was the case with the steps of analysis for utilitarianism, to do all this well takes serious effort and considerable practice. To further complicate things, as an alternative or supplement to these steps, one may sometimes find it advantageous to analyze a problem from the flipside by taking a rights-based perspective.

3. The notion *morally permissible* used here is a very weak one. It amounts to *not forbidden* and comprehends all manner of everyday trivialities (such as wearing a blue shirt, for example) that do not really involve morality at all.
4. If one were comfortable willing that persons always bear to the right in order to avoid head-on collisions, one should be equally comfortable with willing that persons bear to the left. There would be no irrationality in willing either instead of its alternative. Either practice would thus be morally permissible. However, one cannot rationally will *both* practices because they are mutually incompatible. Furthermore, because they are equally rational, rationality offers no preference of one over the other. Arguably, then, one cannot rationally will *either*, and so the issue is not a moral one. Of course, it is desirable to avoid head-on collisions ... but how this is to be done is fundamentally a matter of prudence, not of morality.

Rights-Based Analysis

A **right** is that which is due one or upon which one has a legitimate claim. As we have already seen, rights and duties are correlative. That is, for each right there must be a corresponding duty to deliver or provide whatever is due by that right. Similarly, for every duty there will be a corresponding right. In a sense, my rights establish others' duties, and my duties are established by others' rights. (Of course, if I have a duty to myself, the corresponding right is mine as well.)

In a rather straightforward sense, then, one can think about rights as the flipside of duties, and hence an analysis from the perspective of rights would give the flipside equivalent of a direct analysis of duties.

The correlativity of rights and duties can sometimes help us analyze a particular moral case by giving us the option of looking at the problem from either or both perspectives. Suppose that Mr. Sickman volunteers to participate in a medical trial of an experimental drug intended to arrest the progress of a serious degenerative disease. After several months, it is clear that the drug not only arrests the progress of the disease in Sickman, it actually reverses it. Unfortunately, at the same time, animal studies begin to show that the drug may have dangerous side effects in a significant percentage of those who use it. On that basis (as required by law), the pharmaceutical company terminates the trial. Sickman's degeneration resumes, and he claims that the pharmaceutical company has done him wrong by withdrawing the medication. He says he has a right to health and therefore has a right to the medication.

This may sound reasonable: people do, after all, have a right to be healthy. Or do they? Let us look at this matter from a different perspective. Who is the alleged right to health a right against? That is, who has a duty to provide health? The answer is that no one does because no one can. Health is a condition, not a right. Sickman confuses his strong desire with a right.

Some persons have thought that rights are easier to figure out than duties, and consequently, that we can understand duties better by approaching moral problems from the perspective of rights. However, a comprehensive discussion of the rights theories that are actively in play today is beyond the intended scope of the present work. We'll be happy enough to master the duty perspective.

Applications

Charles Cadwell

Solving Moral Dilemmas

How does one live a good life? We have been trying to understand where the fundamental question of ethics leads us. We have rejected some proposed answers and have found merit in others. We have not yet, however, discovered an ethical theory that everybody accepts as the true foundation of morality. We have, nevertheless, identified two "families" of theories, utilitarian and deontological, that seem to show the most promise for eventually providing a universally recognized, solid foundation upon which we might justify particular claims in normative ethics.

Where, then, does our examination of ethical theory leave us in terms of **practical decision making**? If we can't decide what moral theory is the correct one, what are we to do when we are faced with an ethical dilemma? How can we decide what is morally right and what is morally wrong? Can we find common ground?

Prima Facie Duties

One idea that may achieve this end can be linked to a duty-based analysis that originated with Scottish philosopher **W. D. Ross** (1877–1971) in 1930.[1] Ross saw that some duties—don't murder, tell the truth, help folks out if you can at reasonable cost to you, for example—are commonly recognized as binding so long as no other generally binding duty is in conflict. (These are roughly the sorts of duties that we mentioned in the first step of a Kantian-style deontological analysis.) Ross called such duties **prima facie duties**. (*Prima facie* is Latin for "at first view.") To figure out what duty calls for in any situation where prima facie duties conflict, we must start with philosophical argument to evaluate the relative importance of each duty in the particular situation.

Now, here is an interesting idea: Some thinkers have suggested that "produce the greatest good for the greatest number affected by an action" is a prima facie duty. If so, the notion of prima facie duties can be used to bring utilitarian considerations into a fundamentally deontological approach, giving us a sort of mixed theory. Some thinkers believe that doing so can resolve the seemingly impenetrable barrier between the two families of theories, eliminate the objections particular to each approach as it stands on its own, and give us a way to resolve any moral issue. One problem with this plan may be that it does not provide a clear way to rank obligations when they conflict with each other. Presumably, this ranking must be accomplished by use of philosophical argument, but philosophical argument based upon what?

Prima Facie Principles

Here is an alternative: We have pretty much narrowed the ethical field to two "teams," the deontological (including both duty-based and rights-based analysis) and the utilitarian. If both teams give us the same moral advice in a particular case, we can be pretty sure that that advice is morally warranted, even if we aren't exactly sure what the true nature of that warrant may be. In other words, if we analyze a particular moral problem from both a deontological and a utilitarian perspective, and if each theory yields the same answer, that answer will be the common-ground answer we need.

Of course, going all the way back to the good or any other fundamental theoretical foundation will be a lot of work. Would it be possible to simplify the job by extracting some general principles that flow from *both* utilitarianism and deontology? Taking a hint from Ross, we might call these **prima facie principles**. These would be principles that we could regularly turn to as our primary instrument for moral analysis.

As it happens, there seem to be four such basic moral principles that nearly all moral theories—not just the deontological and utilitarian—support. These prima facie principles focus upon autonomy, nonmaleficence, beneficence, and justice.[2]

---

1. In *The Right and the Good*.
2. Some would add veracity (truth telling), fidelity (promise keeping), and perhaps other duties to this list. Doing so sharpens the focus on these additional principles. I include only four because I am inclined to think that most (if not all) proposed additions are inherent in those four.

Autonomy

The moral principle of **autonomy** tells us that, unless there is an overriding moral reason to do otherwise, we must respect the informed choices of rational, self-governing beings.

What, in this case, does "respect" mean? First, it means that we must not take steps that hinder or prevent a rational, informed agent from carrying out his or her will (unless, of course, carrying out that will would violate autonomy or bring injustice or harm to another). It also means that in our interactions with others we must not conceal factual information that would be relevant and necessary to them to make an informed decision. And finally, it means that we may choose to help others carry out their will. Indeed, the principle of beneficence—see below—encourages us to do so, especially when there would be little or no cost to ourselves.

Deontologists would support the principle of autonomy as an obvious instance of the second form of Kant's Categorical Imperative. Utilitarians would support it on the grounds that one gains utility from doing what one wills to do and suffers when that will is frustrated.

The principle of autonomy has important implications for interactions where one party has expertise or knowledge that the other party does not have and could not easily get. In medicine, for example, the principle demands that patients be given unbiased information about the positive and negative effects of any proposed tests or treatments. In sales and marketing, autonomy requires that products or services, particularly technically advanced products or services, must not be misrepresented to potential customers as to either costs or benefits.

The principle of autonomy also has implications for public policy and civil law. John Stuart Mill captured the idea nicely through the "principle of harm" defended in his treatise, *On Liberty* (1859). Mill asserted that "the only purpose for which power can rightfully be exercised over any member of civilized community, against his will, is to prevent harm to others. His own good, either physical or moral, is not a sufficient warrant ... Over himself, over his own body and mind, the individual is sovereign."

A society—especially a democratic society—must assume that its members make decisions in an informed and rational way. That being the case, society has no right to criminalize or even prohibit any behavior that directly harms no one other than, possibly, the actor. To do so would be to disrespect that actor's autonomy. Having no moral right to restrain "private"—that is, purely personal—behavior, the society is morally prohibited from doing so. This moral restriction on civil lawmaking rises directly from the principle of autonomy as limited by the principle of nonmaleficence.

Nonmaleficence

The moral principle of **nonmaleficence** (non-ma-LEF-i-cence) tells us that, unless there is some overriding reason to do otherwise, one's actions should not inflict evil or harm. Deontologists (who would unquestioningly accept this as a universal law) and utilitarians (who see all evil or harm as contrary to achieving the greatest good) would obviously support this principle.

To practice nonmaleficence, one must avoid the infliction of harm. The challenge therein (and the challenge in any related moral argument) is to determine what would or would not inflict harm ... or, perhaps more fundamentally, what would or would not be a harm. This task would be much easier if we had a clear way to explain just what *harm* is. Unfortunately, we do not.

Consider, for example, the fundamental principle of nonmaleficence directly expressed in the physician's oath, "First, I will do no harm." Suppose a surgeon makes an incision prior to excising an internal cancerous growth. Does that incision do harm? Perhaps it does, but the harm is permissible because of the overriding benefit (removal of a cancer) to follow. On the other hand, even though tissue is damaged, perhaps no harm is done. "Harm" is evidently a normative (rather than a descriptive) term. As such, harm may be highly context dependent, and determining whether harm occurs may require significant normative argument.

It may also be (as the intuitionists claim) that "harm" is, like "red," a primitive term—a term that can be understood but not defined. It seems more likely, however, that "harm" is simply a very hard notion to get a precise handle on. Harm is in some sense the opposite of benefit, but exactly how this might clarify our understanding is elusive. Harm seems somehow linked with damage, but whereas damage can be purely cosmetic, harm cannot. Harm seems also somehow linked with the interests of beings having moral standing: we cannot harm a stone; we can harm a person. This suggests that we must be very careful not to identify any physical change with a harm: a physical change may result in a harm, but the change isn't itself the harm (or the benefit, for that matter).

The concept of *harm* and the principle of nonmaleficence are central to a number of "hot" issues: abortion, euthanasia, capital punishment, and experimental medicine, to name a few.

Nonmaleficence provides a moral foundation for the admonition "Thou shalt not kill." This admonition as stated, as with the traditional formulation of the Golden Rule, must be understood as incomplete. "Kill" is a purely descriptive term. In the food chain, humans are absolute consumers; we cannot live without killing. Normative import comes only when killing incorporates harm, but not all killing harms. This is understood when we "correct" the admonition by appending some phrase like "innocent persons" to it.

"What would be the harm?" "What would make it a harm?" These are the basic questions we must answer as we turn to the principle of nonmaleficence for moral guidance.

Beneficence

The moral principle of **beneficence** tells us that, unless there is some overriding reason to do otherwise, one's actions should serve to provide benefit, whether by promoting good, preventing harm, or removing evil. Any action that supports autonomy would count as a benefit. Thus, for example, autonomy requires that one not conceal factual information that would be relevant and necessary to another person making an informed decision. Beneficence adds a further, positive duty to be sure that all of the information actually necessary to make a rational, well-informed decision be made available. It is, for example, not enough merely to answer a customer's questions honestly; beneficence calls upon us to also answer the questions that the customer does *not* ask ... but should!

The principle of beneficence clearly promotes the utilitarian idea of the greatest good for the greatest number and also coincides nicely with one of Kant's examples of an imperfect duty. It is surely consistent with the Golden Rule of the Christian Gospels: Do unto others as you would have them do unto you.

Beneficence carries the risk that it may be—and perhaps often is—overdone. When someone claims to have done something for someone else's "own good," chances are that the someone else did not wish whatever was done to have been done, and that what was done constituted a violation of autonomy. An alternative form of the Golden Rule, "Do not do unto others that which would be hurtful to you," was perhaps formulated in the negative by an author who recognized the dangers of overextended beneficence.

But even this negative formulation falls short of solving the problem. In both forms, the Golden Rule presupposes that what you and I would desire in a given situation will always be the same. In fact, however, you might find the way that I would wish to be treated were I in your position to be strongly contrary to your wishes or even hurtful to you. This suggests that the Golden Rule should explicitly incorporate **empathy**. Empathy obtains when one has the same thoughts and feelings that another has.

Perhaps, then, as with so many pithy traditional sayings, we must regard the Golden Rule as incompletely stated. A richer formulation would be, "Do unto others as you would have them do unto you *if you were them in their situation*." This expresses the essence of beneficence.

Justice

The moral principle of **justice** tells us that, unless there is some overriding reason to do otherwise, one's actions should serve to bring what is due to whom it is due. This principle closely relates to Kant's idea that duty is tied to moral law and to our earlier observation that the notion of justice arises as a correlative concept coincident with the appearance of the idea of law. Utilitarians would agree that everyone getting what they are due will likely produce the greatest good for the greatest number.

Justice as a political idea (i.e., equal treatment of citizens under the law) naturally extends to a moral ideal: Treat similar kinds in similar situations similarly, without prejudice or bias.

The first practical problem of justice is to determine whether two entities are of similar kinds. Here, **kind** is a moral category comprising all entities with the same moral standing. Whether a particular being is of a particular kind must be determined by what objective qualities that being has and what objective qualities characterize that kind. For moral categories, it is essential that only qualities having basic moral significance—qualities such as the ability to suffer, to reason, and to act upon self-chosen principles—serve to define the category.

Mankind has not always lived up to this standard: Primitive man seems to have granted moral standing only to members of his tribe; for centuries, slaves and women were widely regarded as property with no greater moral standing than other property.

Classifications based on qualities not tied to moral foundations—classifications based on accidents of birth, of gender, of race, of color, or of creed—fundamentally violate the moral principle of justice. Moral growth of and within a society occurs as that society sheds the morally extraneous from those criteria it uses to separate moral kinds.

The other practical problem of justice is to determine the limits of similarity. If we are to treat similar kinds in similar situations similarly, without prejudice or bias, we must determine when two different situations are similar enough to call for similar treatment. Here, judgment is called for. That judgment must be guided by the recognition that equal treatment is not necessarily identical treatment, but rather is treatment based on equal consideration of the interests of all parties involved.

Judgment

Prima facie principles are to be followed except when in conflict with an equal or stronger principle. Clearly, the principles of autonomy, beneficence, nonmaleficence, and justice may in certain circumstances come into conflict. When this happens, we must *judge* what balance best resolves or minimizes the conflict. To a degree, we may be aided by recognizing a prima facie hierarchy. Autonomy surely stands above the others. If an act of beneficence would cause harm, the principle of nonmaleficence holds sway. Justice may be tempered by beneficence, provided, of course, the beneficence is not so excessive as to cause harm. When the combined principles fail to narrow our choices sufficiently, allowing for too many options, one may wish to turn to the principle of utility—a possible fifth prima facie moral principle—for the final refinement.

Judgment may be wise or foolish. In morality, wise judgments come with experience and practice, using calm deliberative reasoning supported by clear concepts, sound moral principles, and open consideration of all relevant facts.

I hope that you will find this hornbook for ethics of lasting value as you face life and seek to make wise moral judgments.

Ethical Foundations of Clinical Practice

Linda Farber Post and Jeffrey Blustein

Linda Farber Post and Jeffrey Blustein, "Ethical Foundations of Clinical Practice," *Handbook for Health Care Ethics Committees*, pp. 3-16. Copyright © 2015 by Johns Hopkins University Press. Reprinted with permission.

As a member of your hospital's ethics committee, you have been called by Dr. Thomas, a second-year surgical resident who was paged for the following consult: Ms. Lawrence is a 23-year-old woman who was returning home from her bridal shower when her car skidded on the ice and hit an oncoming truck. Although her multiple injuries are serious, with immediate surgery and replacement of lost blood, her chances of full recovery are excellent.

Ms. Lawrence is in considerable pain, but she appears coherent and her answers to Dr. Thomas's questions reflect understanding of her condition, the treatment options, and their consequences. Because of her beliefs as a Jehovah's Witness, however, she will not accept blood or blood products and will not consider surgery unless she is promised that it will be done without transfusions.

Dr. Thomas knows that surgical and hemodynamic intervention can prevent this patient's almost certain death. He also knows that saving her life in this way will violate Ms. Lawrence's deeply held religious convictions. What are the conflicting professional, legal, and ethical obligations? What is the role of the ethics committee in resolving this dilemma? What resources are available to help you?

Perhaps the threshold question that should begin our discussion is, what is health care ethics and why does it matter? The short answer is that *health care ethics* is an umbrella term that encompasses a number of subspecialties that address the ethical issues that arise in the health care setting, including clinical ethics, organizational ethics, and research ethics.

As will become clear in the following pages, however, the issues do not lend themselves to short answers, and further clarification and analysis are necessary. The concerns of health care ethics include the well-being and dignity of the patient; matters of choice and decision making; rights and responsibilities of the patient, family, and care team; the responsibilities of health care organizations; access to care; and fairness and justice in health policy.

These matters are neither new nor exotic, but they have become more prominent. Health care has traditionally dealt with the profound moral issues of human existence, including life, self-determination, suffering, and mortality. What has changed are the complexity of medicine; the increased range of choices; and the way care is accessed, delivered, and financed. The ethical implications of these matters have attracted heightened attention, not only from those who make clinical and policy decisions but, especially recently, from those who make legislative and judicial decisions, as well. As ethics has become an integral part of the health care setting, institutional ethics committees have become increasingly visible and active in clinical and organizational decision making. The goal of this [reading] is to help your committee be a knowledgeable, skillful, and effective ethics resource for your institution.

The Role of Ethics in Clinical Medicine

Ethics has a long and distinguished history, grounding both the practice of medicine and the laws related to it. Society considers ethical principles so important that it gives them legal sanction in statutory and case law. Thus, ethical principles, such as respect for autonomy and privacy, are translated into laws about informed consent and confidentiality. Issues related to providing and forgoing health care are governed almost exclusively by state law, however, creating wide variation in the way these matters are handled. For example, decisions about withholding or withdrawing life-sustaining measures might be very different if the patient were being treated in New York or Texas. For this reason, your ethics committee should have some familiarity with how your state laws and regulations address these issues.

While ethics informs all worthy endeavors, it has special significance in the health care professions because of the fiduciary relationship between practitioners and patients. A fiduciary relationship exists when one party, because of superior knowledge, skill, and authority, assumes responsibility for the welfare of another party who is in a position of reliance. In this trust-based relationship, fiduciaries have heightened obligations, including the moral imperative to put the interests of reliant parties ahead of their own interests. Patients, whose illness, injury, disability, pain, or suffering make them vulnerable, place themselves in the hands of health care professionals, based on the confidence that their well-being is the practitioner's highest priority.

Ironically, it is the very technological and medical advances, as well as their promise and potential, which have generated some of the most difficult ethical problems. In critical, acute, and long-term care settings, the very existence of new therapies often creates demand for their use, whether or not they are medically indicated or ethically appropriate. Stage and screen portrayals of brilliant diagnoses and dramatic recoveries have convinced the lay public and, often, clinicians, that everything is curable if enough money and expertise are thrown at it. When that does not happen, when the disease or injury is overwhelming and irreversible, patients and families feel betrayed and practitioners often feel as though they have failed. Likewise, the Internet has become both a help and a hindrance. Patients sometimes come to the therapeutic interaction armed with reams of information about therapies reported to cure their ailments, insisting that they should be tried. In the domain of clinical research, expectations of dramatic breakthroughs are also high, despite the fact that more clinical research results in failure and disappointment than success (Leaf 2013; Bains 2004).

Standing at the intersection of medicine, ethics, and law, health care ethics provides a useful analytic framework for committees charged with thinking through the ethical dilemmas of modern medicine in a rational and responsible manner.

Ethics Committees in the Health Care Setting

The development of bioethics as a powerful influence on the way health care is perceived and practiced was part of a larger social transformation. A hallmark of the latter half of the twentieth century was the heightened notion of individual rights. Virtually every social sphere was affected by the effort to promote equality and redress inequities in race, gender, class, and education. In the context of the various rights movements, including civil, women's, and gay rights, the ethical principle of autonomy became the major support for individual empowerment and self-determination in health care, most prominently in the doctrine of informed consent and the right of refusal. In the process, to a much greater extent than previously, patients became both partners in health care decision making and informed health care consumers.

Ethical, legal, and scientific developments created an obligation to evaluate critically the process of gathering scientific information, translating it into therapeutic applications, and using it responsibly. Advances in medical knowledge and skills generated a new array of treatment options, as well as the concern that the *ability* to intervene could become the *obligation* to intervene. For the first time, questions were raised not only about *how* and *when*, but *whether* to treat. Under what circumstances should therapies be withheld or withdrawn? When does the burden of an intervention outweigh its benefit? How should decisions be made about the allocation of limited medical resources? At the same time, the law was becoming involved in life-and-death matters that used to be confined to the doctor-patient interaction.

Bioethics as a discipline is generally considered to have developed between the 1960s and the 1980s as it became apparent that emerging issues could benefit from thoughtful analysis by people with both clinical and nonclinical perspectives. Philosophers, social scientists, theologians, legal scholars, and biomedical scientists increasingly focused their attention on clinical research, allocation of limited resources, organ transplantation, reproductive technologies, genetic testing and treatment, terminal illness and end-of-life care, and the obligations in the clinical interaction. Clinicians too turned their attention to these matters. These deliberations revealed that ethical analysis had practical application in the research and clinical settings.

The hospital ethics committee was an early institutional effort to bring a formal ethical perspective to the clinical setting, otherwise described as "a politically attractive way for moral controversies to be procedurally accommodated" (Moreno 1995, pp. 93–94). In the early 1980s, hospitals increasingly began to establish ethics committees to answer questions and help make decisions about health care issues with ethical dimensions. These committees had their roots in several types of small decision-making groups, each intended to address specific ethical problems. Sterilization committees, composed mainly of physicians with expertise in psychiatry and psychology, functioned mainly during the 1920s and 1930s to determine which individuals with mental disabilities should be involuntarily sterilized. Abortion selection committees functioned in many hospitals before the 1973 U.S. Supreme Court decision in *Roe v. Wade* legalized abortion. Beginning in 1945, their purpose was to evaluate the requests of women who wished to terminate their pregnancies and determine whether therapeutic abortions were indicated to preserve maternal life or health. Dialysis selection committees emerged during the early 1960s in response to the development of the dialysis machine, the first publicly recognized life-sustaining technology. Made up of lay members of the community, they were charged with choosing among the candidates with end-stage renal disease and determining who would receive chronic hemodialysis.

Beginning in the 1970s, institutional review boards (IRBs) responded to revelations of abuse in medical experimentation by reviewing all government-funded research using human subjects. The 1974 federal mandating of IRBs represented the first codified suggestion of institutional obligation to address ethical concerns. Prognosis committees were occasionally convened by the mid-1970s to assess the projected course of patients' illnesses. In its 1976 ruling in *In re Quinlan*, the New Jersey Supreme Court referred to an article by Dr. Karen Teel and recommended that hospitals have an ethics committee to deal with termination of life-sustaining treatment for incapacitated patients. Although the court used the term *ethics committee*, it was actually suggesting a *prognosis committee* that would render opinions on the likely benefits of continued treatment for patients with grave and irreversible illness.

Infant care review committees began appearing in the wake of the 1982 "Baby Doe" ruling that permitted parents to approve withholding life-saving treatment from a neonate with Down syndrome. These committees, which were intended to review care plans for severely disabled newborns, were also recommended by the President's Commission for the Study of Ethical Problems in Medicine and Behavioral Research in 1983 and endorsed by the U.S. Department of Health and Human Services and the American Academy of Pediatrics. Medical-morals committees met in Catholic hospitals to address sensitive issues, including those related to reproduction, analgesia, and extraordinary interventions at the end of life, in terms of Church doctrine.

Against this backdrop, clinical and administrative staffs began to meet for interdisciplinary deliberations about issues of high-tech care, undertook self-education, and exhibited a growing professional awareness of ethical issues and their implications. During the 1970s and 1980s, hospitals began to establish ethics committees to provide guidance about health care issues with ethical dimensions. Over time, these committees have taken on the additional functions of staff education, clinical guideline development, institutional policy advisement, and clinical case review. Some ethics committees also advise on resource allocation and express or reinforce the institution's commitment to certain values.

Since 1992, the Joint Commission (formerly known as the Joint Commission on Accreditation of Healthcare Organizations, or JCAHO) has required as a condition of accreditation that every health care institution have a standing mechanism to address ethical issues and resolve disputes. In addition, several states, including Massachusetts, New Jersey, Colorado, Mary land, New York, and Texas, have passed statutes requiring hospitals to have ethics committees (Pope 2011). According to a 2007 report of U.S. hospitals, 100% of hospitals with 400 or more beds also have an ethics consultation service, which is commonly part of or allied with an ethics committee (Fox, Myers, and Pearlman 2007). The result is that almost all acute care hospitals, long-term care facilities, hospices, psychiatric institutions, facilities for the developmentally disabled, and other care-providing centers in the United States have ethics committees that meet on a regular or ad hoc basis.

Just as there are different care-providing institutions serving different needs, there are different models of health care ethics committees, based on the size, resources, patient base, type of care delivered, geographic location, community demographics, bud get, consultation needs, and other resources of each facility. Large academic medical centers typically have a multidisciplinary ethics committee that meets monthly and some have additional committees that focus on ethical issues in specific clinical settings, such as pediatrics or neonatology. Many large centers supplement their committees with a full-time bioethicist, who directs the ethics service; conducts or participates in clinical ethics consultation; teaches medical and nursing students, residents, and other staff; and serves as the frontline bioethics resource. Ethics committees in small community hospitals, nursing homes, hospices, and facilities for the developmentally disabled may meet quarterly for education, case review, and policy development, relying on subcommittees or specified individuals to address ethical issues and clinical consultations as the need arises.

Hospice and long-term care ethics committees may be on-site and specific to one institution or provide off-site resources to multiple institutions. These committees typically focus on ethical issues and decisions at the end of life. Ethics committees at psychiatric institutions and facilities for the disabled are also often off-site and serve several facilities.

Ethics consortium committees are off-site resources for multiple institutions that share one or more characteristics or needs. Some focus on specific research, such as stem cell studies, conducted at several centers, while others focus on clinical issues. Some consortium committees address the educational and networking needs of organizations and individuals without offering consultation services, while others provide clinical consultations for practitioners, administrative staff, and the general public. Consortiums may cover a wide range of health care organizations and issues, or they may focus on specific areas, such as research, non-acute care, long-term care, hospice, or particular disease entities or disabilities.

As you read though this [reading], bear in mind that your committee does not own ethics in your institution. The committee should strive to develop ethics expertise, but it would be counterproductive to encourage the notion of ethics exclusivity and the perception that ethics resides only in a select group. Rather, one of your most valuable roles is that of a resource, which, through education, policy development, and consultation, helps clinical and administrative staff to integrate ethics knowledge and skills into their daily practice.

Accordingly, an important committee function is helping staff to identify or anticipate ethical issues and conflicts, develop the skills to handle routine cases in ways that you have modeled in consultation on similar cases, and distinguish complex cases that require the attention of your consultation service. One mark of a successful ethics consultation is when you are stopped in the hall by someone who says, "Remember that case you consulted on two weeks ago? Well, we had another one just like it and we *didn't* have to call you. But now, we've got one that really has us stumped and we need your involvement again."

A crucial task is to make ethics and your committee relevant to the clinical and organizational functioning of your institution. Your clinical consultation and educational strengths will not be solicited if people do not appreciate how what you do can enhance what they do. Make your committee visible by having each interested member regularly attend morning rounds on a particular unit to contribute observations about ethical issues that arise during case discussions. Other members might join select committees—patient safety, institutional review board, conflict of interest—to provide an ethics lens to the deliberations. At the same time, while your committee retains the responsibility to provide ethics expertise, education, and guidance, it is important to reinforce the notions that bioethics is an integral part of the work that health care professionals do every day, and that the health care organization and all those who practice in it are moral agents with ethical obligations that cannot be delegated.

Fundamental Ethical Principles

As you no doubt expected, any discussion of applied bioethics must begin with a review of its theoretical underpinnings. Understanding the key concepts and how they relate to clinical practice is essential to the effective functioning of ethics committees.

The core ethical principles that support the therapeutic relationship and give rise to clinician obligations include

- respecting patient autonomy—supporting and facilitating the capable patient's exercise of self-determination in health care decision making;
- beneficence—promoting the patient's best interest and protecting the patient from harm;
- nonmaleficence—avoiding actions likely to cause the patient harm; and
- justice—allocating fairly the benefits and burdens related to health care delivery.

Respecting Patient Autonomy

Autonomy is the ethical principle widely considered most central to health care decision making. Its prominence here and in other bioethics literature reflects the heightened emphasis typically accorded patient rights, self-governance, and individual choice. Autonomy includes determination of health care goals, power over what is done to one's body, and control of personal information. Only when the individual cannot make decisions are others asked to choose. Autonomy gives priority to personal values and wishes, supporting choices that are informed and uncoerced, and confers the professional obligation to respect patient privacy and confidentiality.

The significance of autonomy to health care decision making is seen in the ethical concepts of decisional capacity, informed consent and refusal, and truth telling. Patients exercise autonomy by making informed care decisions that reflect their goals, values, and preferences. Clinicians demonstrate respect for autonomy by providing information and guidance that enable patients to make knowledgeable decisions, honoring patient choices and implementing them in care plans, preserving patient confidentiality, and protecting the security of patient information.

The notion of autonomy encompasses a range of conceptions, some highly individualistic and somewhat isolating, others more relational and compatible with communitarian values. Criticisms of some versions of the principle of respect for patient autonomy do not invalidate the principle since other versions might be immune to those objections. The search for a full understanding of autonomy has spawned a vast literature and is beyond the scope of this [reading] but, for an ethics committee, the role of autonomy has applied as well as theoretical importance. For example, when considering patient rights and decision making, it is crucial to distinguish autonomy as self-governance according to one's values and principles from the unrestricted liberty to behave entirely according to one's preferences (Gaylin and Jennings 2003). There is also a distinction between negative and positive rights, the former being the right not to have one's self-chosen plan controlled or interfered with, and the latter being a claim on others to behave in certain ways (Takala 2007). This distinction has important implications for patient decisions and clinician obligations. Likewise, while an individualistic conception of autonomy emphasizes each patient's capacity for self-advocacy and self-governance, a relational conception focuses on the conditions, including organizational structure, policy, and process, which either promote or inhibit the exercise of autonomy (Nedelsky 2011).

The heightened emphasis our society customarily places on individualism and independence is a largely Western, and some feminists have argued gendered, phenomenon that is not shared across all cultures or even by all within our culture. Some patients may come from cultures that favor decision making by the family rather than the individual. Even in a culture that prizes self-governance, not everyone is comfortable with or capable of independent decision making. For many patients, authentic decision making is an exercise shared with trusted others and reflects *supported* or *delegated* autonomy. Patients with diminished or fluctuating cognition are likely to rely on spouses or adult children for help in care planning, and even those who are cognitively capable may elect to have others make decisions for them or to consult with them before deciding on a course of action.

Ultimately, respecting patient autonomy does not mean elevating it to a position where it trumps all other considerations. While it is legally and ethically appropriate to honor the wishes of capable patients, it is also necessary to consider the ethical principles that give rise to other, often competing, obligations.

Beneficence

The principle of beneficence underlies obligations to provide the best care for the patient and balance the risks and burdens of care against the benefits. Promoted goods typically include prolonging life, restoring function, relieving pain and suffering, and preventing harm. Beneficence is the principle with arguably the greatest resonance for caregivers, whose traditional mission is to heal and comfort, and notions of nurturing and protecting are reflected in heightened care for those who are most vulnerable. Assessing the patient's "good" is a complex process, however, since perceptions of benefit and best interest are not purely scientific or medical, but involve the patient's expectations, goals, and value judgments. Recognition that patients and their doctors may differ in these assessments has been at least partly responsible for the noticeable shift from physician paternalism to greater emphasis on patient choice and shared decision making.

Nonmaleficence

At the very core of the healing professions is the principle of nonmaleficence, captured in the ancient maxim, "First, do no harm." This principle grounds obligations to avoid the unnecessary infliction of harm or suffering, recognizing that conceptions of harm, as of good, are inextricably tied to individual values and interests. Most, if not all, therapies carry the potential for some risk as well as benefit, and it would not be feasible to limit the therapeutic arsenal to treatments that are entirely benign. Nevertheless, the benefits of recommended treatments are expected to outweigh the possible harms and physicians are required to discuss that calculus with their patients, comparing the burdens and risks to the anticipated goods, being mindful that patients differ in their tolerance of risk. Likewise, the duty to prevent foreseeable harm requires investigators to disclose the benefits and risks of proposed research to potential subjects and IRBs.

Justice

Justice, or equity, refers to those principles of social cooperation that define what each person in the society or member of a group is due or owed. The several types of justice, including distributive, punitive, and compensatory justice, all share the basic notion of treating similar cases similarly and dissimilar cases dissimilarly. In the domain of health care, justice demands that care decisions be based on clinical need rather than ethically irrelevant characteristics, such as race, religion, or socioeconomic status. Most relevant to medical ethics is distributive justice, which concerns the norms and standards for allocating benefits and burdens across a given population. Distributive justice demands that the benefits, risks, and costs of actions—in this case, access to resources related to physical and mental health—be apportioned fairly and without discrimination on both societal and institutional levels. According to the principle of distributive justice, there should be ethically defensible reasons why certain individuals or groups receive benefits or endure burdens that other individuals or groups do not.

Principlism and Alternative Approaches

The four ethical principles discussed above—autonomy, beneficence, nonmaleficence, and justice—have assumed a central place in much of bioethics literature, theory, and clinical analysis. They are used in an attempt to render our moral convictions and the reasons for them coherent. Our very brief tour just touches the surface and you are encouraged to consult Beauchamp and Childress for an in-depth treatment.[...]. As a cautionary note, however, it is important to resist the temptation to employ principles in a mechanical fashion. If used with judgment and sensitivity, they can provide structure and inform sound ethical reasoning. Used rigidly without reference to context and narrative, however, principlist ethics can lead to a distorted and unhelpful analysis.

Challenges to principlist ethics use different theoretical and analytical frameworks in considering ethical issues. Narrative ethics employs the methods and techniques of narrative analysis to provide a richer characterization of ethical problems as a supplement to the dominant principlist approach. Feminist ethics is committed to the view that the moral experience of women, in particular their history of sexual oppression, must be taken seriously in the identification, analysis, and resolution of ethical problems. Virtue ethics gives matters of character, such as courage, loyalty, and compassion, a preeminent place in ethical analysis. Pragmatic ethics stresses the continuity between the methods of problem solving in science and ethics.

It is equally useful in doing ethical analysis to consider clinical situations in terms other than that of ethical principles or analytic frameworks, referring to concepts such as decisional capacity and authority, power imbalances, pain and suffering, confidentiality, truth telling, informed consent, the family's role in decision making, the patient's best interest, forgoing treatment, and quality of life and death. Ethical principles have a foundational role in justifying decisions, but they are given meaning and application by additional considerations. [...]

The Role of Culture, Race, and Ethnicity in Health Care

How people confront decisions about health care is shaped in large part by the beliefs, attitudes, and values inherent in the cultures with the greatest formative influence on them. Choices about advance care planning, approaches to decision making, disclosure of information, life-sustaining interventions, and palliation are often informed by culturally determined notions of self-governance and destiny, truth telling and protection from harm, the power of language to reflect or create reality, filial obligation, the meaning of suffering, religion and spirituality, historical discrimination, and mistrust of health care or the health care system.

The following brief examples are offered to illustrate how culture, race, and ethnicity can influence health care. Studies have found that European Americans, who tend to value independence and self-empowerment, are more likely than others to favor advance directives, full disclosure of health information, and limited treatment at the end of life. In contrast, African Americans have demonstrated reluctance to delegate decision-making authority through advance directives; objection to limiting treatment; and preference for aggressive life-sustaining technology, including cardiopulmonary resuscitation. Hispanics have been shown to defer to physician judgment, value decision making by the family rather than an appointed health care agent, and place great importance on how the family is affected by the patient's illness. Asian and Middle Eastern cultures typically prefer to protect patients from knowledge about serious illness or impending death, and favor family rather than individual decision making. Native American cultures tend to reject advance care discussions because they might bring on the envisioned health problems (Major, Mendes, and Dovidio 2013; Sorkin, Ngo-Metzger, and DeAlba 2010). Similarly, race, culture, ethnicity, and gender inform how pain is experienced, expressed, perceived, and treated, with women receiving less analgesia and more sedation than men, and Hispanics less likely to receive pain management than non-Hispanic white patients. Reports of these studies emphasize the need for balance in interpreting them. Overreliance on the findings risks cultural stereotyping, while failure to attend to cultural distinctions risks assuming that all patients share Western attitudes and values (Morrison and Meier 2004; Kagawa-Singer and Blackhall 2001; Hopp and Duffy 2000; Blackhall et al. 1999; Shepardson et al. 1999; Morrison et al. 1998; Berger 1998; Post et al. 1996; Pellegrino et al. 1992). The same commentators also point out that cultural determinants influence the values and attitudes of physicians as well as those of their patients. The result is the potential for misperception and miscommunication when the parties to the clinical interaction come from different cultural backgrounds.

The extensive literature on cultural influences on health care delivery indicates that, in an increasingly diverse population, multiplicity of languages, socioeconomic inequities, and differing religious beliefs, community values, and cultural traditions may inhibit the provision of clinical services, resulting in widespread disparities in access to and quality of care. These inequities present across the age, geographic, ethnic, nationalistic, and religious spectrums. Increasing the cultural competence of practitioners and care-providing organizations is repeatedly offered as an effective way to diminish these disparities and enhance the quality of care delivered (Aseltine, Katz, and Holmes 2011; Boone 2011; Padela, Imran, and Punekar 2009; Giger et al. 2007; Flores and Lin 2013; Lau et al. 2012).

A valuable ethics committee function is educating care providers about the personal and cultural differences that influence the clinical dynamic and affect patient care. Consider, for example, a series of grand rounds or in-service presentations on how cultural background can inform patient and provider comfort with notions of autonomy, privacy, advance directives, informed consent, and disclosure.

Conflicting Obligations and Ethical Dilemmas

The several ethical principles discussed above confer on clinicians multiple ethical obligations—duties that are grounded in moral norms and must be fulfilled unless there are competing and more compelling obligations. Not surprisingly, these obligations frequently collide, and this is often responsible for the complex character of ethical decision making in health care.

The tension between and among ethical principles may create dilemmas for clinicians when their obligations are in conflict. Ethical dilemmas usually occur in two types of situations. In some instances, an act can be seen as both morally justified and unjustified, but the arguments supporting each position are inconclusive. This makes it difficult for the individual to determine the appropriate course of action. Many commentators have said this about abortion and assisted death, where broad-based social consensus on the ethics of each is lacking. In other instances, an individual may be required to respond to different moral imperatives, each of which is clear, but both of which cannot be discharged at the same time. For example, care professionals are required to respect and promote the autonomy of their patients *and* to protect and enhance their well-being, to provide care to those who need it *and* to be responsible stewards of limited resources, to protect patient confidentiality *and* to alert vulnerable third parties who do not know they are at risk. Resolving these dilemmas requires clinicians and ethics committees to scrutinize carefully the competing interests and obligations, identify the likely consequences of the available choices, and weigh the benefits and risks to those involved.

Let's return to Ms. Lawrence, the patient who is refusing blood transfusion. The dilemma here concerns the tension between Dr. Thomas's obligation to honor his patient's autonomous decision about blood transfusion and his obligations to prevent harm and promote her best interests by providing what he believes is the most beneficial care. On the surface, it seems that he cannot possibly meet one obligation without violating the others, yet he must act. Because both of the principles involved are so central to professional practice and the consequences in this case so profound, the goal must be to protect both Ms. Lawrence's rights and her well-being. The members of your ethics committee can function usefully in a consultative role as these issues are considered.

The first responsibility is to confirm that Ms. Lawrence is capable of making decisions about her care and to ensure that she and Dr. Thomas have clarified the clinical situation, the care goals, the therapeutic options, and their likely consequences. The exercise of patient autonomy through informed consent and refusal depends on the patient's decisional capacity, the quality of the information provided by the physician, and the trust underlying the therapeutic relationship. An ethics consultation can create the opportunity for the patient and appropriate members of the care team to engage in these important discussions.

The next step is to consider the ethical issues, including Ms. Lawrence's right to make care decisions based on her goals and values, and to confirm that her refusal is the product of her deeply held religious convictions rather than coercion or misinformation about blood transfusions. The discussion should explore alternative options and resources, including nonblood therapies and transfer to other institutions that specialize in treatment without transfusion, and their relative risks and benefits. Ms. Lawrence, her family, and the clinical team must be reassured that her refusal will in no way compromise the rest of her care.

Resolving the conflict between the obligation to respect the patient's autonomy and the obligations to promote her best interest and protect her from harm will require a careful collaborative assessment of her decision making, including how she weights the benefits and burdens of the proposed treatment. While it is neither necessary nor appropriate to argue her out of her religious beliefs, the ethics consultant is obliged to be certain that her decision to forgo a life-saving intervention is informed, carefully considered, voluntary, and settled. If Ms. Lawrence genuinely believes that surviving with a blood transfusion would be morally unacceptable, then, for her, the benefits of the intervention would be significantly outweighed by the burdens of the outcome. Under those conditions, her refusal of transfusion should be honored while she receives all other appropriate care and support. In this time-consuming and exacting process, the ethics consultant is a valuable resource, providing all parties with information, ethical analysis, practical guidance, and support.

The patient's autonomy is not the only thing at stake, however. Dr. Thomas and his colleagues also bring to this situation their professional obligations and personal values. Not unreasonably, surgeons and anesthesiologists in this circumstance are likely to be very uneasy about attempting surgery under conditions that restrict their ability to provide optimal care. Even though the patient has agreed to and assumed the risks of surgery without blood transfusions, the doctors will argue that they would be knowingly putting her at what they consider unacceptable risk. Doing so would erode both their competence and professional integrity. Under these restrictive conditions, many surgeons and anesthesiologists may decline to provide care, but they cannot simply abandon the patient. Instead, they must make reasonable efforts to transfer Ms. Lawrence to colleagues or other institutions more comfortable with her limitations, agreeing to operate only if life-saving alternatives were not available.

References

Ahronheim J, Moreno JC, Zuckerman C. 2000. *Ethics in Clinical Practice*. 2nd ed. Gaithersburg, MD: Aspen Publishers.

Annas GJ. 1991. Ethics committees: From ethical comfort to ethical cover. *Hastings Center Report* 21(3):18–21.

Arras JD, Steinbock B, London AJ. 1999. Moral reasoning in the medical context. In Arras JD, Steinbock B, eds. *Ethical Issues in Modern Medicine*. 5th ed. Mountain View, CA: Mayfield Publishing Co., pp. 1–40.

Aseltine RH, Katz MC, Holmes C. 2011. Providing medical care to diverse populations: Findings from a follow-up survey of Connecticut physicians. *Connecticut Medicine* 75(6):337–44.

Bains W. 2004. Failure rates in drug discovery and development: Will we ever get any better? *Business*: 9–18.

Beauchamp TL, Childress JF. 2001. *Principles of Biomedical Ethics*. 5th ed. New York: Oxford University Press.

Beauchamp TL, Walters L, eds. 2003. *Contemporary Issues in Bioethics*. 6th ed. Belmont, CA: Wadsworth-Thomson Learning.

Berger JT. 1998. Culture and ethnicity in clinical care. *Archives of Internal Medicine* 158:2085–90.

Blackhall LJ, Frank G, Murphy ST, Michel V, Palmer JM, Azen SP. 1999. Ethnicity and attitudes towards life sustaining technology. *Social Science & Medicine* 48:1779–89.

Boone S. 2011. A case for diversity, cultural competency and ending disparities in the 21st-century medical practice. *Connecticut Medicine* 75(6):345–46.

Childress, J. 1990. The place of autonomy in bioethics. *Hastings Center Report* 20(1):12–17.

Fletcher JC. 1991. The bioethics movement and hospital ethics committees. *Mary land Law Review* 50:859–94.

Flores G, Lin H. 2013. Trends in racial/ethnic disparities in medical and oral health, access to care, and use of services in U.S. children: Has anything changed over the years? *International Journal for Equity in Health* 12(1):1–16.

Fox E, Myers S, Pearlman RA. 2007. Ethics consultations in United States hospitals: A national survey. *American Journal of Bioethics* 7(2):13–25.

Gaylin W, Jennings, B. 2003. *The Perversion of Autonomy: The Proper Uses of Coercion and Constraints in a Liberal Society.* Washington, DC: Georgetown University Press.

Giger J, et al. 2007. American Academy of Nursing Expert Panel report: Developing cultural competence to eliminate health disparities in ethnic minorities and other vulnerable populations. *Journal of Transcultural Nursing* 18(2):95–102.

Hopp FP, Duffy SA. 2000. Racial variations in end-of-life care. *Journal of the American Geriatrics Society* 48(6):658–63.

In re Quinlan, 70 N.J. 10, 355 A.2d 647 (1976).

Joint Commission on Accreditation of Healthcare Organizations. 1999. *Comprehensive Accreditation Manual for Hospitals.* Oakbrook Terrace, IL: Joint Commission on Accreditation of Healthcare Organizations.

Jonsen AR. 1998. *The Birth of Bioethics.* New York: Oxford University Press.

Kagawa-Singer M, Blackhall LJ. 2001. Negotiating cross-cultural issues at the end of life: "You've got to go where he lives." *Journal of the American Medical Association* 286(23):2992–3001.

Lau M, Lin H, Flores G. 2012. Racial/ethnic disparities in health and health care among U.S. adolescents. *Health Services Research* 47(5):2031–59.

Leaf C. 2013. Do clinical trials work? *The New York Times Sunday Review*, July 13.

Levine RJ. 2003. Informed consent: Some challenges to the universal validity of the Western world. In Beauchamp TL, Walters L, eds. *Contemporary Issues in Bioethics.* 6th ed. Belmont, CA: Wadsworth-Thomson Learning, pp. 150–55.

Lo B. 2000. *Resolving Ethical Dilemmas: A Guide for Clinicians.* 2nd ed. Philadelphia: Lippincott Williams & Wilkins, pp. 140–46.

Major B, Mendes WB, Dovidio JF. 2013. Intergroup relations and health disparities: A social psychological perspective. *Health Psychology* 32(5):514–24.

Mappes TA, Degrazia D. 2001. *Biomedical Ethics.* 5th ed. Boston: McGraw-Hill, pp. 1–55.

May L, Hua L, Glenn F. 2012. Racial/ethnic disparities in health and health care among US adolescents. *Health Services Research* 47(5):2031–59.

Miller B. 1995. Autonomy and the refusal of life-sustaining treatment. In Arras JD, Steinbock B, eds. *Ethical Issues in Modern Medicine.* 4th ed. Mountain View, CA: Mayfield Publishing Co., pp. 202–11.

Moreno JD. 1995. *Deciding Together: Bioethics and Moral Consensus.* New York: Oxford University Press.

Moreno JD. 1998. Ethics committees and ethics consultants. In Kuhse H, Singer P, eds. *A Companion to Bioethics.* Malden, MA: Blackwell Publishers, pp. 475–84.

Morrison RS, Meier DE. 2004. High rates of advance care planning in New York City's elderly population. *Archives of Internal Medicine* 164(22):2421–26.

Morrison RS, Zayas LH, Mulvihill M, Baskin SA, Meier DE. 1998. Barriers to completion of health care proxies: An examination of ethnic differences. *Archives of Internal Medicine* 158(22):2493–97.

Nedelsky J. 2011. *Law's Relations: A Relational Theory of Self, Autonomy, and Law.* New York: Oxford University Press.

O'Neill O. 2002. *Autonomy and Trust in Bioethics.* Cambridge: Cambridge University Press.

Padela AI, Imran RA, Punekar BS. 2009. Emergency medical practice: Advancing cultural competence and reducing healthcare disparities. *Academic Emergency Medicine* 16(1):69–75.

Pearson SD, Sabin J, Emanuel EJ. 2003. *No Margin, No Mission: Health-Care Organizations and the Quest for Ethical Excellence.* New York: Oxford University Press.

Pellegrino ED. 1992. Intersections of Western biomedical ethics and world culture. In Pellegrino ED, Mazzarella P, Corsi P, eds. *Transcultural Dimensions in Medical Ethics.* Frederick, MD: University Publishing Group.

Pope TM. 2011. Legal briefing: Healthcare ethics committees. *Journal of Clinical Ethics* 22(1):74–93.

Post LF, Blustein J, Gordon E, Dubler NN. 1996. Pain: Ethics, culture, and informed consent to relief. *Journal of Law, Medicine & Ethics* 24:348–59.

Powell T, Lowenstein B. 1996. Refusing life-sustaining treatment after catastrophic injury: Ethical implications. *Journal of Law, Medicine & Ethics* 24:54–61.

Protection of Human Subjects, 45 CFR 47.107; see also 45 CFR 46.112 (1990).

Rosner F. 1985. Hospital medical ethics committees: A review of their development. *Journal of the American Medical Association* 253(18):2693–97.

Ross JW, Glaser JW, Rasinski-Gregory D, Gibson JM, Bayley C. 1993. *Health Care Ethics Committees: The Next Generation.* Chicago: American Hospital Publishing.

Ross JW, Michel V, Pugh D. 1986. *Handbook for Hospital Ethics Committees.* Chicago: American Hospital Publishing.

Rothman DJ. 1991. *Strangers at the Bedside: A History of How Law and Bioethics Transformed Medical Decision Making.* New York: Basic Books.

Schneider CE. 1998. *The Practice of Autonomy: Patients, Doctors, and Medical Decisions.* New York: Oxford University Press.

Shepardson LB, Gordon HS, Ibrahim SA, Harper DL, Rosenthal GE. 1999. Racial variation in the use of do-not-resuscitate orders. *Journal of General Internal Medicine* 14(1):15–20.

Solomon MZ. 2005. Realizing bioethics goals in practice: Ten ways "is" can help "ought." *Hastings Center Report* 35:40–47.

Sorkin DH, Ngo-Metzger Q, DeAlba I. 2010. Racial/ethnic discrimination in health care: Impact on perceived quality of care. *Journal of General Internal Medicine* 25(5):390–96.

Spencer EM, Mills AE, Rorty MV, Werhane PH. 2000. *Organization Ethics in Health Care.* New York: Oxford University Press.

Takala T. 2007. Concepts of "person" and "liberty," and their implications to our fading notions of autonomy. *Journal of Medical Ethics* 33(4):225–28.

Teel K. 1975. The physician's dilemma: A doctor's view. What the law should be. *Baylor Law Review* 27:6–9.

Thomasma DC. 1993. Assessing bioethics today. *Cambridge Quarterly of Healthcare Ethics* 2:519–27.

Thomasma DC, Monagle JF. 1998. Hospital ethics committees: Roles, membership, structure, and difficulties. In Monagle JF, Thomasma DC, eds. *Health Care Ethics: Critical Issues for the 21st Century.* Gaithersburg, MD: Aspen Publishers, pp. 460–70.

Toulmin S. 1981. The tyranny of principles. *Hastings Center Report*: 31–39.

Wear S, Katz P, Andrzejewski B, Haryadi T. 1990. The development of an ethics consultation service. *HEC Forum* 2:75–87.

Wolf SM. 1991. Ethics committees and due process: Nesting rights in a community of caring. *Maryland Law Review* 50:798–858.

Unit II

Moral Virtue

Selections from "Virtue of Character

Aristotle; trans. Terence Irwin

How a Virtue of Character Is Acquired

Virtue, then, is of two sorts, virtue of thought and virtue of character. Virtue of thought arises and grows mostly from teaching; that is why it needs experience and time. Virtue of character [i.e., of *ethos*] results from habit [*ethos*]; hence its name 'ethical', slightly varied from 'ethos'.

§2 Hence it is also clear that none of the virtues of character arises in us naturally. For if something is by nature in one condition, habituation cannot bring it into another condition. A stone, for instance, by nature moves downwards, and habituation could not make it move upwards, not even if you threw it up ten thousand times to habituate it; nor could habituation make fire move downwards, or bring anything that is by nature in one condition into another condition. §3 And so the virtues arise in us neither by nature nor against nature. Rather, we are by nature able to acquire them, and we are completed through habit.

§4 Further, if something arises in us by nature, we first have the capacity for it, and later perform the activity. This is clear in the case of the senses; for we did not acquire them by frequent seeing or hearing, but we already had them when we exercised them, and did not get them by exercising them. Virtues, by contrast, we acquire, just as we acquire crafts, by having first activated them. For we learn a craft by producing the same product that we must produce when we have learned it; we become builders, for instance, by building, and we become harpists by playing the harp. Similarly, then, we become just by doing just actions, temperate by doing temperate actions, brave by doing brave actions.

§5 What goes on in cities is also evidence for this. For the legislator makes the citizens good by habituating them, and this is the wish of every legislator; if he fails to do it well he misses his goal. Correct habituation distinguishes a good political system from a bad one.

§6 Further, the sources and means that develop each virtue also ruin it, just as they do in a craft. For playing the harp makes both good and bad harpists, and it is analogous in the case of builders and all the rest; for building well makes good builders, and building badly makes bad ones. §7 Otherwise no teacher would be needed, but everyone would be born a good or a bad craftsman.

It is the same, then, with the virtues. For what we do in our dealings with other people makes some of us just, some unjust; what we do in terrifying situations, and the habits of fear or confidence that we acquire, make some of us brave and others cowardly. The same is true of situations involving appetites and anger; for one or another sort of conduct in these situations makes some temperate and mild, others intemperate and irascible. To sum it up in a single account: a state [of character] results from [the repetition of] similar activities.

8§ That is why we must perform the right activities, since differences in these imply corresponding differences in the states. It is not unimportant, then, to acquire one sort of habit or another, right from our youth. On the contrary, it is very important, indeed all-important.

Habituation

Our present discussion does not aim, as our others do, at study; for the purpose of our examination is not to know what virtue is, but to become good, since otherwise the inquiry would be of no benefit to us. And so we must examine the right ways of acting; for, as we have said, the actions also control the sorts of states we acquire.

§2 First, then, actions should accord with the correct reason. That is a common [belief], and let us assume it. We shall discuss it later, and say what the correct reason is and how it is related to the other virtues.

§3 But let us take it as agreed in advance that every account of the actions we must do has to be stated in outline, not exactly. As we also said at the beginning, the type of accounts we demand should accord with the subject matter; and questions about actions and expediency, like questions about health, have no fixed answers.

§4 While this is the character of our general account, the account of particular cases is still more inexact. For these fall under no craft or profession; the agents themselves must consider in each case what the opportune action is, as doctors and navigators do. §5 The account we offer, then, in our present inquiry is of this inexact sort; still, we must try to offer help.

§6 First, then, we should observe that these sorts of states naturally tend to be ruined by excess and deficiency. We see this happen with strength and health—for we must use evident cases [such as these] as witnesses to things that are not evident. For both excessive and deficient exercise ruin bodily strength, and, similarly, too much or too little eating or drinking ruins health, whereas the proportionate amount produces, increases, and preserves it.

§7 The same is true, then, of temperance, bravery, and the other virtues. For if, for instance, someone avoids and is afraid of everything, standing firm against nothing, he becomes cowardly; if he is afraid of nothing at all and goes to face everything, he becomes rash. Similarly, if he gratifies himself with every pleasure and abstains from none, he becomes intemperate; if he avoids them all, as boors do, he becomes some sort of insensible person. Temperance and bravery, then, are ruined by excess and deficiency, but preserved by the mean.

§8 But these actions are not only the sources and causes both of the emergence and growth of virtues and of their ruin; the activities of the virtues [once we have acquired them] also consist in these same actions. For this is also true of more evident cases; strength, for instance, arises from eating a lot and from withstanding much hard labor, and it is the strong person who is most capable of these very actions. §9 It is the same with the virtues. For abstaining from pleasures makes us become temperate, and once we have become temperate we are most capable of abstaining from pleasures. It is similar with bravery; habituation in disdain for frightening situations and in standing firm against them makes us become brave, and once we have become brave we shall be most capable of standing firm. [...]

Virtuous Actions versus Virtuous Character

Someone might be puzzled, however, about what we mean by saying that we become just by doing just actions and become temperate by doing temperate actions. For [one might suppose that] if we do grammatical or musical actions, we are grammarians or musicians, and, similarly, if we do just or temperate actions, we are thereby just or temperate.

§2 But surely actions are not enough, even in the case of crafts; for it is possible to produce a grammatical result by chance, or by following someone else's instructions. To be grammarians, then, we must both produce a grammatical result and produce it grammatically—that is to say, produce it in accord with the grammatical knowledge in us.

§3 Moreover, in any case, what is true of crafts is not true of virtues. For the products of a craft determine by their own qualities whether they have been produced well; and so it suffices that they have the right qualities when they have been produced. But for actions in accord with the virtues to be done temperately or justly it does not suffice that they themselves have the right qualities. Rather, the agent must also be in the right state when he does them. First, he must know [that he is doing virtuous actions]; second, he must decide on them, and decide on them for themselves; and, third, he must also do them from a firm and unchanging state.

As conditions for having a craft, these three do not count, except for the bare knowing. As a condition for having a virtue, however, the knowing counts for nothing, or [rather] for only a little, whereas the other two conditions are very important, indeed all-important. And we achieve these other two conditions by the frequent doing of just and temperate actions.

§4 Hence actions are called just or temperate when they are the sort that a just or temperate person would do. But the just and temperate person is not the one who [merely] does these actions, but the one who also does them in the way in which just or temperate people do them.

§5 It is right, then, to say that a person comes to be just from doing just actions and temperate from doing temperate actions; for no one has the least prospect of becoming good from failing to do them.

§6 The many, however, do not do these actions. They take refuge in arguments, thinking that they are doing philosophy, and that this is the way to become excellent people. They are like a sick person who listens attentively to the doctor, but acts on none of his instructions. Such a course of treatment will not improve the state of the sick person's body; nor will the many improve the state of their souls by this attitude to philosophy.

Virtue of Character: Its Genus

Next we must examine what virtue is. Since there are three conditions arising in the soul—feelings, capacities, and states—virtue must be one of these.

2§ By feelings I mean appetite, anger, fear, confidence, envy, joy, love, hate, longing, jealousy, pity, and in general whatever implies pleasure or pain. By capacities I mean what we have when we are said to be capable of these feelings—capable of being angry, for instance, or of being afraid or of feeling pity. By states I mean what we have when we are well or badly off in relation to feelings. If, for instance, our feeling is too intense or slack, we are badly off in relation to anger, but if it is intermediate, we are well off; the same is true in the other cases.

§3 First, then, neither virtues nor vices are feelings. For we are called excellent or base insofar as we have virtues or vices, not insofar as we have feelings. Further, we are neither praised nor blamed insofar as we have feelings; for we do not praise the angry or the frightened person, and do not blame the person who is simply angry, but only the person who is angry in a particular way. We are praised or blamed, however, insofar as we have virtues or vices. §4 Further, we are angry and afraid without decision; but the virtues are decisions of some kind, or [rather] require decision. Besides, insofar as we have feelings, we are said to be moved; but insofar as we have virtues or vices, we are said to be in some condition rather than moved.

§5 For these reasons the virtues are not capacities either; for we are neither called good nor called bad, nor are we praised or blamed, insofar as we are simply capable of feelings. Further, while we have capacities by nature, we do not become good or bad by nature; we have discussed this before.

§6 If, then, the virtues are neither feelings nor capacities, the remaining possibility is that they are states. And so we have said what the genus of virtue is.

Virtue of Character: Its Differential

But we must say not only, as we already have, that it is a state, but also what sort of state it is.

§2 It should be said, then, that every virtue causes its possessors to be in a good state and to perform their functions well. The virtue of eyes, for instance, makes the eyes and their functioning excellent, because it makes us see well; and similarly, the virtue of a horse makes the horse excellent, and thereby good at galloping, at carrying its rider, and at standing steady in the face of the enemy. §3 If this is true in every case, the virtue of a human being will likewise be the state that makes a human being good and makes him perform his function well.

§4 We have already said how this will be true, and it will also be evident from our next remarks, if we consider the sort of nature that virtue has.

In everything continuous and divisible we can take more, less, and equal, and each of them either in the object itself or relative to us; and the equal is some intermediate between excess and deficiency. §5 By the intermediate in the object I mean what is equidistant from each extremity; this is one and the same for all. But relative to us the intermediate is what is neither superfluous nor deficient; this is not one, and is not the same for all.

§6 If, for instance, ten are many and two are few, we take six as intermediate in the object, since it exceeds [two] and is exceeded [by ten] by an equal amount, [four]. §7 This is what is intermediate by numerical proportion. But that is not how we must take the intermediate that is relative to us. For if ten pounds [of food], for instance, are a lot for someone to eat, and two pounds a little, it does not follow that the trainer will prescribe six, since this might also be either a little or a lot for the person who is to take it—for Milo [the athlete] a little, but for the beginner in gymnastics a lot; and the same is true for running and wrestling. §8 In this way every scientific expert avoids excess and deficiency and seeks and chooses what is intermediate—but intermediate relative to us, not in the object.

§9 This, then, is how each science produces its product well, by focusing on what is intermediate and making the product conform to that. This, indeed, is why people regularly comment on well-made products that nothing could be added or subtracted; they assume that excess or deficiency ruins a good [result], whereas the mean preserves it. Good craftsmen also, we say, focus on what is intermediate when they produce their product. And since virtue, like nature, is better and more exact than any craft, it will also aim at what is intermediate.

§10 By virtue I mean virtue of character; for this is about feelings and actions, and these admit of excess, deficiency, and an intermediate condition. We can be afraid, for instance, or be confident, or have appetites, or get angry, or feel pity, and in general have pleasure or pain, both too much and too little, and in both ways not well. §11 But having these feelings at the right times, about the right things, toward the right people, for the right end, and in the right way, is the intermediate and best condition, and this is proper to virtue. §12 Similarly, actions also admit of excess, deficiency, and an intermediate condition.

Now virtue is about feelings and actions, in which excess and deficiency are in error and incur blame, whereas the intermediate condition is correct and wins praise, which are both proper to virtue. §13 Virtue, then, is a mean, insofar as it aims at what is intermediate.

§14 Moreover, there are many ways to be in error—for badness is proper to the indeterminate, as the Pythagoreans pictured it, and good to the determinate. But there is only one way to be correct. That is why error is easy and correctness is difficult, since it is easy to miss the target and difficult to hit it. And so for this reason also excess and deficiency are proper to vice, the mean to virtue; 'for we are noble in only one way, but bad in all sorts of ways.'

§15 Virtue, then, is a state that decides, consisting in a mean, the mean relative to us, which is defined by reference to reason, that is to say, to the reason by reference to which the prudent person would define it. It is a mean between two vices, one of excess and one of deficiency.

§16 It is a mean for this reason also: Some vices miss what is right because they are deficient, others because they are excessive, in feelings or in actions, whereas virtue finds and chooses what is intermediate.

§17 That is why virtue, as far as its essence and the account stating what it is are concerned, is a mean, but, as far as the best [condition] and the good [result] are concerned, it is an extremity.

§18 Now not every action or feeling admits of the mean. For the names of some automatically include baseness—for instance, spite, shamelessness, envy [among feelings], and adultery, theft, murder, among actions. For all of these and similar things are called by these names because they themselves, not their excesses or deficiencies, are base. Hence in doing these things we can never be correct, but must invariably be in error. We cannot do them well or not well—by committing adultery, for instance, with the right woman at the right time in the right way. On the contrary, it is true without qualification that to do any of them is to be in error.

§19 [To think these admit of a mean], therefore, is like thinking that unjust or cowardly or intemperate action also admits of a mean, an excess and a deficiency. If it did, there would be a mean of excess, a mean of deficiency, an excess of excess and a deficiency of deficiency. §20 On the contrary, just as there is no excess or deficiency of temperance or of bravery (since the intermediate is a sort of extreme), so also there is no mean of these vicious actions either, but whatever way anyone does them, he is in error. For in general there is no mean of excess or of deficiency, and no excess or deficiency of a mean.

The Particular Virtues of Character

However, we must not only state this general account but also apply it to the particular cases. For among accounts concerning actions, though the general ones are common to more cases, the specific ones are truer, since actions are about particular cases, and our account must accord with these. Let us, then, find these from the chart.

§2 First, then, in feelings of fear and confidence the mean is bravery. The excessively fearless person is nameless (indeed many cases are nameless), and the one who is excessively confident is rash. The one who is excessive in fear and deficient in confidence is cowardly.

§3 In pleasures and pains—though not in all types, and in pains less than in pleasures—the mean is temperance and the excess intemperance. People deficient in pleasure are not often found, which is why they also lack even a name; let us call them insensible.

§4 In giving and taking money the mean is generosity, the excess wastefulness and the deficiency ungenerosity. Here the vicious people have contrary excesses and defects; for the wasteful person is excessive in spending and deficient in taking, whereas the ungenerous person is excessive in taking and deficient in spending. §5 At the moment we are speaking in outline and summary, and that is enough; later we shall define these things more exactly.

§6 In questions of money there are also other conditions. Another mean is magnificence; for the magnificent person differs from the generous by being concerned with large matters, while the generous person is concerned with small. The excess is ostentation and vulgarity, and the deficiency is stinginess. These differ from the vices related to generosity in ways we shall describe later.

§7 In honor and dishonor the mean is magnanimity, the excess something called a sort of vanity, and the deficiency pusillanimity. §8 And just as we said that generosity differs from magnificence in its concern with small matters, similarly there is a virtue concerned with small honors, differing in the same way from magnanimity, which is concerned with great honors. For honor can be desired either in the right way or more or less than is right. If someone desires it to excess, he is called an honor-lover, and if his desire is deficient he is called indifferent to honor, but if he is intermediate he has no name. The corresponding conditions have no name either, except the condition of the honor-lover, which is called honor-loving.

This is why people at the extremes lay claim to the intermediate area. Moreover, we also sometimes call the intermediate person an honor-lover, and sometimes call him indifferent to honor; and sometimes we praise the honor-lover, sometimes the person indifferent to honor. §9 We will mention later the reason we do this; for the moment, let us speak of the other cases in the way we have laid down.

§10 Anger also admits of an excess, deficiency, and mean. These are all practically nameless; but since we call the intermediate person mild, let us call the mean mildness. Among the extreme people, let the excessive person be irascible, and his vice irascibility, and let the deficient person be a sort of inirascible person, and his deficiency inirascibility.

§11 There are also three other means, somewhat similar to one another, but different. For they are all concerned with common dealings in conversations and actions, but differ insofar as one is concerned with truth telling in these areas, the other two with sources of pleasure, some of which are found in amusement, and the others in daily life in general. Hence we should also discuss these states, so that we can better observe that in every case the mean is praiseworthy, whereas the extremes are neither praiseworthy nor correct, but blameworthy. Most of these cases are also nameless, and we must try, as in the other cases also, to supply names ourselves, to make things clear and easy to follow.

§12 In truth-telling, then, let us call the intermediate person truthful, and the mean truthfulness; pretense that overstates will be boastfulness, and the person who has it boastful; pretense that understates will be self-deprecation, and the person who has it self-deprecating.

§13 In sources of pleasure in amusements let us call the intermediate person witty, and the condition wit; the excess buffoonery and the person who has it a buffoon; and the deficient person a sort of boor and the state boorishness.

In the other sources of pleasure, those in daily life, let us call the person who is pleasant in the right way friendly, and the mean state friendliness. If someone goes to excess with no [ulterior] aim, he will be ingratiating; if he does it for his own advantage, a flatterer. The deficient person, unpleasant in everything, will be a sort of quarrelsome and ill-tempered person.

§14 There are also means in feelings and about feelings. Shame, for instance, is not a virtue, but the person prone to shame as well as [the virtuous people we have described] receives praise. For here also one person is called intermediate, and another—the person excessively prone to shame, who is ashamed about everything—is called excessive; the person who is deficient in shame or never feels shame at all is said to have no sense of disgrace; and the intermediate one is called prone to shame.

§15 Proper indignation is the mean between envy and spite; these conditions are concerned with pleasure and pain at what happens to our neighbors. For the properly indignant person feels pain when someone does well undeservedly; the envious person exceeds him by feeling pain when anyone does well, while the spiteful person is so deficient in feeling pain that he actually enjoys [other people's misfortunes.]

§16 There will also be an opportunity elsewhere to speak of these. We must consider justice after these. Since it is spoken of in more than one way, we shall distinguish its two types and say how each of them is a mean. Similarly, we must also consider the virtues that belong to reason.

Relations between Mean and Extreme States

Among these three conditions, then, two are vices—one of excess, one of deficiency—and one, the mean, is virtue. In a way, each of them is opposed to each of the others, since each extreme is contrary both to the intermediate condition and to the other extreme, while the intermediate is contrary to the extremes.

§2 For, just as the equal is greater in comparison to the smaller, and smaller in comparison to the greater, so also the intermediate states are excessive in comparison to the deficiencies and deficient in comparison to the excesses—both in feelings and in actions. For the brave person, for instance, appears rash in comparison to the coward, and cowardly in comparison to the rash person; the temperate person appears intemperate in comparison to the insensible person, and insensible in comparison with the intemperate person; and the generous person appears wasteful in comparison to the ungenerous, and ungenerous in comparison to the wasteful person. §3 That is why each of the extreme people tries to push the intermediate person to the other extreme, so that the coward, for instance, calls the brave person rash, and the rash person calls him a coward, and similarly in the other cases.

§4 Since these conditions of soul are opposed to each other in these ways, the extremes are more contrary to each other than to the intermediate. For they are further from each other than from the intermediate, just as the large is further from the small, and the small from the large, than either is from the equal.

§5 Further, sometimes one extreme—rashness or wastefulness, for instance—appears somewhat like the intermediate state, bravery or generosity. But the extremes are most unlike one another; and the things that are furthest apart from each other are defined as contraries. And so the things that are further apart are more contrary.

§6 In some cases the deficiency, in others the excess, is more opposed to the intermediate condition. For instance, cowardice, the deficiency, not rashness, the excess, is more opposed to bravery, whereas intemperance, the excess, not insensibility, the deficiency, is more opposed to temperance.

§7 This happens for two reasons: One reason is derived from the object itself. Since sometimes one extreme is closer and more similar to the intermediate condition, we oppose the contrary extreme, more than this closer one, to the intermediate condition. Since rashness, for instance, seems to be closer and more similar to bravery, and cowardice less similar, we oppose cowardice, more than rashness, to bravery; for what is further from the intermediate condition seems to be more contrary to it. This, then, is one reason, derived from the object itself.

§8 The other reason is derived from ourselves. For when we ourselves have some natural tendency to one extreme more than to the other, this extreme appears more opposed to the intermediate condition. Since, for instance, we have more of a natural tendency to pleasure, we drift more easily toward intemperance than toward orderliness. Hence, we say that an extreme is more contrary if we naturally develop more in that direction; and this is why intemperance is more contrary to temperance, since it is the excess [of pleasure].

How Can We Reach the Mean?

We have said enough, then, to show that virtue of character is a mean and what sort of mean it is; that it is a mean between two vices, one of excess and one of deficiency; and that it is a mean because it aims at the intermediate condition in feelings and actions.

§2 That is why it is also hard work to be excellent. For in each case it is hard work to find the intermediate; for instance, not everyone, but only one who knows, finds the midpoint in a circle. So also getting angry, or giving and spending money, is easy and everyone can do it; but doing it to the right person, in the right amount, at the right time, for the right end, and in the right way is no longer easy, nor can everyone do it. Hence doing these things well is rare, praiseworthy, and fine.

§3 That is why anyone who aims at the intermediate condition must first of all steer clear of the more contrary extreme, following the advice that Calypso also gives: 'Hold the ship outside the spray and surge.' For one extreme is more in error, the other less. §4 Since, therefore, it is hard to hit the intermediate extremely accurately, the second-best tack, as they say, is to take the lesser of the evils. We shall succeed best in this by the method we describe.

We must also examine what we ourselves drift into easily. For different people have different natural tendencies toward different goals, and we shall come to know our own tendencies from the pleasure or pain that arises in us. §5 We must drag ourselves off in the contrary direction; for if we pull far away from error, as they do in straightening bent wood, we shall reach the intermediate condition.

§6 And in everything we must beware above all of pleasure and its sources; for we are already biased in its favor when we come to judge it. Hence, we must react to it as the elders reacted to Helen, and on each occasion repeat what they said; for if we do this, and send it off, we shall be less in error.

§7 In summary, then, if we do these things we shall best be able to reach the intermediate condition. But presumably this is difficult, especially in particular cases, since it is not easy to define the way we should be angry, with whom, about what, for how long. For sometimes, indeed, we ourselves praise deficient people and call them mild, and sometimes praise quarrelsome people and call them manly.

§8 Still, we are not blamed if we deviate a little in excess or deficiency from doing well, but only if we deviate a long way, since then we are easily noticed. But how great and how serious a deviation receives blame is not easy to define in an account; for nothing else perceptible is easily defined either. Such things are among particulars, and the judgment depends on perception.

§9 This is enough, then, to make it clear that in every case the intermediate state is praised, but we must sometimes incline toward the excess, sometimes toward the deficiency; for that is the easiest way to hit the intermediate and good condition.

The Individual Virtues of Character

Aristotle; trans. Terence Irwin

Aristotle, Selections from "Virtue of Character," *Nichomachean Ethics*, trans. Terence Irwin, pp. 40-49. Copyright © 1999 by Hackett Publishing Company, Inc. Reprinted with permission.

Bravery; Its Scope

First let us discuss bravery. We have already made it apparent that there is a mean about feelings of fear and confidence. §2 What we fear, clearly, is what is frightening, and such things are, speaking without qualification, bad things; hence people define fear as expectation of something bad.

§3 Certainly we fear all bad things—for instance, bad reputation, poverty, sickness, friendlessness, death—but they do not all seem to concern the brave person. For fear of some bad things, such as bad reputation, is actually right and fine, and lack of fear is shameful; for if someone fears bad reputation, he is decent and properly prone to shame, and if he has no fear of it, he has no feeling of disgrace. Some, however, call this fearless person brave, by a transference of the name; for he has some similarity to the brave person, since the brave person is also a type of fearless person.

§4 Presumably it is wrong to fear poverty or sickness or, in general, [bad things] that are not the results of vice or caused by ourselves; still, someone who is fearless about these is not thereby brave. He is also called brave by similarity; for some people who are cowardly in the dangers of war are nonetheless generous, and face with confidence the [danger of] losing money.

§5 Again, if someone is afraid of committing wanton aggression on children or women, or of being envious or anything of that sort, that does not make him cowardly. And if someone is confident when he is going to be whipped for his crimes, that does not make him brave.

§6 Then what sorts of frightening conditions concern the brave person? Surely the most frightening; for no one stands firmer against terrifying conditions. Now death is most frightening of all, since it is a boundary, and when someone is dead nothing beyond it seems either good or bad for him any more. §7 Still, not even death in all conditions—on the sea, for instance, or in sickness—seems to be the brave person's concern.

§8 In what conditions, then, is death his concern? Surely in the finest conditions. Now such deaths are those in war, since they occur in the greatest and finest danger. §9 This judgment is endorsed by the honors given in cities and by monarchs. §10 Hence someone is called fully brave if he is intrepid in facing a fine death and the immediate dangers that bring death. And this is above all true of the dangers of war.

§11 Certainly the brave person is also intrepid on the sea and in sickness, but not in the same way as seafarers are. For he has given up hope of safety, and objects to this sort of death [with nothing fine in it], but seafarers' experience makes them hopeful. §12 Moreover, we act like brave men on occasions when we can use our strength, or when it is fine to be killed; and neither of these is true when we perish from shipwreck or sickness.

Bravery; Its Characteristic Outlook

Now what is frightening is not the same for everyone. We say, however, that some things are too frightening for a human being to resist; these, then, are frightening for everyone, at least for everyone with any sense. What is frightening, but not irresistible for a human being, varies in its seriousness and degree; and the same is true of what inspires confidence.

§2 The brave person is unperturbed, as far as a human being can be. Hence, though he will fear even the sorts of things that are not irresistible, he will stand firm against them, in the right way, as reason prescribes, for the sake of the fine, since this is the end aimed at by virtue.

§3 It is possible to be more or less afraid of these frightening things, and also possible to be afraid of what is not frightening as though it were frightening. §4 The cause of error may be fear of the wrong thing, or in the wrong way, or at the wrong time, or something of that sort; and the same is true for things that inspire confidence.

§5 Hence whoever stands firm against the right things and fears the right things, for the right end, in the right way, at the right time, and is correspondingly confident, is the brave person; for the brave person's actions and feelings accord with what something is worth, and follow what reason prescribes.

§6 Every activity aims at actions in accord with the state of character. Now to the brave person bravery is fine; hence the end it aims at is also fine, since each thing is defined by its end. The brave person, then, aims at the fine when he stands firm and acts in accord with bravery.

§7 Among those who go to excess the excessively fearless person has no name—we said earlier that many cases have no names. He would be some sort of madman, or incapable of feeling distress, if he feared nothing, neither earthquake nor waves, as they say about the Celts.

The person who is excessively confident about frightening things is rash. §8 The rash person also seems to be a boaster, and a pretender to bravery. At any rate, the attitude to frightening things that the brave person really has is the attitude that the rash person wants to appear to have; hence he imitates the brave person where he can. §9 That is why most of them are rash cowards; for, rash though they are on these [occasions for imitation], they do not stand firm against anything frightening. §12 Moreover, rash people are impetuous, wishing for dangers before they arrive, but they shrink from them when they come. Brave people, on the contrary, are eager when in action, but keep quiet until then.

§10 The person who is excessively afraid is the coward, since he fears the wrong things, and in the wrong way, and so on. Certainly, he is also deficient in confidence, but his excessive pain distinguishes him more clearly. §11 Hence, since he is afraid of everything, he is a despairing sort. The brave person, on the contrary, is hopeful, since [he is confident and] confidence is proper to a hopeful person.

§12 Hence the coward, the rash person, and the brave person are all concerned with the same things, but have different states related to them; the others are excessive or defective, but the brave person has the intermediate and right state.

§13 As we have said, then, bravery is a mean about what inspires confidence and about what is frightening in the conditions we have described; it chooses and stands firm because that is fine or because anything else is shameful. Dying to avoid poverty or erotic passion or something painful is proper to a coward, not to a brave person. For shirking burdens is softness, and such a person stands firm [in the face of death] to avoid an evil, not because standing firm is fine.

Conditions That Resemble Bravery

Bravery, then, is something of this sort. But five other sorts of things are also called bravery.

The bravery of citizens comes first, since it looks most like bravery. For citizens seem to stand firm against dangers with the aim of avoiding reproaches and legal penalties and of winning honors; that is why the bravest seem to be those who hold cowards in dishonor and do honor to brave people. §2 That is how Homer also describes them when he speaks of Diomede and Hector: 'Polydamas will be the first to heap disgrace on me', and 'For some time Hector speaking among the Trojans will say, "The son of Tydeus fled from me."' §3 This is most like the [genuine] bravery described above, because it results from a virtue; for it is caused by shame and by desire for something fine, namely honor, and by aversion from reproach, which is shameful.

§4 In this class we might also place those who are compelled by their superiors. However, they are worse to the extent that they act because of fear, not because of shame, and to avoid pain, not disgrace. For their commanders compel them, as Hector does; 'If I notice anyone shrinking back from the battle, nothing will save him from being eaten by the dogs.' §5 Commanders who strike any troops who give ground, or who post them in front of ditches and suchlike, do the same thing, since they all compel them. The brave person, however, must be moved by the fine, not by compulsion.

§6 Experience about a given situation also seems to be bravery; that is why Socrates actually thought that bravery is scientific knowledge. Different people have this sort [of apparent courage] in different conditions. In wartime professional soldiers have it; for there seem to be many groundless alarms in war, and the professionals are the most familiar with these. Hence they appear brave, since others do not know that the alarms are groundless. §7 Moreover, their experience makes them most capable in attack and defense, since they are skilled in the use of their weapons, and have the best weapons for attack and defense. §8 The result is that in fighting nonprofessionals they are like armed troops against unarmed, or trained athletes against ordinary people; for in these contests also the best fighters are the strongest and physically fittest, not the bravest.

§9 Professional soldiers, however, turn out to be cowards whenever the danger overstrains them and they are inferior in numbers and equipment. For they are the first to run, whereas the citizen troops stand firm and get killed; this was what happened at the temple of Hermes. For the citizens find it shameful to run, and find death more choiceworthy than safety at this cost. But the professionals from the start were facing the danger on the assumption of their superiority; once they learn their mistake, they run, since they are more afraid of being killed than of doing something shameful. That is not the brave person's character.

§10 Spirit is also counted as bravery; for those who act on spirit also seem to be brave—as beasts seem to be when they attack those who have wounded them—because brave people are also full of spirit. For spirit is most eager to run and face dangers; hence Homer's words, 'put strength in his spirit,' 'aroused strength and spirit,' and 'his blood boiled.' All these would seem to signify the arousal and the impulse of spirit.

§11 Now brave people act because of the fine, and their spirit cooperates with them. But beasts act because of pain; for they attack only because they have been wounded or frightened, (since they keep away from us in a forest). They are not brave, then, since distress and spirit drives them in an impulsive rush to meet danger, foreseeing none of the terrifying prospects. For if they were brave, hungry asses would also be brave, since they keep on feeding even if they are beaten; and adulterers also do many daring actions because of lust.

§12 Human beings as well as beasts find it painful to be angered, and pleasant to exact a penalty. But those who fight for these reasons are not brave, though they are good fighters; for they fight because of their feelings, not because of the fine nor as reason prescribes. Still, they have something similar [to bravery]. The [bravery] caused by spirit would seem to be the most natural sort, and to be [genuine] bravery once it has also acquired decision and the goal.

§13 Hopeful people are not brave either; for their many victories over many opponents make them confident in dangers. They are somewhat similar to brave people, since both are confident. But whereas brave people are confident for the reason given earlier, the hopeful are confident because they think they are stronger and nothing could happen to them; §14 drunks do the same sort of thing, since they become hopeful. When things turn out differently from how they expected, they run away. The brave person, on the contrary, stands firm against what is and appears frightening to a human being; he does this because it is fine to stand firm and shameful to fail.

§15 Indeed, that is why someone who is unafraid and unperturbed in emergencies seems braver than [someone who is unafraid only] when he is warned in advance; for his action proceeds more from his state of character, because it proceeds less from preparation. For if we are warned in advance, we might decide what to do [not only because of our state of character, but] also by reason and rational calculation; but in emergencies [we must decide] in accord with our state of character.

§16 Those who act in ignorance also appear brave, and indeed they are close to hopeful people, though inferior to them insofar as they lack the self-esteem of hopeful people. That is why the hopeful stand firm for some time, whereas if ignorant people have been deceived and then realize or suspect that things are different, they run. That was what happened to the Argives when they stumbled on the Spartans and took them for Sicyonians.

§17 We have described, then, the character of brave people and of those who seem to be brave.

Feelings Proper to Bravery

Bravery is about feelings of confidence and fear—not, however, about both in the same way, but more about frightening things. For someone is brave if he is undisturbed and in the right state about these, more than if he is in this state about things inspiring confidence.

§2 As we said, then, standing firm against what is painful makes us call people brave; that is why bravery is both painful and justly praised, since it is harder to stand firm against something painful than to refrain from something pleasant. §3 Nonetheless, the end that bravery aims at seems to be pleasant, though obscured by its surroundings. This is what happens in athletic contests. For boxers find that the end they aim at, the crown and the honors, is pleasant, but, being made of flesh and blood, they find it distressing and painful to take the punches and to bear all the hard work; and because there are so many of these painful things, the end, being small, appears to have nothing pleasant in it.

§4 And so, if the same is true for bravery, the brave person will find death and wounds painful, and suffer them unwillingly, but he will endure them because that is fine or because failure is shameful. Indeed, the truer it is that he has every virtue and the happier he is, the more pain he will feel at the prospect of death. For this sort of person, more than anyone, finds it worthwhile to be alive, and knows he is being deprived of the greatest goods, and this is painful. But he is no less brave for all that; presumably, indeed, he is all the braver, because he chooses what is fine in war at the cost of all these goods. §5 It is not true, then, in the case of every virtue that its active exercise is pleasant; it is pleasant only insofar as we attain the end.

§6 But presumably it is quite possible for brave people, given the character we have described, not to be the best soldiers. Perhaps the best will be those who are less brave, but possess no other good; for they are ready to face dangers, and they sell their lives for small gains.

§7 So much for bravery. It is easy to grasp what it is, in outline at least, from what we have said.

Temperance; Its Scope

Let us discuss temperance next; for bravery and temperance seem to be the virtues of the nonrational parts. Temperance, then, is a mean concerned with pleasures, as we have already said; for it is concerned less, and in a different way, with pains. Intemperance appears in this same area too. Let us, then, now distinguish the specific pleasures that concern them.

§2 First, let us distinguish pleasures of the soul from those of the body. Love of honor and of learning, for instance, are among the pleasures of the soul; for though a lover of one of these enjoys it, only his thought, not his body, is at all affected. Those concerned with such pleasures are called neither temperate nor intemperate. The same applies to those concerned with any of the other nonbodily pleasures; for lovers of tales, storytellers, those who waste their days on trivialities, are called babblers, but not intemperate. Nor do we call people intemperate if they feel pain over money or friends.

§3 Temperance, then, will be about bodily pleasures, but not even about all of these. For those who find enjoyment in objects of sight, such as colors, shapes, a painting, are called neither temperate nor intemperate, even though it would also seem possible to enjoy these either rightly or excessively and deficiently. §4 The same is true for hearing; no one is ever called intemperate for excessive enjoyment of songs or playacting, or temperate for the right enjoyment of them.

§5 Nor is this said about someone enjoying smells, except coincidentally. For someone is called intemperate not for enjoying the smell of apples or roses or incense, but rather for enjoying the smell of perfumes or cooked delicacies. For these are the smells an intemperate person enjoys because they remind him of the objects of his appetite. §6 And we can see that others also enjoy the smells of food if they are hungry. It is the enjoyment of the things [that he is reminded of by these smells] that is proper to an intemperate person, since these are the objects of his appetite.

§7 Nor do other animals find pleasures from these senses, except coincidentally. What a hound enjoys, for instance, is not the smell of a hare, but eating it; but the hare's smell made the hound perceive it. And what a lion enjoys is not the sound of the ox, but eating it; but since the ox's sound made the lion perceive that it was near, the lion appears to enjoy the sound. Similarly, what pleases him is not the sight of 'a deer or a wild goat', but the prospect of food.

§8 The pleasures that concern temperance and intemperance are those that are shared with the other animals, and so appear slavish and bestial. These pleasures are touch and taste.

§9 However, they seem to deal even with taste very little or not at all. For taste discriminates flavors—the sort of thing that wine tasters and cooks savoring food do; but people, or intemperate people at any rate, do not much enjoy this. Rather, they enjoy the gratification that comes entirely through touch, in eating and drinking and in what are called the pleasures of sex. §10 That is why a glutton actually prayed for his throat to become longer than a crane's, showing that he took pleasure in the touching. And so the sense that concerns intemperance is the most widely shared, and seems justifiably open to reproach, since we have it insofar as we are animals, not insofar as we are human beings.

§11 To enjoy these things, then, and to like them most of all, is bestial. For indeed the most civilized of the pleasures coming through touch, such as those produced by rubbing and warming in gymnasia, are excluded from intemperance, since the touching that is proper to the intemperate person concerns only some parts of the body, not all of it.

Temperance; Its Outlook

Some appetites seem to be shared [by everyone], while others seem to be additions that are distinctive [of different people]. The appetite for nourishment, for instance, is natural, since everyone who lacks nourishment, dry or liquid, has an appetite for it, sometimes for both; and, as Homer says, the young in their prime [all] have an appetite for sex. Not everyone, however, has an appetite for a specific sort of food or drink or sex, or for the same things. §2 That is why an appetite of this type seems to be distinctive of [each of] us. Still, this also includes a natural element, since different sorts of people find different sorts of things more pleasant, and there are some things that are more pleasant for everyone than things chosen at random would be.

§3 In natural appetites few people are in error, and only in one direction, toward excess. Eating indiscriminately or drinking until we are too full is exceeding the quantity that accords with nature; for [the object of] natural appetite is the filling of a lack. That is why these people are called 'gluttons', showing that they glut their bellies past what is right; that is how especially slavish people turn out.

§4 With the pleasures that are distinctive of different people, many make errors and in many ways; for people are called lovers of something if they enjoy the wrong things, or if they enjoy something in the wrong way. And in all these ways intemperate people go to excess. For some of the things they enjoy are hateful, and hence wrong; distinctive pleasures that it is right to enjoy they enjoy more than is right, and more than most people enjoy them.

§5 Clearly, then, with pleasures excess is intemperance, and is blameworthy. With pains, however, we are not called temperate, as we are called brave, for standing firm against them, or intemperate for not standing firm. Rather, someone is intemperate because he feels more pain than is right at failing to get pleasant things; and even this pain is produced by the pleasure [he takes in them]. And someone is temperate because he does not feel pain at the absence of what is pleasant, or at refraining from it.

§6 The intemperate person, then, has an appetite for all pleasant things, or rather for the most pleasant of them, and his appetite leads him to choose these at the cost of the other things. That is why he also feels pain both when he fails to get something and when he has an appetite for it, since appetite involves pain. It would seem absurd, however, to suffer pain because of pleasure.

§7 People who are deficient in pleasures and enjoy them less than is right are not found very much. For that sort of insensibility is not human; indeed, even the other animals discriminate among foods, enjoying some but not others. If someone finds nothing pleasant, or preferable to anything else, he is far from being human. The reason he has no name is that he is not found much.

§8 The temperate person has an intermediate state in relation to these [bodily pleasures]. For he finds no pleasure in what most pleases the intemperate person, but finds it disagreeable; he finds no pleasure at all in the wrong things. He finds no intense pleasure in any [bodily pleasures], suffers no pain at their absence, and has no appetite for them, or only a moderate appetite, not to the wrong degree or at the wrong time or anything else at all of that sort. If something is pleasant and conducive to health or fitness, he will desire this moderately and in the right way; and he will desire in the same way anything else that is pleasant, if it is no obstacle to health and fitness, does not deviate from the fine, and does not exceed his means. For the opposite sort of person likes these pleasures more than they are worth; that is not the temperate person's character, but he likes them as correct reason prescribes.

Intemperance

Intemperance is more like a voluntary condition than cowardice; for it is caused by pleasure, which is choiceworthy, whereas cowardice is caused by pain, which is to be avoided. §2 Moreover, pain disturbs and ruins the nature of the sufferer, while pleasure does nothing of the sort; intemperance, then, is more voluntary. That is why it is also more open to reproach. For it is also easier to acquire the habit of facing pleasant things, since our life includes many of them and we can acquire the habit with no danger; but with frightening things the reverse is true.

§3 However, cowardice seems to be more voluntary than particular cowardly actions. For cowardice itself involves no pain, but the particular actions disturb us because of the pain [that causes them], so that people actually throw away their weapons and do all the other disgraceful actions. That is why these actions even seem to be forced [and hence involuntary].

§4 For the intemperate person the reverse is true. The particular actions are the result of his appetite and desire, and so they are voluntary; but the whole condition is less voluntary [than the actions], since no one has an appetite to be intemperate.

§5 We also apply the name of intemperance to the errors of children, since they have some similarity. Which gets its name from which does not matter for our present purposes, but clearly the posterior is called after the prior.

§6 The name would seem to be quite appropriately transferred. For the things that need to be tempered are those that desire shameful things and tend to grow large. Appetites and children are most like this; for children also live by appetite, and desire for the pleasant is found more in them than in anyone else.

§7 If, then, [the child or the appetitive part] is not obedient and subordinate to its rulers, it will go far astray. For when someone lacks understanding, his desire for the pleasant is insatiable and seeks indiscriminate satisfaction. The [repeated] active exercise of appetite increases the appetite he already had from birth, and if the appetites are large and intense, they actually expel rational calculation. That is why appetites must be moderate and few, and never contrary to reason. §8 This is the condition we call obedient and temperate. And just as the child's life must follow the instructions of his guide, so too the appetitive part must follow reason.

§9 Hence the temperate person's appetitive part must agree with reason; for both [his appetitive part and his reason] aim at the fine, and the temperate person's appetites are for the right things, in the right ways, at the right times, which is just what reason also prescribes.

So much, then, for temperance.

Virtue

Piers Benn

Much of our discussion so far has been centred around two important issues in moral theory: that of whether there can be any objective basis for our judgements of right and wrong, and good and bad, and that of whether there is any credible theory that can determine what we ought to do. The first question is metaethical: it asks about the status of moral claims. Can they be literally true or false? If not, is there some other way in which they can be justified? Can there be a moral system which is objectively binding on all people in all places and at all times? The second question, as we have seen, concerns moral theory. Is there some theory—for example, "always promote the greatest happiness of the greatest number"—that can determine our duty? Both these questions have taken us to the heart of contemporary moral philosophy, and both leave us with seemingly intractable puzzles. On the one hand, it is initially hard to understand how evaluative judgements can be objectively true; on the other hand, even leaving the objectivity question aside, it is hard to see much resemblance between dominant theories like utilitarianism and the way most of our moral reasoning actually proceeds in everyday life. For most of us, the important moral questions we face are not about what to do when faced with the choice between causing one death and causing five, or between torturing a terrorist to gain life-saving information, and refusing to torture the terrorist at the risk that his hidden bomb goes off. They are really more like: should I open a bottle of wine tonight, or finish this chapter? Should I, out of benevolence, omit an unflattering detail about someone in a reference I write for her? What might be useful is some credible account both of the nature of morality and the nature of the good life that can speak to ordinary life.

It is in this spirit that from about the late 1950s there has been a revival of interest in specific *virtues and vices* and the centrality of virtue in moral philosophy. In what follows we shall be guided mainly by the question of whether virtue theory, as it is sometimes called, can contribute anything to morality that cannot be captured by some other approach. We should also bear in mind problems about the objectivity of morality. For it is possible that a theory of the virtues, and the good life virtues make possible, can provide the kind of objectivity we were seeking for moral claims. Whether this is so is a question we shall postpone until the end.

Aristotle's Ethics

Virtue theorists place a special emphasis on virtues and vices and give relatively little explicit attention to moral rules and principles. For this reason we might contrast virtue theory with *action-based theory*. Whereas for the Kantian, the central question of morality is "what ought I to do", for the virtue theorist, the really important question is "what kind of person ought I be?" This is not to say there is any strict incompatibility between these two approaches. Indeed, the extent to which they are in conflict is an intriguing question to which we shall return. For the moment, let us just say that there is a difference of emphasis and priority. Our task is to see if anything interesting comes out of the idea of the virtues.

Contemporary virtue theory is greatly inspired by the Greek philosopher Aristotle (384–322 BC). For it is in Aristotle's *Nicomachean ethics*[1] that we find a highly detailed yet lucid treatment of the subject. In contrast to Kantian and utilitarian approaches, Aristotle is not concerned to discover a supreme practical principle telling us what to do, or to derive any secondary moral rules from such a principle. He is concerned with the sort of people we must be if we are to live the good life. If we can become like this, through proper moral education and practice in making right decisions, then we shall live the good life.

But what is this good life? Here we need to introduce Aristotle's account of human nature and human fulfilment. The opening words of the *Nicomachean ethics* are "Every art and every inquiry, and similarly every action and pursuit, is thought to aim at some good; and for this reason the good has rightly been declared to be that at which all things aim." Some goods are chosen for the sake of other goods, and these in turn may be chosen for the sake of yet other goods. But it cannot be that everything is chosen only for the sake of something else—that way the whole process goes on to infinity. There must be something that is chosen for its own sake, and this must be the chief good. To know the nature of this good is the aim of all ethical enquiry. Since it is the chief good, it is nonsensical to go on asking why it should be pursued; someone who needs to ask that question has not understood what it is. However, it may not be possible, on the spot, to give to someone who does not recognize that good a reason why he should pursue it. To

---

1. Modern Aristotelians would accept that most or all of what Aristotle says about the good life for "men" applies to women as well. However, Aristotle himself is referring to a life that he thinks is appropriate mainly for males of high standing. I therefore shall often use the masculine pronoun in my discussion of Aristotelian ethics.

know what the good consists of, you must have received the right kind of moral education and formed your character in the right way. This is a long-drawn out process that centres on the education of desire.

The Good for Man: Happiness

According to Aristotle, the chief good for man is *eudaimonia*, which is usually translated as *happiness*.[2] It is something "final and self-sufficient, and is the end of action".[3] It is desired for itself alone, and cannot be made better by the addition of any other good. This eudaimonia is not exactly a psychological state, such as a feeling of euphoria, but is really a condition of well-being, or faring well. No doubt there is a connection between feeling happy and having your life go well. But it is the idea of your life going well that captures the idea of eudaimonia; we might say that in such a state you flourish.

Of what does such flourishing consist? The answer to this is found by discovering the function that man uniquely performs, and that sets him apart from all other living creatures. This brings to light an important element in Aristotle's philosophy; everything in nature has a function or characteristic activity, and man is no exception. The function of the eye is to see, the hand to hold, similarly each part of the body has a function, or is "for something". Aristotle thinks that man's function cannot be mere biological living, since animals and plants also do this. It cannot consist in perception either, since some animals also are perceivers. It must, says Aristotle, consist in that which is unique to us, as human beings. This is the life of our rational element. It is "activity of soul exhibiting excellence, and if there be more than one excellence, in accordance with the best and the most complete".[4] For only human beings enjoy this.

The connection between man's function and his good (or happiness) is this: that just as an eye flourishes if it does well that which it is for, so a man flourishes and is happy if he does well that for which he is for. This is brought out in a slightly opaque way, as follows: "... if we say 'a so-and-so' and 'a good so-and-so' have a function which is the same in kind, e.g. a lyre-player and a good lyre-player ... if this is the case ... human good turns out to be an activity of soul exhibiting excellence...".[5] For every activity there is an appropriate excellence, and all activity aims not only to perform its appropriate function, but to perform it as well as possible.

Some Initial Difficulties

Before linking this with a theory of the virtues, it is worth giving Aristotle's theory a helping hand by first conceding certain well-known criticisms of it, and then trying to show how something important may still be retained in spite of them.

A first, obvious objection is to the idea that man is *for* something; that he has a function. True (the critic says), there are things that man does, and many of these are guided by some kind of reasoning.

---

2. See Aristotle, Nicomachean ethics, trans. W.D. Ross (Oxford: Oxford University Press, 1980).

3. Aristotle, ibid., I.7, p. 12.

4. Aristotle, ibid., 1.7, p. 14.

5. Aristotle, ibid., 1.7, p. 13.

But this is no ground for thinking that this is his function, independently of the plans and activities that he actually values. In other words, the mere fact that there are certain thing she can do and sometimes does, is a poor ground for thinking this is what he *should* be doing. Secondly, even if we allow that man does have a function in this sense, it by no means follows that it is an activity that is unique to him. The mere fact that man alone lives according to a rational principle does not imply that this is what he is for, and that his good consists in doing this well. Thirdly (the critic continues), it is obvious that men do many things, apart from thinking, that no other creature can do. Competition, sport, artistic endeavour, as well as less edifying activities like mass murder and torture are also unique to the human race. Why should the life of the rational element in us be given special importance? Either we include all these activities under the heading of *rational activity*, in which case the idea becomes vacuous, because it leaves too many different activities from which to choose, or we narrowly restrict the activities that are to count as exhibiting man's rational function, in which case we are still left with many other activities apart from rational ones, each of which can claim to constitute the function of man, since no other creature can engage in them.

Aristotelian Rejoinders

These points have some merit. But they do not fatally damage Aristotle's theory. The first criticism gains particular plausibility from Darwin's theory of evolution by natural selection, which has forced us to be more careful than Aristotle could be in claiming that anything in nature literally has a purpose. Modern Aristotelians should accept this theory, or lose entitlement to serious consideration. The explanation for the existence of eyes and ears is not literally given in goal-directed terms. Eyes did not literally develop *in order* to see; they *exist*, and they *do* see (or better, enable their bearers to see). They are the product of hundreds of millions of years of adaptation, which itself may not be guided by any purpose at all. However, even admitting this, it is clear that the distinct causal contribution of the eye is that it enables vision, and it seems appropriate to talk of eyes that do not enable vision as being defective or damaged. Seeing is what eyes do best, at least relative to human interests. So there might likewise be something that humans do best, such that they flourish when they do it well.

What this thing is could be linked, moreover, to our interests as rational beings and not only to our interests as biological beings. Aristotle gets his ideas about function from his metaphysical biology, but it is important not to construe his ideas about human well-being in purely biological terms. Our rational capacities owe their existence to biological evolution, but once they are in place, they can generate rational interests that can even go against our interests as biological entities. Self-sacrifice, for instance, might be in our interests as rational beings, even if our chief biological drive is to survive.

The second point perhaps has more force—it is difficult to see why the function of man (even allowing that there is one) must consist in what is unique to him. However, we may be understanding the idea of a *rational principle* somewhat too narrowly in making this criticism. Thinking is not to be sharply opposed to perceiving or experiencing emotions and sensations. Perception itself essentially involves understanding as well as raw experience, and emotions also can have a rational element, in that they are often *about* something. So although both humans and animals perceive and feel, humans' way of doing all these things might be unique. It is oversimple to say that humans and animals enjoy roughly similar sense experiences and differ only in the ability to reason. For the rationality that is distinctive of humanity pervades all aspects of our lives and is not limited to purely abstract reasoning. This does not make the idea of the rational principle vacuous through being too inclusive. The fact that rationality is manifested in such a variety of activities does not imply that the concept of rationality itself is vague or over-inclusive. Aristotle's theory, incidentally, backs this up: in fact he goes on to say that even if the best life is one of contemplation, you can lead a good life just by displaying practical reason in all your many types of dealing.

Virtues and Needs

We can return to the idea of man's function and good to see how these ideas connect with Aristotle's account of the virtues. One important point is that virtues are not just *good* or *admirable* in some abstract way; they are needs. We all need the virtues—that is, we need to possess them ourselves, rather than merely profit from the possession of them by others. For Aristotle, they are needed in order to be happy. Happiness, he tells us, is an activity of soul in accordance with perfect virtue. To lack virtue is therefore to lack happiness, which is the good.

What is meant, in general, by saying that one thing is needed for something else? Sometimes there is a straightforward means-end relation. A man might, in this sense, need to be hard-working in order to realize his ambition to be rich or famous. What he values is the end result alone, but he knows that he will not get it unless he cultivates a habit of work. In this case, he does not value industriousness for itself—he may prefer, other things being equal, to do as little as possible. So in this case, there is only an accidental relationship between the means and the desired end; if he could attain the end without the bother of working, he would do so. But it is not in this sense that we need the virtues in the Aristotelian scheme. Rather, there is an internal relationship between virtue and happiness; virtue is a *part of happiness*. Virtue is needed for happiness, but not in a simple means-end way: there could not, even in principle, be any happiness apart from virtue. The good for man—happiness—is to live according to a rational principle. Virtue is a disposition to choose well, according to this rational principle. Man fares well—in a state of eudaimonia—when he lives and chooses according to it.

The Virtues and the Mean

Virtue, says Aristotle, is a state of character. It is not a passion, like anger or fear, or a faculty, like the capacity for anger or fear. Neither is it virtuous or vicious—*per se*—to feel such emotions. The important thing is that in respect of these feelings, virtue is the *mean state* between excess and deficiency. This is Aristotle's famous *doctrine of the mean*. At times he calls virtue the intermediate state between too much and too little, but makes it clear that this is not a matter of being literally at the mid-point between two extremes. Rather, where the mean is to be found depends on the circumstances and must be discerned by careful judgement.

Some examples should illustrate this well. Anger, for instance, can be virtuous, provided that it is experienced in the right degree, towards the right object and at the right time. Pleasure, too, is virtuous when taken in the right things and in the right degree. Aristotle calls the *excess*, the *deficiency* and the *mean* by different names. Thus liberality is the mean with regard to disposing of money, while prodigality is the excess and meanness the deficiency. In matters of honour and dishonour, "the excess is known as a sort of 'empty vanity', and the deficiency is undue humility".[6] With respect to courage, the excess is rashness and the deficiency cowardice.

The nature of the virtues in Aristotle's ethical theory has sparked off much controversy. The basic virtues of courage, justice, temperance and wisdom (what medieval thinkers called the *cardinal* virtues) have an important place both in Aristotle's scheme and in later Christian and secular thought. To get on in life we all need these virtues: courage because we could all face dangerous and fearful challenges, temperance because the ability to forswear or postpone the gratification of desire is essential to getting what we really want, and to lasting happiness. There are other virtues noted by Aristotle, such as *megalopsuchia*, often translated as *pride*, which are not valued by later thought. Aristotle does not value humility, though he does condemn boastfulness. Medieval Christian philosophy condemned pride as one of the seven deadly sins, though megalopsuchia is not the Christian sin of pride, which requires the Christian God as its context. Perhaps it is closer to the modern managerial virtue of *assertiveness*, much extolled today. It is also important to note that Aristotle's system takes hierarchy, including slavery, for granted. The highest virtue could be possessed only by males of a high social standing, and signs of such virtue apparently included a measured pace and a bass voice. But these outrages against the spirit of modernity should not prevent fruitful discussion of the content and structure of Aristotle's theories.

Pleasure and Desire

The rational principle that determines the mean, however, cannot be reduced to specific moral rules, or even general principles like "always treat others as ends" or "maximize the good". Right decisions depend on perception of individual circumstances. This does not mean that there are no absolutely forbidden actions, such as murder or adultery. However, we do not become virtuous (and therefore happy) by learning rules for bidding these actions. We gain virtue, and hence learn to make right decisions, by cultivating certain dispositions—and in particular by educating our desires.

Aristotle describes desires and appetites as an irrational element in the soul, but this is interestingly qualified. For although our desires do not in themselves grasp a rational principle, they can nevertheless respond to it. Moral virtue is a state of character that is acquired by moulding one's desires in the right way. It is not a matter of reason overriding desire or trying to ignore it. On the contrary, for Aristotle, the motive to all action, whatever its moral character, is desire. Virtue is fundamentally a matter of having the right desires, towards the right objects and in the right degree. This explains why Aristotle makes a distinction between acting virtuously, and acting in conformity with virtue. "Actions, then, are just and temperate when they are such as the just or the temperate man would do; but it is not the man who does these that is just and temperate, but the man who also does the mas just and temperate men do them".[7] In other words, the agents must be in the right condition when they do them—in particular, action must spring from a firm character of the proper kind. Virtuous deeds must be second nature. They must have firm dispositions to the right kind of choices, and these dispositions are expressed in their desires.

---

6. Aristotle, ibid., II.7, p. 41.

7. Aristotle, ibid., TI.5. p. 35.

From this we can see the importance of the education of character—the acquisition of these firm dispositions. According to Aristotle, this does not come naturally but must be taught. To this extent, there is some similarity between acquiring virtue and acquiring skills such as mastery of a musical instrument; both require practice before the appropriate habits are acquired. You get the dispositions by first of all acting as if you already had them—you train yourself to do the right things, and gradually you gain a standing disposition to do them. When you have this disposition, it will be second nature to choose according to the rational principle that defines the good life. Reason and desire will be in harmony, and inner conflict (which, incidentally, is plausibly regarded as a major cause of unhappiness) will have been removed. Moreover, a sign that the virtuous disposition has been acquired is that you take *pleasure* in performing virtuous deeds and are repelled by the thought of vicious ones. This attractive doctrine is in stark contrast to that of Kant, who insisted that pleasure in right action contributes in no way to its moral worth, and that no action with genuine moral worth can be explained solely by reference to the desires of the agent. It is surely better to take Aristotle's position on this, for much as we can muster some admiration for those who act solely out of a sense of duty and take no pleasure in doing their duty, we tend to think better of agents who like to do what they ought, because their good deeds express their real character.

What this suggests is that the fundamental question of morality, for virtue theory, is not: what ought I to do? but rather: what dispositions should I acquire? Once we have answered the second question, we may be able to answer the first. When confronted with a certain choice—say, between divulging a friend's confidence in order to be entertaining, or keeping quiet—the crucial question concerns what the person with the relevant virtue would do. Loyalty is an indispensable part of friendship, for it is the virtue that makes friendship possible. So the question would be: what would a loyal person do? Surely such a person would already have acquired certain desires and dispositions that would totally rule out breaking trust, at least for this sort of reason. Now it may well be that some of us, those of us who have not cultivated these dispositions throughout our lives, do not have a present reason to act as the loyal person would. We cannot immediately acquire such a reason, since we cannot immediately acquire the requisite desires. Given our actual desires, we lack a reason to be loyal. But Aristotle would still insist that we have reason to acquire the right dispositions and desires, because without them we cannot attain complete happiness, the human good. We do not function well as rational beings if our desires are not moulded in the light of a rational principle.

Is Virtue Theory Trivial?

This, then, is the Aristotelian background to modern virtue theory, which of course has acquired a life of its own. Whatever we say in praise of various virtues—in particular, the cardinal virtues of courage, justice, temperance and wisdom—there is an awkward problem. With what, exactly, is virtue theory being contrasted? Can it say anything true and important that other moral theories are unable to say?

Consider the idea that there are certain praiseworthy and blameworthy actions, and that a virtuous person (one, that is, with well-ingrained dispositions towards certain kinds of behaviour) would do the good things and shun the bad. Still, why shouldn't the good and the bad themselves be understood in terms of an action-based (non-virtue-based) theory such as utilitarianism? Suppose that what we ought to do is promote the greatest happiness of the greatest number. Why not then say that a virtuous person is one who has a standing disposition to promote the greatest happiness of the greatest number? Benevolence is the specific virtue that comes closest to such a disposition, so perhaps we should call it a utilitarian virtue. Talk of virtue, on this account, contributes nothing distinctive. Calling people virtuous is just shorthand for saying that they are disposed to do what is right—and the content of what is right could be given in purely utilitarian terms.

A similar criticism of virtue theory could, of course, be made by a Kantian, who might say that virtuous people are those whose characters dispose them to act on principles they can will to become universal laws. In fact, those who believe that there are morally obligatory and forbidden actions will want to define virtue as a disposition to do what is required and refrain from what is forbidden (whatever these may be). In other words, perhaps virtue theory is not a viable replacement for action-based theories of moral obligation (be they utilitarian, Kantian, or whatever). We cannot eliminate the idea of right and wrong conduct, and replace it with virtue concepts, to do with good and bad character.

This criticism of virtue theory contains an important truth. There do seem to be indispensable principles and duties, respect for which cannot be understood simply in terms of the exercise of some specific virtue. It is often pointed out that the Aristotelian idea of the virtues is incompatible with modern democratic notions (although which should be abandoned, Aristotle's ideas or the modern democratic notions is something that might still be discussed). Aristotle thought that the highest virtue could be possessed only by those of an elevated social standing; thus he is really talking about appropriate behaviour for an Athenian gentleman. However, virtue theory need not endorse all of Aristotle's ideas about the specific virtues, or those of the Greeks generally. The important criticism is that the concept of the virtues makes little sense apart from the idea that a virtuous individual is disposed to do the right things—and we seem to need some other account that can tell us what the right things are.

Virtue Theory's Reply

The best reply the virtue theorist can make is this. No doubt there are right and wrong actions, and perhaps some of these are so absolutely, on account of their *intrinsic nature*. But virtue theory can shed light on these moral constraints. For example, whereas an action-based theory might ask, "How is the world improved or made worse by such and such an action?", a virtue theorist might ask what the doing of this action would reveal about the one who does it. Is this the action of a just, courageous or temperate person? If we think in this way, we end up with a set of moral concerns that is more plausible than anything that can be delivered by purely action-based accounts. In particular, it can offer telling criticisms of both utilitarian and contractualist approaches.

Suppose we accept that benevolence is an important virtue, being a disposition to be moved by sympathy for others and to act for the good of others, even when there is no special relationship in place and no prior agreement to help them. We then remember that utilitarianism makes much of benevolence—indeed its governing conception of morality is that of the impartial benevolent spectator. So when we contemplate some course of action, we ask whether it would be recommended by this hypothetical figure. Now, as we saw earlier, utilitarianism allows that some individuals could be morally obliged to devote substantial effort to producing what is intrinsically evil, in order to maximize the good. The question that will be asked by one of the few people chosen to produce the evil, as small cogs in the smoothly benevolent utilitarian machinery, is: could a truly benevolent person do this? Whatever the overall net good produced (if this even makes any sense), is my production of something intrinsically bad, consistent with my possessing all the important virtues? This consideration reminds us of earlier discussions of integrity. We can now link the idea of integrity with virtue theory—for integrity purports to be a virtue, or even virtue as such.

As we saw earlier, the familiar utilitarian answer is that this is a mere rhetorical assertion. Whereas before, it seemed as though we just had a stand-off with one side saying "yea" and the other "nay" to this utilitarian implication, asking what it is to possess a virtue may get us further. If Aristotle is right, virtues are deep dispositions acquired by training and habituation. It is psychologically highly unlikely that people habituated in the ways of benevolence, with a deeply ingrained disposition to concern for others, will be able to give up this concern upon calculating that more overall good would accrue if they did so. Although, for Aristotle, virtue involves the exercise of judgement in order to see what is required by the particular situation, it is unlikely that the proper exercise of such judgement by virtuous people could ever dictate the sustained infliction of suffering on a few people, to benefit the many. That would be radically contrary to the benevolent disposition. Human nature being what it is, it is very difficult to have kind or loyal dispositions, which operate when they are needed, but which are simply abandoned when utility so requires. To demand that we become like this is to fail to take account of what we actually are. As things are, the genuinely benevolent person never, or at most very rarely, does this sort of thing. Most or all of those who have urged atrocities for the "greater good"—notably revolutionary dictators such as Hitler, Lenin and Mao Tse-tung—have actually turned out to be men of extraordinary cruelty.

The question "would a virtuous person do this?" also has implications for the adequacy of purely contractualist theories. There seem to be actions to which we reasonably take exception, but which do not appear to be forbidden by a contractualist approach. Suppose that someone goes into a cemetery one night, making sure that no one can see him, and then spits on graves. This seems to be wantonly disrespectful and offensive. But to whom? Who is hurt or harmed? If we do not believe the dead can be hurt or harmed (since they no longer exist), and if the perpetrator does his deed in secret so that others cannot be upset, it is hard to answer these questions. Yet one might object just on grounds of character. To spit on graves is a sign of a bad character, a disrespectful disposition, and a virtuous person would not dream of doing it. These considerations are perhaps not decisive, but they do present a challenge pointing to the validity of appealing to virtues and vices to explain the moral nature of acts.

Virtue and Motives

In fact, this kind of case leads to more general considerations about character and motive that seem to lend credibility to virtue theory. It is sometimes said that the main deficiency of purely action-based theories is that they have nothing to say about the moral dimensions of motives. They seem, according to these critics, to be saying that you are morally all right if you simply do the right thing, whatever went on in your mind when you did it. I suggest that there is something to be said for this criticism of action-based theory.

Some qualifications must be made, however, for motives do have a kind of importance in both Kantian and some utilitarian approaches. Indeed, for Kant, motive is indispensable—actions possess moral worth only if they are (a) in accordance with the categorical imperative, and (b) performed from the motive of duty. However, Kant's view on this is absurdly restrictive: he is right that we sometimes should admire people who act well from a sense of duty, especially when they do not feel like acting well—but it is surely wrong to withhold moral praise from those who are prompted only by native kindness. In fact, when we praise dutiful people who lack natural sympathy, we are really praising them for one virtue, strength of will, which operates to counter-act a deficiency in other virtues, such as instinctive kindness. We should likewise exonerate utilitarianism of the charge of disregarding the importance of motive and character. Most utilitarians would insist that they are important—if only because a standing disposition towards benevolence, or even towards respecting certain moral rules, has a long-term utilitarian value. *Rule utilitarians* are among those who emphasize the importance of character training; it is better have a disposition to keep certain rules even when breaking them seems to bring some immediate utilitarian benefit, than not abide by these rules and risk losing the long term benefit they bring.

The real trouble with these action-based concessions to character and virtue theory is that they have latched onto the wrong reasons for valuing good character—or at least have failed to capture the most fundamental ones. Consider how we might morally assess the following things: a habit of daydreaming about others praising you; fantasies of revenge; sexual fantasies about a person you know to be unavailable; wallowing in contemptuous thoughts about someone you consider a loser; feeling happy when someone you envy suffers a setback. This sort of list could go on indefinitely. What seems common to all the items is that they may well not issue in any wrong action. Merely entertaining thoughts of revenge will not necessarily result in acting on those thoughts, and wallowing in sexual fantasies about someone else's partner need not result in any attempt to seduce that partner. In consequence, a commonly held view is that there is nothing wrong with these thoughts; provided no one else is harmed, there is no objection to entertaining them.

But is this really so obvious? There are complex questions about the relationship between fantasy and genuine desire. Many people, for example, would not opt for all their sexual fantasies to become real even if they were offered the choice. However at least some private wallowing in fantasy of various kinds expresses real desire and character. An envious person might do spiteful things, but perhaps more often he will simply have envious thoughts, nursing his unhappiness that someone else has something he has not (and perhaps does not even want). Even when he does do spiteful deeds, much of what is wrong with them is precisely that they are prompted by envy. *Motives* (e.g. envy, jealousy) are often what gives our actions their moral complexion, and motives are born from our characters, from our individual sets of virtues and vices. This goes against the common assumption that the only thing to worry about, with respect to certain private imaginings, is that they might be acted out. There is as much truth in the reverse; if they are acted out, much of what is objectionable about the actions is the motive and state of character from which they spring.

An important contribution of virtue theory, therefore, is not that it does away with moral principles, but that it helps shape them. Rather than merely telling us not to steal, lie and so on, it tells us more generally to act justly, wisely, courageously and temperately. To act justly will usually entail not lying or stealing. But, to revert to Aristotle, we display virtue in doing the right thing only if the act springs from a standing disposition of character. To have this character will exclude not only the doing of unjust or disrespectful acts when these acts have victims, but also when they do not—as in the example of spitting on graves or wallowing in envious thoughts. The job of moral philosophy is largely concerned with asking how our characters should develop and what particular dispositions we should have.

More generally, and less negatively, consideration of the virtues can help shape principles of action by bringing a certain explanatory simplicity to them. Sometimes we get a sense of the moral shape of an action if we can detect in it a general similarity to other acts whose moral complexion we already understand. The use of virtue terms is a good way to describe this similarity. Thus, we might want to say that what deception, cheating, stealing and fraud have in common is that they are dishonest and, more generally, unjust. (In fact, words like *dishonest* play a more central role in everyday moral talk than words like *wrong*). The concept of justice is the bridging idea here. If I am wondering whether I can justify a certain course of action towards another, I have a better grip on the problem if I ask whether the behaviour is just, kind, honest, and so on, than if I vaguely ask whether it is right or ethical. Again, this is not to say that we can dispense with the idea of right and wrong, or reduce it all to talk of virtue. It does say that a grasp of virtues can help us classify individual acts and make their rightness or wrongness intelligible and explicable.

The Unity of the Virtues

But discussion of virtue raises an important difficulty that troubled Plato and Aristotle. Is it possible to display a virtue in an action that also displays a vice? If an action manifests one virtue, can it also be contrary to another? Cases that come to mind are the apparent courage of a terrorist in planting bombs that harm innocent people, or the apparent benevolence of the Robin Hood thief who steals lawfully gained property in order to help the poor. Is the terrorist courageous? He might be thought so if he carries bombs that could go off prematurely and kill him, and if he knows that if he is caught he will be tortured, imprisoned or killed. Is the thief benevolent? His thieving certainly seems to be motivated by sympathy for the poor in their plight.

The problem is not to do with whether one individual's character can contain both virtuous and vicious traits. For surely almost everyone's character has both. The question is whether a particular benevolent act can also be unjust, or a courageous act also cruel. (If you think these are bad examples of virtues or vices, replace them with others).

Start from the plausible idea that each virtue is something everybody should cultivate to the fullest possible extent. We should try not only to be *reasonably* honest, or *moderately* benevolent, but completely so. After all, it is not as if Aristotle, in proposing the doctrine of the mean, was saying that the good life is the mean between vice and virtue, and that too much virtue could be a bad thing! Each virtue is a mean state between two opposing vices, one of excess and the other of deficiency, but there can be no such thing as an excess of virtue itself. However, if we also allow that the more heedless of human suffering the terrorist is, the more courage he shows, we are implying that if he becomes more compassionate he also becomes less courageous. If he ought to have as much courage as possible, it would be hard to avoid calling this decrease in courage a moral deficiency. Similarly, if we allow that it is better to be perfectly benevolent than only moderately so, and allow that the man who steals to help the poor shows more benevolence than one who refuses to steal, then we seem committed to saying that (at least in respect of one virtue) the one who steals or kills should be admired more.

These implications do not seem edifying. Don't we want to say that Virtues like justice and benevolence never truly conflict and that a perfectly benevolent person always acts within the constraints of justice? You do not always become more benevolent in direct proportion to the amount of happiness you create, because even if it is better, *ceteris paribus*, to create more rather than less happiness, it still seems to be usually wrong (because unjust) to steal or cheat.

According to one theory, the reason the specific virtues never conflict is that all virtues are ultimately different facets of one and the same thing—perhaps some master virtue, or *virtue* itself. This notion is called the theory of the *unity of the virtues*. Thus Plato[8] discusses whether all virtue is really knowledge, that is, whether courage, temperance, justice and wisdom are all ultimately kinds of knowledge. The supposition that you can display courage on some particular occasion but show a lack of wisdom, would entail that on this occasion you both possess and lack knowledge, which seems contradictory. I shall not pursue this idea, however. For there is a more promising solution, which comes from Philippa Foot's article, "Virtues and Vices."[9]

Foot acknowledges, as we have just done with respect to the courageous terrorist and the benevolent thief, that there is something wrong with praising people whose apparent courage leads them to ever bolder crimes, or whose seeming benevolence leads them to unjust acts like theft. However, there is still something implausible about flatly denying that the criminal is courageous or the thief benevolent. Part of the difficulty with such denial (though this is not how she puts it) is that the courage shown in the pursuit of noble ends and the courage (or "courage") shown in the pursuit of bad ones seem to be exactly the same except in respect of their ends. Although the selection of the unworthy end may spring from a deficiency of some virtue, it does not seem to come from a deficiency of courage. To deny that courage is shown in the bad act is to define the word "courage" arbitrarily; we are merely deciding to use the *word* "courage" when we happen to approve of the end, but not use it otherwise. This is what is known as a "persuasive definition".

A good example of persuasive definition is in the dispute between those who would call the terrorist a freedom-fighter and those who would call him a terrorist. Often the use of such terms is purely persuasive or emotive. If you approve of him, you use one term and if you disapprove you use another, even if there is no descriptive difference that explains the difference in the terminology. Freedom-fighters might slaughter innocent people as a means to freedom; terrorists do exactly the same. In the cases of courage and benevolence being displayed in bad pursuits, what we should say (according to Foot) is that although courage, benevolence, etc., are indeed displayed, *they do not operate as virtues* in these cases. Although courage is *by nature* a virtue, things do not always operate according to their natures. Analogously, a solvent, by nature, dissolves in water—but there can be special circumstances that prevent it from doing so. Prudence is also a virtue and normally operates as such, but not in people who are so obsessed with danger that they never take even rational risks. Such people, in fact, lack courage. Industriousness usually acts as a virtue, but not in people who neglect their families to advance their careers. These states of character are virtues because they are what a normal human needs to get through life and flourish, yet there can still be times when they do not operate as virtues.

8. Plato, Meno, in W.K Guthrie, trans., Plato, Protagoras and Meno (Harmondsworth: Penguin, 1956).
9. See P. Foot, Virtues and Vices, in P. Foot, Virtues and Vices (Oxford: Blackwell, 1978). This succinct and seminal article should be studied carefully by anyone wishing to pursue virtue theory.

This is a promising line of argument. However, it must be admitted that this explanation may not apply to all virtues, but only to the "executive" ones like courage and industriousness. It is harder to claim that there are occasions when justice does not operate as a virtue. But Foot's account is at least a plausible partial solution to the problem, even though it seems to leave some problems unanswered.

We have suggested that investigation of the kind of people we should be, and not just of how we should act, is an important part of moral philosophy, and that it can help us determine how we should behave. We also saw that we cannot replace action-talk with virtue-talk. We cannot get rid of the concept of right and wrong action. In fact, the more plausible virtue-based approaches do not suggest that we can—rather, they justify their views on what is right and wrong in terms of virtues. Thus, they might tell us not to cheat because it is dishonest, and not to bully others because it is cruel.

This raises another problem, however. Although there is rhetorical resonance in words like *dishonest*, *cruel*, *dishonourable* and so on, that might sometimes have an effect on behaviour when words like *wrong* and *immoral* do not, we still need some reason why we should value these virtues. What is so good about honesty? Questions like this become even more pressing when it comes to alleged virtues that do not relate to behaviour that is widely valued. The admonition to avoid casual sex because it is *unchaste*—chastity being a specifically sexual virtue—is unlikely, at least in a libertarian culture such as our own, to convince many people. What is so admirable about chastity? How can appealing to this concept, without further explanation, provide a good reason for sexual restraint?

Questions like this are perfectly legitimate, whether or not true answers to them will gain much acceptance. They become more urgent when two different virtues come into apparent conflict. Suppose loyalty impels me not to inform on my friend who is fraudulently drawing state benefit, but that a sense of justice impels me to do so. How do we adjudicate between these virtues, once we have decided that it is these virtues that are in play?

It is here that Aristotle's conception of virtue is relevant. For him, a virtue is a constitutive part of living well—of eudaimonia. Living well means living in accordance with our nature. Now, obviously enough, there is much diversity among people, for example in the way of talents, interests or occupations. Such differences indicate that, in many ways, the good life for one person is not the good life for another. But we can get the *structure* of an answer from Aristotelian virtue theory—we do not need to agree with all his claims about human nature and the content of the virtues. What we get, in essence, is plausible: that we are social beings who form plans, enjoy intimate relationships, have ambitions and pleasures—and that there are more and less fulfilling ways of going about these things. If we cultivate the virtues internal to friendship we are likely to have satisfactory and life-enhancing friendships, and if we have the virtues internal to work, our work is likely to be fulfilling. As we mentioned earlier, it is best to think of the virtues as needs. They are needed for the satisfactory fulfilment of the activities in which we characteristically engage.

This leaves many questions unanswered, of course. We cannot claim to have a blueprint for answering all moral problems or resolving dilemmas. What we do have is an idea of the sort of thing we should be looking for when we try to solve such problems.

Virtues, Strange Obligations and Moral Objectivity

There is another advantage in virtue theory, which is that even if it is vague in its prescriptions, it can rule out certain things as morally unimportant. Writers like Foot[10] and Anscombe[11] stress that anything that can be called a moral requirement must be related to human good and harm. Hence it would not merely be eccentric, but incoherent, to posit as amoral principle that you should clap your hands repeatedly, or run around trees anticlockwise. Of course, if these activities have some meaning in a given context, then they may have amoral dimension—maybe the hand-clapping is applause that you politely offer to your neighbour's dismally untalented child at a school concert. But handclapping cannot in itself have any moral value. This is because it is intrinsically unrelated to human good and harm. We can make no sense of hand-clapping as a moral obligation. This is not so of all moral theories and supposed obligations that we reject. For example, although we might regard utilitarianism as substantially misguided, we can still recognize its claim to be a moral doctrine as coherent and intelligible because it aims to produce happiness, which is a good.

If the virtues are human needs relating to a flourishing life, then we can make the above point by saying that hand-clapping is entirely unrelated to any virtue or vice. We need a disposition to face danger when necessary, and we call this courage. We need a disposition to restrain our impulses at times, and we call this temperance. That we need these things is the reason why they are virtues, but we do not need a disposition to run around trees a certain way, or clap our hands. We do not think that such activities make us good people.

This brings us back to the Aristotelian conception of a good person and its relation to human function. As we saw, Aristotle thought that everything in nature had a function and that a condition of flourishing for a living being is that it should live in accordance with that function. Thinking was man's distinctive function, so he lived well if he lived in accordance with a *rational principle*. (He also believed that an even higher activity than practical reasoning was theoretical reasoning, and that consequently the best life was the purely contemplative one. The cultivation of intellectual virtues as well as moral ones contributed to the good life. For reasons of simplicity I have not discussed this aspect of his theory). Thinking well was the essence of being a good man. This idea has considerable theoretical attractions, both for answering questions about the content of morality and its objectivity. It seems to make moral truth into a kind of *naturalistic* truth; we are supposed to discern whether a man is living well simply by seeing whether he is living according to his function. Similarly, we can see whether a certain boat is a good boat by observing whether it floats, moves smoothly across water, and so on—in other words, by observing whether or not it fulfils the function of boats. If it is beautiful and expertly crafted, but cannot stay afloat, then in spite of these merits it is not a good boat.

"Good" as a Descriptive Term

This fact leads us to notice something quite important about the way the word "good" is used in such examples. In saying that a vessel is a good boat, we are not saying simply that it is *both* good *and* a boat.

10. See for example P. Foot, Goodness and Choice, in P. Foot, Virtues and Vices (Oxford: Blackwell 1978). See many other articles in that book as well.
11. See a landmark article of G.E.M. Anscombe, Modern moral philosophy, Philosophy 33 (1958), pp. 1–19.

We are saying that it is good *as* a boat. Analogously, for Aristotle, to speak of a good man (feminism was not around, though women were believed to exist), is to speak of somebody who is good as a man, who discharges the function characteristic of man.[12]

Other examples will clarify the way "good" is used here. A good knife is not a thing which is *both* good *and* a knife. That idea is nonsense. It is just a good knife, a knife that performs the function of a knife well. Similarly, a small buffalo is not a thing which is small and a buffalo; it is small *as* a buffalo, that is, small by the standards of buffaloes. A small buffalo is bigger than a big cat. By contrast, a rectangular table is *just* something that is a table and rectangular.

The suggestion, then, is that goodness in men may be a matter of being "good men", that is, good as far as men go. This means that the term "good" is not just a term of approval: it is descriptive. Certain descriptions must be satisfied if the term "good" is to be correctly applied. The criteria for such goodness are decided according to man's function. If we can discern man's function, and discern who is living according to it, we have an objective, descriptive answer to questions about goodness in men. Correspondingly, actions performed by men are right or wrong according to whether they incline them towards, or away from, the fulfilment of their function. Furthermore (and here we return to an earlier concern) if we really can construe human goodness in this way, then certain puzzles about the objectivity of such goodness appear to have been solved, at least up to a point. There is no need to invoke mysterious action-guiding properties, or strange non-natural entities; values are instead both objective and naturalistic. We can find out whether a person is good by looking and seeing, in a wholly non-mysterious way.

Some Problems

Some difficulties, however, diminish the force of this suggestion. Whereas the example of the eye's function suggests that good eyes are those that see well, and defective ones those that do not, it is unclear that people have functions so specific that we can identify the good life as the fulfilment of it. We allowed that there is something important and true in the idea that the good life is connected to the rational faculty, but there are problems in trying to identify this completely with the *moral* life. No doubt there is *some* connection between the flourishing of our most distinctive qualities, and the possession of moral virtue. However, people display many distinctively human excellences, and not all of them are moral virtues. Aristotle himself distinguishes moral from intellectual virtue, and we can mention many other kinds as well: social virtues (like being good at conversation), creativity, artistic talent, humour, physical strength, endurance, beauty. We certainly value these things in ourselves and others, and many of them are unique to humans. Activities in accordance with these have as much claim to define the function of man as the life of moral virtue. Sometimes they even conflict with moral virtue. Unusual creativity might bring with it a certain moral indifference, and a bit of malice and intolerance can contribute to the social virtues of being funny and interesting.

Aristotle does mention some of these non-moral virtues and does regard some of them as part of the

---

12. Aristotle did in fact think there was such a thing as being a good woman, that is, good as a woman but it was not his concern to elaborate this in his Nicomachean ethics.

good for man. He attaches value to the social virtues and treats artistic talent in his *Poetics*. He also regards endurance as meritorious. This tends to illustrate that our modern notion of virtue is different in many ways from that of Aristotle. For him, there is a far less pronounced distinction between what we call moral virtue and other excellences. This observation does not so much detract from Aristotle's theory of the good life, as from the attempt to use Aristotelian ideas to back up a narrow, modern account of the moral life. For Aristotle, flourishing as a human being is not just a matter of possessing the moral virtues. Nevertheless, if we bear this caution in mind, we are still able to derive some substantial guidance as to the moral life from Aristotle's ideas about function. Virtues like temperance really are crucial to our flourishing, and we understand the nature of temperance and our need of it if we reflect on what happens to people who lack it. There is, indeed, evidence that children who are able to defer gratification of immediate impulses become more successful and happy as adults than those who lacked this ability as children. This accords with Aristotle's advice that habituation in the virtues must begin at an early age.

A more serious objection to Aristotelian ethics is that there may be no more than a loose connection between the life that benefits us and the moral life. This brings us to a theme that occupies Plato, in his *Republic*: namely, does it pay to lead to moral life? Certainly, the virtues generally help our lives to go well—but the life that is good for us (i.e. the life that benefits us) and the morally virtuous life are not the same thing. Utilitarians, for all their faults, are right to urge that our duties of concern for strangers extend beyond what most of us like to think; that serious sacrifices to the quality of our lives may be required by morality. No doubt some self-sacrificing people, such as Christian ascetics, would urge that we *really* lead the good life if we make these sacrifices. There is some truth in this, in that, for example, too many material possessions can be a burden, but unless their fundamental religious beliefs are true, it is surely an overstatement. It is more credible to say that a certain sacrifice of genuine well-being, of the good life for us, is necessary if we are to act well.

As far as the question of the objectivity of human goodness is concerned, we can offer the following summary of virtue theory's contribution to the problem. There is considerable plausibility in the claim that actions that are morally right spring from the exercise of specific moral virtues, and that contemplation of the virtues (and indeed vices) therefore helps us determine the content of morality. It is also plausible that virtues are both a means to well-being (or human flourishing) and, in some way, a part of that flourishing. Thus morality appears at its core to be essentially connected to human good and harm, and this suggests that certain actions simply could not be accounted right or wrong in themselves, if they have no connection to human good and harm. This in turn partially breaks down the "fact-value distinction'. This distinction clearly breaks down in the case of the good knife, because not just any knife can count as a good one; only a knife that cuts well (i.e. performs the proper function of knives) can count as a good knife. Thus, certain evaluations of knives (like good, reasonable and useless) are logically tied to certain descriptive properties of them. In the same way, there is a limited sense in which not just any style of living could count as human flourishing, and not just any action could count as morally right. So far, then, there is much of importance in the Aristotelian way of looking at things.

For the reasons given above, this theory won't solve all our problems, either concerning the content of morality or its objectivity. Morality is only part of human well-being, and perhaps not the most significant part. To a great extent, a wealthy aesthete who lacks a social conscience, and who surrounds himself with fine things and refined human company, does lead the good life—he does flourish. But the demands of morality, perhaps of a Kantian or utilitarian kind, still generate objective practical reasons for him to attend to more impartial concerns. If, as is plausible, such moral concerns can override the importance of the good life he leads, then there is a way in which the objectivity of these concerns cannot be entirely captured in an Aristotelian account of moral objectivity. Virtue theory, for all its virtues, does not have the last or only word on these things.

Selections from "Codes of Ethics in Health Care: Virtues Versus Rules"

Dennis Sansom

The Crisis in Codes of Ethics

Talk of the crisis in codes of ethics has become commonplace. Such codes are said to be ineffective, little understood or used, and not nearly as influential as one's own personal values. For instance, in 2009 D.C. Mallory, P. Sevigny, et al. questioned eleven focus groups of physicians in six culturally different countries concerning their perceptions of their profession's code of ethics. The findings were not optimistic about the influence of the codes. They state,

> Two findings were particularly interesting. The first was the apparent emphasis placed on personal values and the perceived impact of culture on the interpretation of these codes. The second was that at no time did any of the respondents from these international focus groups put forward the view that their specific medical code of ethics, in particular, was helpful in clarifying the unknown or ambiguous—at best, medical ethics codes were

tolerated, as they did not seem to interfere with the predetermined ethical intent of the physician.[1]

This lack of effectiveness on the part of the physicians' code does not lead Mallory, Sevigny, et al. to conclude that the physicians are not interested in ethical guidelines, however. In fact, they find that physicians looking for ways to explain and justify their actions appeal to the ethical guidelines laid out by their culture or their own consciences, but they do not look to the medical codes for instruction or illumination in their daily practice unless such codes match their own value system. In light of their research, it is fitting for Mallory, Sevigny, et al. to close their article with the admonition that "This finding points to the need to re-evaluate the purpose, content, and delivery of codes, value statements, missions, and credos, in order for them to be more functional tools in the promoting ethical conduct."[2]

Sarah Cox, Douglas Cripps, et al. reach a similarly sobering conclusion. Relying on previous data (some of which comes from the above mentioned article), they find that most practitioners in therapeutic recreation (the area of their specialty) do not consult their professional codes. Instead, the practitioners see their professional codes as, at best, "artifacts of professional status."[3] If professional codes are viewed merely as artifacts they certainly fail as informative and descriptive ethical guidelines. The "speculative" quality of the codes, the way in which they function as something the professional looks at but does not integrate into its practice, became obvious to Cox, Cripps, et al. in their own focus group study. They asked the participants, "to what extent does [the] code of ethics assist you in your ethical deliberations?" The data fell into three themes: 1). a lack of awareness of the code, 2). a lack of education/training in ethical treatment of patients, and 3). other codes supersede the professional one. From these themes, they conclude, "a code of ethics has very little use in practice."[4]

Pessimism concerning the effectiveness of codes of ethics is not limited to medicine and other health care professions, it is seen across the board in other professions as well. John Dobson has analyzed the effectiveness of codes of ethics in business and other disciplines. He believes that such codes lack effectiveness because they are trumped by the more powerful and underlying influence of neo-classical utilitarianism. It is assumed that people always act according to their self-interests and that, hence, people's personal codes are more likely to be shaped by consequentialist reasoning than by the principles laid out in professional codes of ethics. In fact, Dobson reasons, the professional codes "may be no more than a legalistic gloss over the real ethos that pervades the organization."[5] Furthermore, because they act as a gloss at best, professionals are somewhat schizophrenic about which code truly represents their activity—the rationalistic and lofty ideals of the profession and organization's code of ethics or the

1. Malloy, D. C., Sevigny, P., et al. "Perceptions of the Effectiveness of Ethical Guidelines: An International Study of Physicians". *Medicine, Health Care, and Philosophy,* 2009;12: 380

2. Ibid. 382

3. Cox, Sarah, Cripps, Douglas, Lee, Yongho, and Malloy, David C. "Code of Ethics: Is It Time to Reconsider?" *Annual in Therapeutic Recreation.* 2011; 19: 140

4. Ibid. 143

5. Dobson, John. "Why Ethics Codes Don't Work," *Financial Analysts Journal.* 2003. November/December: 29

pervasive "neoclassical economic rationality" which most people have acculturated as their real ethical guideline.[6]

Dobson's observations raise an important question: why should the professions write codes of ethics and expect them to be obeyed if such codes are not only ineffective in shaping actual ethical actions but are also unable to challenge an underlying rationality that can possibly shape the practitioner in ways somewhat contrary to the ethical purposes of medicine and health care? If codes truly function as more artifact than ethical curriculum and are superseded in relevance by other values systems, perhaps the reason for their ineffectiveness lies in how they are conceived. Codes typically present themselves as sets of principles that represent proper behavior in certain situations, and as such they attempt to provide a manual for professional behavior. Thus, when we use a code as a manual we intend it to be practically useful. However, if the above commentators are correct, most practitioners already follow a *de facto* operating manual (i.e., utilitarianism), which may or may not be consistent with the moral purposes of their profession. We must examine critically whether codes of ethics should even be conceived, written, and applied as steps in a manual, for, if we truly treat codes in this way, they become rules to follow rather than descriptions of the kind of person who would want to be ethical in the practice of their profession. Some insights from Tom Beauchamp and James Childress will help us make clear this distinction.

Statutory Rules Versus Virtues

Beauchamp and Childress highlight a fault in the use of professional codes. Though they admit that professions "often transmit moral guidelines," which are used to "specify and enforce obligations for their members," the professions hope that their members will be "competent and trustworthy." Thus, "[t]o avoid moral confrontation and legal struggles, some professions codify their standards in order to reduce [conflicts over professional standards or with persons outside the professions]."[7]

Yet, Beauchamp and Childress think that the codes tend to oversimplify moral requirements and try to safeguard the professional from culpability and legal reactions. The idea is that if practitioners follow the codes, we (as practitioners) are ethically and, consequently, legally safe from criticism and reprisal if the practice goes wrong. They then assert the challenging conclusion that "The pursuit of professional norms in these circumstances may do more to protect the profession's interests than to introduce a broad and impartial moral viewpoint."[8]

Beauchamp and Childress express a legitimate concern about the formation and implementation of codes of ethics—do we comply with codes because they are rules that protect us against challenges (litigious or otherwise) or because they nurture individuals to embody the virtues necessary to carry on in morally difficult professions? For some, the codes exist "to protect the profession's interests," while for others they represent "impartial moral viewpoints."[8] This contrast marks a serious divide between two different ways of estimating the role of ethical codes. If codes serve only as protection, they act as statutory

6. Ibid. 30
7. Beauchamp, Tom L., Childress, James F. *Principles of Biomedical Ethics, Fifth Edition.* Oxford: Oxford University Press; 2001: 6
8. Ibid. 7

rules. If codes express a moral viewpoint, they explain the character of a certain kind of moral person. Consider the following contrast between codes as statutory rules and moral virtues:

1. Codes as Statutory Rules:
   a. are restrictive about what should not be done;
   b. if broken, punished by reprimand, exclusion from membership, fine, or imprisonment;
   c. compliance motivated by desire to avoid reprisals;
   d. failure to comply can lead to malpractice and possibly criminality;
   e. backed by an authoritarian enforcer;
   f. presuppose obedience by the participant;
   g. the ideal compiler is the autonomous agent who assents to their necessity.
2. Codes as Moral Virtues:
   a. are constructive concerning what should be done;
   b. if broken, one feels shame for letting down the profession;
   c. compliance is motivated by desire to contribute to the honor of the profession;
   d. failures are accidents within a difficult profession;
   e. are backed by the moral force of an honorable profession;
   f. presuppose a coherent moral tradition;
   g. the ideal compiler is the noble professional who embodies the virtues.

The two justifications for the codes differ greatly in their purposes and motives.

First, consider a justification for codes as statutory rules. This justification draws its power in society from an underlying metaphor: the body is a machine and health care is a contractual transaction. Codes seen as statutory rules rely upon a legalistic understanding of the codes to account for why we should hold such codes to be binding upon their subjects. Within this justification, codes are like contract laws, which hold people accountable to agreements and promises. Though these laws are not immutable and do not necessarily rest upon a sense of natural law, they are authoritative because they reveal a significant aspect of our society—the force of the market. Of course, the word market is large and often ambiguous, but it generally refers to the way people conduct interactions and exchanges according to a particular quantifiable measurement of social power, i.e. money. As soon as money becomes part of the agreement and contract, people act to protect and guarantee their interests as much as possible.

Codes as statutory rules reflect this sense of contractual arrangements. That is, just as we expect to know whether a mechanic or auto-dealer will provide the services and products we desire, we want to know whether a physician or pharmacist will do the same. We assume that they will honor their perceived end of the contract and bargain, and we expect codes to assure us of that assumption.

It is certainly reasonable to expect contracts and negotiations to abide by acceptable rules, and it is desirous for a stable society to insist that providers honor their contractual obligations and promote themselves as faithful and truthful people with regard to these contracts. However, something is left out if we apply this metaphor to health care. The issues of health, whether physical, emotional, or social, are not so transactional. Though we know, for example, that automobile and home repairs rest on mechanistic rules and that, hence, it makes sense to hold those who provide these services accountable for knowing the rules and assuring their results, issues of human health are far more complex than can be explained in this way. Health cannot be characterized by a machine, which is governed by causal laws of clear cause and effect. The unpredictable and unfortunate happen to the human body and psyche not only because mistakes happen here as they would to operating or repairing a machine, but because of the nature of human identity as body and soul.[9] I do not mean to imply that we have two substances, one material and the other an immaterial soul, and that, consequently, we can scientifically explain the first but not the second. Rather, because a mechanistic and materialistic explanation does not sufficiently explain the human experience, it is more accurate to account for our identity as humans in terms of both body and soul rather than as body only. I do not pretend that the word soul is free of ambiguity (and, frankly, the word body is also ambiguous), but I do think it is useful (just as the word body is useful). The admission that we are also a soul recognizes that elements of our identity exist which escape a mechanistic, materialistic explanation. Society is growing in scientific and medical knowledge of what it means to be human, and this growth comes from empirical research, but we are also more aware of what we do not know and what we cannot predict about the human experience, particularly in relation to human health.

This is why treating codes for health care as statutory rules misses the mark. Its underlying metaphor does not allow us to admit the existence of inexplicable and the unintended consequences. Our experiences of health, illness, and dying do not conform to mechanistic rules; our bodies are not cars in need of repair. Hence, it follows that we cannot manage or control the issues of health care as though they were merely contracts and power negotiations.

Consider a justification for Codes as Moral Virtues. Its appeal comes from the way it expresses its underlying metaphor—that of a covenant. I use the word virtue in the narrow, Aristotelian sense of referring to the particular human characteristics necessary to fulfill human purpose within a community. These characteristics are honed out of trial and error in accordance with what actually fulfills the human goal and desire of reaching life's completion as a person in community. Of course, some communities do not foster this sense of virtue, though they may require certain dutiful behaviors (for example, a mob family may require loyalty, but this would not be a virtue because the family itself could not be virtuous. It does not contribute to a good greater than its own greed and dominance). However, a community of honor and nobility is committed to a good that, in principle, enables all people within the community to reach a sense of purpose and fulfillment. Such a community would be virtuous, engendering and requiring virtuous people to enact its moral purpose.

What keeps a virtuous community cohesive and committed to its own perpetuity is an understanding of the nature of a covenant as something that works toward the moral good of all. A covenant community

9. I am aware that for many the body is a machine and can be explained according to mechanistic laws. We can call this view the Hobbesian Person. Just as all reality is but matter in motion, understandable according to mechanistic laws, so too are people and human health. Though such a view does provide for a necessary explanation of our physical experience, I reject it as a sufficient explanation of the human experience. It would take a long essay to prove this claim, but I think it is defensible. However, by this, I do not dismiss or discredit the empirical basis of medical research and the need for observable and scientifically tested protocols in medicine. What I reject is the assumption that just because an empirical finding can provide a necessary explanation for what is physically assessable that therefore a materialistic-mechanistic accounting can provide a comprehensive, sufficient explanation of the human experience.

presupposes that certain people take upon themselves tasks and assignments that express the moral purposes of the community. We typically call such tasks and assignments "professions", rather than simply "jobs". Professions express the community's moral goals and, hence, are accountable to the larger calling of the society's existence as a moral reality (promoting a sense of good as well as human purpose). Not only do they perform highly technical skills, they reflect the moral underpinnings of society.

A sense of professional vocation has characterized the practice of health care since the time of the Hippocratic oath. Health care is more than a job requiring certain skills; it is a necessary function within society that helps it to achieve its moral purpose, the promotion of human health and well-being. We not only expect health care providers to be interested in contracts and negotiations, but we also expect them to be interested in the totality of the human experience, for it is intertwined with the provision of health care. Because the human experience can be neither reduced to algorithmic, causal rules nor managed by mechanistic laws, health care providers must be committed to goals larger than the mere exercise of their skills. In other words, they must be people who understand and are committed to the professional nature of their work and the way that work promotes the health and well-being of persons in society.

The above list of Codes as Statutory Rules does not express this sense of professional calling. However, the list of Codes as Virtues does. The common thread among the statements in the second list is the force of a community held together by a moral covenant that requires certain portions of its populace to perform necessary and highly trained tasks so that people can reach their comprehensive purposes in life. Such a code cultivates the kind of person necessary to support a covenant-community. Such a community is then enabled to establish and promote human fulfillment and well-being.

Of course, the way I have explained the two estimations of codes of ethics makes the Codes as Moral Virtues the more attractive list, but there is a good reason for this—the covenant metaphor better expresses what we experience as persons with comprehensive goals in a community than does the metaphor of a machine. We need such a code to prepare and sustain its adherents to perform and persevere in a profession that inevitably experiences tragedy, not necessarily because of mistakes, but rather because of the natural limitations of dealing with illness and morality.

The Tragic Dimension of Health Care

The inevitability of non-culpable errors in the practice of the health care professions indicates a tragic dimension to their practice. The word tragedy has several meanings, but I use it to refer to those grievous situations in which bad outcomes result from good people's good decisions. This happens in the medical professions.

Consider the contrast between such non-culpable inevitability and medical malpractice. Practitioners who commit malpractice are guilty of not providing the service that they were expected to provide. Courts determine malpractice guilt when practitioners perform medical care badly, not merely because bad results follow from their actions. Proper medical practice is typically established by what is called the "standard of care." This phrase has technical meanings, both legal and professional, and refers to what a prudent practitioner would do under certain circumstances. Here, a prudent practitioner would not simply make defensible judgments, but would base such judgments on the precedence of previous medical practice in similar circumstances. The profession does not base its standard of care upon guaranteed results but upon the best, established practices. It is instructive to note that health care rests its norms of practice upon the best possible way (based upon practice and research) to treat a situation, rather than upon the assurance that results will always follow. Such a course of action knows that unforeseen and unpredictable results can follow even from what has been established as the best possible standard of care. What determines good medicine is not elimination of the possibility of tragic consequences, but the performance of acceptable and tested practices.

For example, we do not (or at least should not) assume that medicine fails because cancer patients die after taking chemotherapy. It is our common experience that such unwelcomed and grievous deaths occur in spite of the best that medicine can provide. However, we would think doctors fail if they do not practice what has been accepted as the standard of care in such circumstances. Sometimes the best professionals, acting according to their best knowledge and skills, cannot prevent unintended and deleterious situations from occurring. Each branch of health care can tell countless stories in which the practitioner follows the dictates of established and best care and still causes unwanted conditions, either directly or indirectly. Because the stakes are so high in health care, the emotional toll on a practitioner can be enormously heavy. It takes someone with courage, fortitude, patience, and practical wisdom to join and contribute to such professions.

Stanley Hauerwas, Richard Bondi, and David Burrell aptly describe the tragic dimension to the practice of medicine. For them, medicine is a "moral art" that is difficult to categorize as either care for the patient or faithful application of knowledge and technology. However, the most forceful aspect of medicine as a moral art is "that medicine is moral art because it must be guided by convictions that sustain the effort to care in the face of death."[10] There are natural, temporal, and economic limits to involvement with the caring for and curing of patients that even sophisticated and powerful modern technology cannot remove. In fact, this limitation characterizes all people before death. Medicine has to face this tragic dimension as a profession.

Because of this natural limitation, we should not expect more of medicine than it can provide. It cannot remove the tragic nature of life from our experience and, thus, it cannot remove tragedy from its own professional purpose. If a patient dies or suffers a disease, health care has not necessarily failed. Furthermore, we assume too much of medicine if we guarantee success in every effort. Patients and diseases do not necessarily follow simple, mechanistic, causal patterns. They have histories that are filled with unpredictable occurrences and idiosyncrasies. No one person can map out all the forces and aspects that come to bear on a patient, and it is hubris to believe one can.

Moreover, medical codes of ethics do not require the professional to be omniscient or omnipotent. They do, however, require that the practitioner uphold the honor of the profession and respect the patient's dignity. One must have a certain kind of courage, fortitude, and patience to endure in a profession that overtly intends to care and cure the patient, but which also naturally loses patients. Thus, medicine holds both great opportunities and built-in disadvantages, and it takes a moral community that is committed to its moral art to nurture professionals to persevere in such a demanding and troubling profession.

At this point, Hauerwas, Bondi, and Burrell are apprehensive: "For if medicine requires a moral

---

10. Hauerwas, Stanley, Bondi, Richard, and Burrell, David B. *Truthfulness and Tragedy: Further Investigations in Christian Ethics.* Notre Dame: University of Notre Dame Press; 1977: 186

community sufficient to sustain it as a tragic profession, then no such community seems to exist. In other words, I am suggesting that no moral community exists to provide medicine with a story sufficient to guide and sustain its activities."[11] This is a troubling assessment, since codes as virtues presuppose moral practitioners, who, in turn, presuppose a moral community that knows how to teach the virtues.

Though the Hippocratic Oath is often extolled as the paragon and paradigm of medical ethical codes, we should not treat it as though it represents a set of abstract ethical principles that are either pertinent for all time or readily applicable to all ethical dilemmas in medicine and health care. Rather than a set of abstract principles exemplifying universal ethical truths, the code originally represented the requirements of a certain community of people who called themselves doctors and who were committed to the art of health care. The moral demands of the health care professions called for a code of ethics around which the professionals could learn how to act as the kind of moral beings they should be in the practice of their particular work. The codes did not, and do not now, create the moral demands of the professions. They express the professions' compelling moral forces.

Charles Hemingway and Douglas Querin capture this relationship clearly when they say, "[Codes] are not simply boilerplate documents that exist in the abstract. They are living, breathing documents with real-world implications."[12] Hemingway and Querin reach this conclusion after demonstrating the inadequacy of assuming that codes function in the same way as criminal, civil, and administrative laws. Laws operate under the warrant of the state's authority and are indifferent to the specific necessities of the profession. According to Hemingway and Querin, to treat the codes of ethics as though they had the precedence and power of coercion of criminal, civil, and administrative laws is a mistake and misuse of the codes. Rather than treating the codes as laws, we should understand and handle codes of ethics as "consensus standards of conduct, reflecting the aspirations, expectations and obligations of each profession."[13] That is, the codes do not create the ethics of the profession. Instead, the real-life moral obligations of the profession's practice create the need to articulate codes expressive of the profession's moral purpose. We write codes of ethics so that we can retain and be faithful to the compelling moral practices of the profession.

For this reason, it is more consistent with the practice of medicine and health care to see codes as inspirational of human performance in the actual practice of medicine rather than as prescriptive of the correct procedural steps needed to assure success and to safeguard against mistakes.[14] They are inspirational because they represent the kind of person the practitioner should be when she or he functions according to the best purposes of the profession. Codes of ethics should codify the necessary requirements for practitioners to carry on the continual learning, wisdom, and skill of a profession that is not reducible to a set of abstract, prescriptive rules. They must express what has been learned in the maturation of a profession designed to help patients overcome their illnesses, maintain their health,

11. Ibid. 202

12. Hemingway, Charles H, and Querin, Douglas S. "Ethics Codes and the Law: Code Provisions Often Have Relevance Well Beyond the Group Establishing the Code." *Addiction Professional.* 2011; March-April: 20

13. Ibid. 19

14. Farrell, Brian J. Cobbin, Deirdre M., and Farrell, Helen M. "Codes of Ethics: Their Evolution, Development and Other Controversies." *The Journal of Management Development.* 2002; 21: 152–163

and come as close as possible to live out a natural course of life. The codes should become clarions for vocational integrity rather than merely safeguards against mistakes, legal challenges, and social opprobrium. They should express the moral qualities of those people who can carry on in a tragic profession whose aims for healing and health sometimes go unmet. Though it is necessary to include within a professional code regulative rules that guide practitioners in specific concerns and dilemmas, they must be couched within the larger and more important concern of describing the kind of person who must sustain a profession that inevitably deals with the tragic consequences it creates.

[...]

Conclusion

I have tried to show that the codes of ethics for the medical professions should be treated as the necessary virtues needed to fulfill the purposes of the professions. Medicine demands a great deal from the character of its practitioners. They must not only master certain knowledge and technical skills, but they must also be able to endure in a tragic profession. Furthermore, since tragedy befalls all lives, we can learn from the moral arts of medicine how to cultivate the necessary virtues to preserve and remain committed to a morally purpose-driven life. Other professions may provide similar modeling (teaching and ministry for example), but in dealing with matters of health, life, and death, medicine does so in a particularly poignant way, that is, when it uses its codes as virtues and not merely as statutory rules.

The Qualities of a Compassionate Nurse According to the Perceptions Of Medical-Surgical Patients

Diane Domine Kret

Diane Domine Kret, "The Qualities of a Compassionate Nurse According to the Perceptions Of Medical-Surgical Patients," *Medsurg Nursing*, vol. 20, no. 1, pp. 29-36. Copyright © 2011 by Anthony J. Jannetti, Inc. Reprinted with permission. Provided by ProQuest LLC. All rights reserved.

Compassion is thought of as a nursing quality that impacts patient care. Research to describe compassion among nurses is nonexistent. In this study, the complexities of compassion, its effect on patient care, and the historical roots of compassion are explored. Attempts are made to measure levels of compassion rendered by the health care team, including physicians, physician's assistants, and nurses. This descriptive study is designed to explore the qualities of compassionate nurses as perceived by patients in medical-surgical units.

Compassion is considered a nursing quality that impacts patient care. Literature contains many descriptions of what compassion is and does for the patient, but none of these descriptors is uniform. Understanding begins with the derivation of the word *compassion*. According to McNeill, Morrison, and Nouwen (1982),

The word compassion is derived from the Latin words *pati* and *cum*, which together mean "to suffer with." Compassion challenges us to cry out with those in misery, to mourn with those who are lonely, to weep with those in tears. Compassion requires us to be weak with the weak, vulnerable with the vulnerable, and powerless with powerless. Compassion means full immersion in the condition of being human. (p. 4)

This definition illustrates the depth and emotion involved in being a compassionate individual. It also shows the sacrifice required to understand the complexity of emotions a person may have.

Compassion is developed through a connection between two individuals. It is evoked by a deep understanding of another person's suffering and pain. According to Morse, Bottorff, Anderson, O'Brien, and Solberg (1992),

Compassion is a strong emotion or sentiment stimulated by the presence of suffering that evokes recognition and mutual sharing of the despair or pain of the sufferer. The compassionate caregiver echoes the sufferer's sentiment and shares in the suffering. In sharing in the other's suffering, the caregiver expresses compassion that strengthens and comforts the sufferer. (p. 814)

The compassionate nurse thus is challenged to share in the suffering of the patient.

The relationship between the nurse and the patient is vital because the nurse has the most direct contact with the patient. As stated by Dietze and Orb (2000), "If the nurse is able to develop a relationship of confidence and trust with the patient, not only will healing occur, but the patient's spiritual, emotional and other needs can be effectively addressed" (p. 172). Compassion provides the nurse with awareness of the suffering the patient may experience. Through this awareness, the patient's emotional and physical needs are met more fully.

Compassion is a reaction of emotion felt by an individual witnessing another person's plight or misfortune. "Compassion connotes sorrow or pity excited by the distress or misfortunes of another" (Forsyth, 1980, p. 39). Compassion and empathy are related very closely, but the two terms cannot be used synonymously. According to Benbassat and Baumal (2004),

Empathy begins with gaining an insight into the patient's concerns, feelings and sources of distress. In turn, this produces compassion, i.e., a feeling of discomfort produced by the distress of another person. Compassion leads to a desire to remove the cause of distress or at least to alleviate it. (p. 833)

Compassion is therefore a reaction to empathy. A better understanding of the patient must be reached in order for the nurse to care for the patient in an effective, meaningful way. "To empathize means to share and experience the feelings of the patient. The main motive of empathizing is to achieve an understanding of the patient" (Ehmann, 1971, pp. 75–76). In this understanding, an individual can serve better and be more sensitive to a suffering person in the time of need.

Care is another component of compassion. As Wollenburg (2004) noted, "Compassion indicates that we care deeply about others, particularly those who are suffering or in trouble" (p. 1785). Care is an important attribute to compassion because the action of caring has the potential to alleviate an individual's suffering. Care is the "actions and activities directed toward assisting, supporting, or enabling another individual or group with evident or anticipated needs to ameliorate or improve a human condition or lifeway or to face death" (Gaut & Leininger, 1991, p. 46). It has a direct relationship to curing and healing. George (1995) identified it as one of the dominating concepts in nursing, stating, "Care is assumed to be a distinct, dominant, unifying and central focus of nursing, and, while curing and healing cannot occur effectively without care, care may occur without cure" (p. 376). In addition, care is nondiscriminatory, rooted in a person's "sense of another human person in need of someone" (Roach, 1991, p. 15).

Compassion is intrinsic in nursing practice because through compassion the patient's suffering is alleviated in a meaningful and effective way, which also empowers the nurse through his or her compassionate actions toward the patient. According to Dietze and Orb (2000),

> Compassionate care ... is not simplistically about taking away another person's pain or suffering, but is about entering into that person's experience so as to share their burden in solidarity with them and hence enabling them to retain their independence and dignity. (p.169)

Discernment of compassionate care first needs to be based on a clear understanding of the concept of compassion expressed by nurses and perceived by patients. In addition, understanding the perceptions of patients provides insight concerning their care expectations.

Review of Literature

Research linking compassion and nursing is minimal (Fogarty, Curbow, Wingard, McDonnell, & Somerfield, 1999; Screeche-Powell, 2004; Skaff, Toumey, Rapp, & Fahringer, 2003).

Ten components of compassion among physicians' assistants (PAs) were investigated by Skaff and coauthors (2003). The components included forbearance, consideration, explanatory communication, concern, honoring the person, attentive listening, attention to detail, general compassion, patience, and familiarity. Findings showed only 3 of 10 components (forbearance, consideration, explanatory communication) were validated by patients. Although patients gave positive responses on their PAs' communication skills, they did not validate the components more associated with empathy and compassion, such as patience and concern. Findings also demonstrated patients who were handed the survey by their PAs responded more positively then those surveyed over the phone.

Screeche-Powell (2004) studied a compassionate nursing intervention given to patients on coronary artery bypass graft (CABG) waiting lists. A cardiac clinical nurse specialist was designated to be the "cardiac outreach sister" to customize, complete, and evaluate a pre-surgical intervention to improve the experience of patients waiting for CABG and provide emotional support throughout their waiting period. Limitations to the study included the failure to identify compassion specifically, with its presence only inferred by compassionate actions, the omission of the control group for ethical reasons, and the lack of discussion regarding reliability and validity of the tool. In addition, 40% of patients who were offered a home visit refused it for various reasons. The study did suggest, however, many of the patients indicated the telephone call from the cardiac outreach sister showed this nurse was compassionate toward them and provided the attention they needed to undergo this difficult waiting period. The patients believed they were not alone but had "someone to turn to" with their problems or concerns, even if questions seemed trivial. Patients identified the sister's compassionate interventions as her active listening skills, continuation of care by providing answers to specific questions they had concerning the surgery, additional reading material given to reinforce previous information, and emotional support during the preoperative waiting time.

The only study that provided a tool to measure compassion was conducted by Fogarty and colleagues (1999). For the purposes of Fogarty's study, the definition of compassion from Webster's II New Riverside University Dictionary (1988) was used: "Sympathetic concern for the suffering of another, together with the inclination to give aid or support or show mercy" (p. 225). Researchers questioned whether watching a 40second video demonstrating compassion by a medical doctor would reduce the anxiety of patients with breast cancer. Two tapes were created in this study: the standard videotape and the enhanced compassion videotape. In the standard videotape, a dramatized oncologic consultation was recorded to include the physician giving the patient two choices of treatment for metastatic breast cancer; risks, benefits, and side effects of treatment; and probability of short-term versus long-term survival. The enhanced compassion video provided the same dramatized oncologic consultation with the exception of two short segments in which the physician displayed concern for the patient's emotional distress by first recognizing her distress and then comforting the patient by touching her hand. The measures used in this study included a compassion scale assessing the physician's compassion; a State-Trait Anxiety Inventory Scale (STAI-S), which measured the patients' anxiety; and a treatment information recall score, which measured the amount of information the patient retained and understood after the physician discussed the treatment options. The STAI-S was given as a pretest before the enhanced compassion and standard videos, and was repeated as a post-test after the video was viewed. The study found patients who viewed the enhanced compassion video had a higher average total compassion score (mean 220) compared to patients who viewed the standard video (mean 137).

Although all patient participants experienced anxiety, patients who watched the enhanced compassion video were significantly less anxious than patients who saw the standard video (Fogarty et al., 1999). Mean post-test STAI-S scores of patients who viewed the enhanced video were 40.0, compared to 44.7 for patients who viewed the standard video ($p = 0.011$); this suggested patients who watched the enhanced video were less anxious than patients who viewed the standard video. The study also showed patients who viewed the enhanced compassion video rated their physicians higher than the standard video viewers on other positive attributes, such as the belief the doctor cared about the patient ($p < 0.001$), acknowledged patient's emotions ($p < 0.001$), encouraged the patient's questions ($p = 0.011$), encouraged patient's participation in treatment ($p = 0.004$), and wanted what was best for the patient ($p = 0049$).

For the study, Fogarty and colleagues (1999) developed a compassion scale to measure the degree to which the physician displayed compassion and credibility, and the variability that occurred with the different video interventions. The compassion scale used "a semantic differential format" (p. 373) that included five pairs of characteristics: *warm/cold, pleasant/unpleasant, compassionate/distant, sensitive/insensitive,* and *caring/uncaring.* Each pair of characteristics was presented along a 10-cm line. Study participants were in structed to put an X on the line to indicate their perceptions of the physician on the continuum. "The distance of the X from the left anchor was calculated in millimeters, such that each item had a possible range of 0–100" (p. 373). The closer the X was to the characteristic, the more the physician displayed the characteristic. If the participant placed the X closest to the characteristics *warm, pleasant,* compassionate, sensitive, and caring, the physician was seen as highly compassionate. The scale items were developed to measure the degree to which the physician displayed compassion and credibility, and the variability that occurred with the different video manipulations. The items within the scale were analyzed using principal axis factoring and oblique rotation. According to Fogarty (1996),

> Two subscales were created using the factor analysis solution summing all items loading over.55 on each factor. Five items were included in the "compassion" subscale, which had alpha coefficient of.92. Four items were in the "credibility" subscale, which had an alpha coefficient of.83. (p. 14)

The alpha coefficient is a reliability coefficient with a normal range between 0.00 and +1.00 (Polit & Beck, 2004b). The compassion subscale had an alpha coefficient of.92, indicating it had a high reliability. Fogarty (1996) developed the content validity of this scale through a previous pilot study examining the reactions of women watching the compassion-enhanced videos. The items for the compassion scale were drawn from in-depth interviews with women describing specific characteristics within the videos. A limitation of this compassion scale was that it was used only twice in Fogarty's own studies (Fogarty, 1996; Fogarty et al., 1999). In addition, compassion was included as one of the items in the scale. Despite these limitations, this scale was the only tool found in the literature and was applied to the current study.

Purpose of the Study

In this descriptive study, the complexities of compassion and its effect on patient care, the historical roots of compassion, and attempts to measure levels of compassion rendered by the health care team, including nurses, physicians, and physician's assistants were explored. The study was designed to examine the qualities of compassionate nurses perceived by patients in medical-surgical units. The study addressed the following questions:

- Do medical-surgical patients perceive their nurses as compassionate?
- What are the most frequently occurring qualities of compassion perceived by the medical-surgical patients?

Design/Methods

Consultation with a bio-statistician determined 100 nurses were needed for the study. Initial consideration by the hospital institutional review board (IRB) led to a recommendation to use random rather than convenience sampling for the study. During the first 3 months of the study, every third nurse was selected from a roster of all medical-surgical nurses within the hospital. However, data collection proved to be difficult due to the availability of the selected nurses. Many of the randomly selected nurses had moved to critical care units or other specialty areas within the hospital or outside the facility. Due to this difficulty, the IRB approved a change to convenience sampling, in which any nurse who agreed to participate in the study was included, and the protocol eventually was extended to 2 years to allow sufficient time for data collection.

Study #_____

Directions: Rate your nurse by placing an X on each line. (Each line represents one quality.) Then on the next page, list qualities that you feel a compassion nurse should have.

cold   warm

| 0 | 2.5 | 5 | 7.5 | 10 |

unpleasant   pleasant

| 0 | 2.5 | 5 | 7.5 | 10 |

distant   compassionate

| 0 | 2.5 | 5 | 7.5 | 10 |

insensitive   sensitive

| 0 | 2.5 | 5 | 7.5 | 10 |

uncaring   caring

| 0 | 2.5 | 5 | 7.5 | 10 |

Figure 2.5.1   Compassion Scale

Fogarty et al., 1999. Used with permission.

To facilitate study completion in 2 years, the author recruited nurses who volunteered to participate as data collectors. These nurses were required to complete a training day to ensure consistency in the data collection. They received information about the compassion study, and learned the process of interviewing patients and nurses to obtain the necessary data.

First, a data collector approached an assigned nurse on the medical-surgical unit and gave a brief summary of the compassion study with an invitation to participate in the study. Of the 105 nurses asked to participate in the study, five nurses refused because they did not want to take the time away from their work. The remaining 100 nurses completed informed consent and demographics forms and identified the district in which they worked. Patients then were chosen using convenience sampling. The first patient within that nurse's district who agreed to participate in the study was asked to sign informed consent and demographic forms. Of 112 patients asked to participate in the study, only 12 refused. Only one patient per nurse was used in this study because it provided an opportunity for 100 different nurses to be rated on their compassion by 100 different patients. To be included in the study, a patient had to be awake, alert, and oriented; able to read English; and able to provide consent. To protect the nurses' and patients' confidentiality, sequential numbers identified the compassion scale to link it to the demographic sheet. No names, dates, or patient identifying information appeared on the demographic sheets.

Patients from medical-surgical units were asked to rate their nurses' level of compassion (see Figure 2.5.1) by placing an X on each line that included a quality of compassion. For the purposes of this study, the characteristics used from the 1999 study by Fogarty and colleagues only included the compassion scale, applied it to the nurse, and included measurable increments to provide descriptors for a nurse for each of the five pairs of compassion characteristics. Patients then were asked to state something their nurses did they thought was compassionate.

Permission was granted by the author for use of the compassion scale. The Cronbach's alpha/ Coefficient alpha test was used to test for internal consistency reliability for this study. As the value gets closer to +1.00, a higher internal consistency of the tool was reflected. The compassion scale had a Cronbach's alpha of 0.939, which indicated a high reliability. An instrument that has high internal reliability shows the variables used within the tool or instrument measured the same trait (Polit & Beck, 2004b).

With the use of Spearman's rho, a strong relationship was identified among psychosocial variables in which r was equal or greater than 0.7. "… for most psychosocial variables (e.g. stress and severity of illness), an r of.70 is high; correlations between such variables are typically in the.10 to.40 range" (Polit & Beck, 2004a, p. 469). As shown in the correlation matrix in Table 2.5.1, all variables within the compassion scale had strong relationships with each other. The strong relationship among the variables within the compassion scale implied the variables had a strong relationship with the trait of compassion. With this strong relationship with compassion, the same variables could be used to measure compassion effectively. Because the correlation was high among the variables, a future study can use this compassion scale on a different population.

Data Analysis

The biostatistician analyzed the data using the Statistical Analysis System (SAS), which is a statistical software. The analyses were performed using version 9.1 of SAS (SAS Institute Inc., Cary, NC) (Delwiche & Slaughter, 2008). Kendall Tau-b Correlation Coefficients were computed for demographics, including patient age, nurse age, nurse years of experience, nurse hours worked per week, and hours assigned to the patient. The CORR procedure with the software computed Pearson correlation coefficients, three nonparametric measures of association, and the probabilities associated with these statistics. The software's FREQ procedure was used to correlate frequency scores of the compassion scale to various demographic elements for the patient and the nurse. The FREQ procedure also produced contingency tables that examined the relationships among classification variables (Rosner, 2000).

Table 2.5.1. Correlation Among Variables within Compassion Scale

Spearman Correlation Coefficients (N = 100) Prob > |r| under H0: Rho=0					
	Cold_Warm	Unpleasant_Pleasant	Distant_Compassionate	Insensitive_Sensitive	Uncaring_Caring
Cold_Warm	1.00000	0.71913 <0.0001	0.76808 <0.0001	0.75110 <0.0001	0.72158 <0.0001
Unpleasant_Pleasant	0.71913 <0.0001	1.00000	0.76119 <0.0001	0.78967 <0.0001	0.73366 <0.0001
Distant_Compassionate	0.76808 <0.0001	0.76119 <0.0001	1.00000	0.81732 <0.0001	0.80344 <0.0001
Insensitive_Sensitive	0.75110 <0.0001	0.78967 <0.0001	0.81732 <0.0001	1.00000	0.78229 <0.0001
Uncaring_Caring	0.72158 <0.0001	0.73366 <0.0001	0.80344 <0.0001	0.78229 <0.0001	1.00000

Association of compassion rating with continuous characteristics was estimated by Kendall Tau-b Correlation Coefficients, a correlation index used for ordinal variables (Polit & Beck, 2004a). The association of compassion rating with categorical nurse characteristics was estimated by Cochran-Armitage Trend Test, which was used to examine trends among groups (Corcoran & Mehta, 2001). To adjust the possible co-variates, ordinal logistic regression was used. Correlation among the variables within the compassion scale was estimated by Spearman's rho, which is a correlation index utilized in ordinal-level measures (Polit & Beck, 2004a).

Nurses' characteristics identified by patients were categorical characteristics. Patients were asked to describe nurses' compassionate qualities. Only 68 of 100 patients completed the section that required them to write descriptors of compassion displayed by their nurses. These were grouped into common themes, which were tallied into frequency of occurrences.

Results

Of patients involved in the study, 47% (n = 47) were ages 56–75 and 41% (n = 41) were ages 67–95; 9% (n = 9) were 36–35; 2% (n = 2) were < 35; and 1% (n = 1) was > 95. Nurse participants worked either day shift (61%, n = 61) or night shift (39%, n = 39). Most of them had 0–4 years of experience (76%, n = 76); 24% (n = 24) had 5 or more years of experience. More specifically 12% (n = 12) had 5–9 years of experience and the other 12% (n = 12) had 10+ years of experience. In addition, 46% (n = 46) worked 36 hours a week while 45% (n = 45) worked more than 36 hours week; the remaining 9% (n = 9) worked less than 36 hours. Finally, the hours assigned to the patient were as follows: 38% (n = 38) worked 9–12.5 hours with the patient; 31% (n = 31) worked 5–8 hours with the patient; 23% (n = 23) worked more than 12.5 hours with the patient; and 8% (n = 8) worked 4 hours or less with the patient.

Examination of the simple statistics indicated the mean scores in the compassion ratings showed little variability. The median score of 10 that the compassion ratings had in common from the simple statistics (see Table 2.5.2) showed some collinearity, which was attributed to the fact these characteristics occurred within the same scale developed to measure compassion.

For the Kendall Tau-b Correlation Coefficients, statistical significance was identified when p was less than 0.05 (Munro, 2005). The Kendall Tau-b Correlation Coefficients was ap plied to the statistical data of this compassion study; statistical significance was shown (see Table 2.5.3) in the age of the patient with the compassion ratings of unpleasant-pleasant ($p = 0.0131$), distant-compassionate ($p = 0.0183$), and uncaring-caring ($p = 0.0250$). Statistical significance also was shown in the years of experience of the nurse and the compassion rating of cold-warm ($p = 0.0378$).

Similar to the Kendall Tau-b Cor relation Coefficients, the Cochran-Armitage test statistical significance was identified when p was less than 0.05 (Corcoran & Mehta, 2002). Statistical significance was found with the nurses' shift (day or night) and the compassion ratings of unpleasant-pleasant ($p = 0.0233$) and distant-compassionate ($p = 0.0178$) (see Tables 2.5.4 & 2.5.5).

In the qualitative analysis, patients were asked to describe nurses' compassionate qualities. The compassion themes found within the written descriptors included caring (54), attentive (35), dedicated (13), approachable (11), professional (9), and keeping the patient informed (7).

Discussion

In this study, patients from medical-surgical units were asked to evaluate their nurses' level of compassion and then identify a compassionate behavior demonstrated by their nurses. The perceived level of nurses' compassion was compared to patient and nurse demographics to elicit any statistical significance. The answer to the first question (Do medical-surgical patients perceive their nurses as compassionate?) was "yes." Little variability was shown in the mean scores of the compassion ratings, which implied nurses were very compassionate. A ceiling effect was assumed here due to the high mean scores, but the results were believed to be genuine because of the true compassion displayed by the nurses. The qualitative analysis addressed characteristics of compassion in response to the second question. Most frequently occurring themes of compassion were caring (54) and attentive (35).

Table 2.5.2. Simple Statistics

Variable	N	Mean	Standard Deviation	Median	Minimum	Maximum
AgePt	100	3.30000	0.73168	3.00000	1.00000	5.00000
AgeNurse	100	1.77000	0.52905	2.00000	1.00000	3.00000
YrsExperience	100	1.36000	0.68931	1.00000	1.00000	3.00000
HrsPerWk	100	2.36000	0.64385	2.00000	1.00000	3.00000
HrsAssigned	100	2.76000	0.90028	3.00000	1.00000	4.00000
Cold_Warm	100	9.36600	1.08881	10.00000	5.00000	10.00000

Table 2.5.2. Simple Statistics

Unpleasant_Pleasant	100	9.53100	0.92558	10.00000	5.00000	10.00000
Distant_Compassionate	100	9.32600	1.48621	10.00000	2.50000	10.00000
Insensitive_Sensitive	100	9.45400	1.18615	10.00000	2.50000	10.00000
Uncaring_Caring	100	9.60200	0.95779	10.00000	5.00000	10.00000

Table 2.5.3. Continuous Characteristics in Compassion Scale

	Kendall Tau-b Correlation Coefficients (N = 100)				
	Cold_ Warm	Unpleasant_ Pleasant	Distant_ Compassionate	Insensitive_ Sensitive	Uncaring_ Caring
AgePt	0.12980 0.1478	0.22530 0.0131	0.21355 0.0183	0.14980 0.0981	0.20514 0.0250
AgeNurse	−0.08267 0.3682	−0.10622 0.2535	−0.08427 0.3635	−0.10763 0.2459	0.01409 0.8806
YrsExperience	−0.18927 0.0378	−0.14651 0.1123	−0.16759 0.0684	−0.12582 0.1715	−0.11175 0.2296
HrsPerWk	0.01096 0.9038	0.12928 0.1592	0.10013 0.2741	0.00825 0.9282	0.05001 0.5891
HrsAssigned	0.12778 0.1416	0.13575 0.1231	0.06704 0.4449	0.14814 0.0915	0.08490 0.3387

For the Kendall Tau-b Correlation Coefficients, statistical significance was identified when p was less than 0.05 (Munro, 2005). The statistical significance shown between patient age and compassion ratings of unpleasant-pleasant (p = 0.0131), distant-compassionate (p = 0.0183), and uncaring-caring (p = 0.0250) may be attributed to the increased attention and care needed by aging patients. Older patients perceived their nurses to be pleasant, compassionate, and caring.

Statistical significance seen between years of experience of the nurse and the compassion rating of cold-warm (p = 0.0378) implied the more experienced nurse may be colder toward the patient. This finding unfortunately implied the vigor and passion demonstrated by the newer nurse may diminish as the nurse becomes more experienced. This may be attributed to compassion fatigue. According to Bush (2009),

> Nurses who are idealistic, highly motivated, and committed also are at high risk to experience burnout and compassion fatigue, possibly the result of the cumulative losses they experience that cause disappointment and despair or if they perceive that they are not moving toward their care goals and do not feel effective in changing the environment to do so. (p. 26)

Table 2.5.4. Unpleasant_Pleasant by Shift

Unpleasant_Pleasant	Shift		Total	
Frequency Col Pct	1	2		
5	1 1.64	0 0.00	1	
7.5	8 13.11	1 2.56	9	
8	1 1.64	0 0.00	1	
8.5	5 8.20	2 5.13	7	
9	3 4.92	2 5.13	5	
9.5	2 3.28	1 2.56	3	
9.8	1 1.64	0 0.00	1	
9.9	1 1.64	1 2.56	2	
10	39 63.93	32 82.05	71	
Total	61	39	100	

Bush indicated all caregivers, especially nurses, are at risk for compassion fatigue due to high-stress environments that include high nurse-patient ratios, little to no administrative and peer support, and demands to provide the same high quality of care when working with fewer resources.

Similar to the Kendall Tau-b Correlation Coefficients, the Cochran-Armitage test statistical significance was identified when p is less 0.05 (Corcoran & Mehta, 2001). Statistical significance was shown between the nurses' shift (day or night) and the compassion ratings of unpleasant-pleasant (p = 0.0233) and distant-compassionate (p = 0.0178). This statistical significance implied patients perceived their nurses were pleasant and compassionate, regardless of whether their nurses worked a day or night shift. This may be attributed to the fact that the nurses who took care of them were perceived to be consistently compassionate and pleasant towards their patients.

Table 2.5.5. Distant_Compassionate by Shift

Distant_Compassionate	Shift	Total

Table 2.5.5. Distant_Compassionate by Shift

Frequency Col Pct	1	2	
2.5	3 4.92	0 0.00	3
7.5	11 18.03	1 2.56	12
7.6	1 1.64	0 0.00	1
8	0 0.00	1 2.56	1
8.5	1 1.64	1 2.56	2
9	3 4.92	2 5.13	5
9.5	2 3.28	2 5.13	4
9.8	1 1.64	1 2.56	2
9.9	1 1.64	0 0.00	1
10	38 62.30	31 79.49	69
Total	61	39	100

Study Limitations

An uneven distribution of the day shift (61%) and night shift (39%) occurred due to the availability of data collectors. Another limitation was the majority of nurses within this study had 0–4 years of experience (76%). Contributing to this result is that a medical-surgical unit is often the point of professional entry for many new nurses. A further study may include the increase or decrease in compassion as nurses move through the continuum of novice to expert.

Another limitation to this study was the lack of correlation between time spent with the patient and the compassion perceived by the patient. Although the hours the nurse was assigned to the patient was one variable in the study related to compassion, no statistical significance was noted. Further studies are needed to explore the difference between the quality of time and the length of time spent with the patient, and the perception of compassion. Also, because the study found older adults perceived their nurses as pleasant, compassionate, and caring, further study may include the special needs of older adult patients and how compassion can play a part in their healing process or recovery in the hospital.

Perhaps the most important limitation is the inclusion of compassion as one of the qualities in the compassion tool. This provided a description of the abstract term that could have been explained better with addition of an adjective, instead of using the word compassion. Additional research is needed to develop a tool that would describe the complexity of compassion and measure compassion with cognitively impaired patients. Another addition to this may include developing a new tool that combines these qualities with the frequently occurring themes of compassion found in this study.

Nursing Implications

Compassion is considered one of the qualities of an exemplary nurse, and understanding the meaning of compassion is important to nursing professionals. In the conclusion of her concept analysis of compassion, Schantz (2007) stated, "… nothing less than compassion can empower nursing to assume major roles in solving or preventing problems afflicting the global community" (p. 54). In an effort to include compassion in health care reform, Youngson (2008) developed an organization called the Centre for Compassion in Healthcare. The key points of the action plan for this organization are to "declare 'compassion' as a core value; hone communication and relationship skills; challenge models of professionalism; and declare compassion as a management and leadership competence" (p. 3). As Youngson suggested "Investing time up front to check a patient's need [for compassion] increases efficiency, safety, and patient satisfaction" (p. 4).

Conclusion

Although this study provided insight into patients' perceptions of medical-surgical nurses' compassion, the concept of compassion remains elusive in its complexity as evidenced by the many unanswered questions. Intrinsic to nursing, compassion will remain a quality patients will always expect from their nurses and health care providers. Additional research will lead to a better understanding of what it means to be a compassionate nurse.

References

Benbassat, J., & Baumal, R. (2004). What is empathy, and how can it be promoted during clinical clerkships? *Academic Medicine: Journal of the Association of Medical Colleges, 79*(9), 832–839.

Bush, N.J. (2009). Compassion fatigue: Are you at risk? *Oncology Nursing Forum, 36*(1), 24–28.

Corcoran, C.D., & Mehta, C.R. (2001). *Exact level and power of permutation, bootstrap and asymptotic tests of trend.* Retrieved from http://biostats.snu.ac.kr/cda2002_1/monteboot.pdf

Delwiche, L., & Slaughter, S. (2008). *The little SAS book* (4th ed.). Cary, NC: SAS Publishing.

Dietze, E.V., & Orb, A. (2000). Compassionate care: A moral dimension of nursing. *Nursing Inquiry, 7*(3), 166–174.

Ehmann, V.E. (1971). Empathy: Its origin, characteristics, and process. *Perspectives in Psychiatric Care, 9*(2), 72–80.

Fogarty, L.A. (1996). Message, source and person factors in breast cancer treatment decision making. *Dissertation of Physician Rating. Baltimore*, MD: School of Public Health, John Hopkins University.

Fogarty, L.A., Curbow, B.A., Wingard, J.R., McDonnell, K., & Somerfield, M.R. (1999). Can 40 seconds of compassion reduce patient anxiety? *Journal of Clinical Oncology*, 17(1), 371–379.

Forsyth, G.L. (1980). Analysis of the concept of empathy: Illustration of one approach. *Advances in Nursing Science*, 2(2), 33–42.

Gaut, D., & Leininger, M.M. (1991). *Care: The compassionate healer*. New York: National League for Nursing.

George, J.B. (1995). Madeleine M. Leininger. In J.B. George (Ed.), *Nursing theories: The base for professional nursing practice* (4th ed) (pp. 373–389). Norwalk, CT: Appleton & Lange.

McNeill, D.P., Morrison, D.A., & Nouwen, H.J.M. (1982). *Compassion, a reflection on the Christian life*. Garden City, NY: Doubleday & Company, Inc.

Morse, J.M., Bottorff, J., Anderson, G., O'Brien, B., & Solberg, S. (1992). Beyond empathy: Expanding expressions of caring. *Journal of Advanced Nursing*, 17(7), 809–821.

Munro, B.H. (2005). *Statistical methods for healthcare research*. Philadelphia: Lippincott Williams & Wilkins.

Polit, D.F., & Beck, C.T. (2004a). Analyzing quantitative data: Descriptive statistics. In D.F. Polit & C.T. Beck (Eds.), *Nursing research: Principles and methods* (pp. 451–476). Philadelphia: Lippincott Williams & Wilkins.

Polit, D.F., & Beck, C.T. (2004b). Assessing data quality. In D.F. Polit, & C.T. Beck (Eds.), *Nursing research: Principles and methods* (pp. 413–447). Philadelphia: Lippincott Williams & Wilkins.

Roach, S.M.S. (1991). The call to consciousness: Compassion in today's health world. In D.A. Gaut & M.M. Leininger (Eds.), *Caring: The compassionate healer* (pp. 7–17). New York: National League for Nursing Press.

Rosner, B. (2000). *Fundamentals of biostatistics* (5th ed.). New York: Duxbury Press.

Schantz, M.L. (2007). Compassion: A concept analysis. *Nursing Forum*, 42(2), 48–55.

Screeche-Powell, C. (2004). A nurse-led intervention for patients on CABG waiting lists. *Nursing Times*, 100(8), 32–35.

Skaff, K.O., Toumey, C.P., Rapp, D., & Fahringer, D. (2003). Measuring compassion in physician assistants. *Journal of the American Academy of Physician Assistants*, 16, 31–37.

Webster's Riverside (1988). Compassion. *Webster's II New Riverside University Dictionary* (2nd ed., vol. 1). Boston: Houghton Mifflin.

Wollenburg, K. (2004). Leadership with conscience, compassion, and commitment. *American Journal of Health-System Pharmacy: Official Journal of the American Society of Health*, 61(17), 1785–1791.

Youngson, R. (2008). *Compassion in healthcare: The missing dimension of healthcare reform?* Retrieved from http://www.compassioninhealthcare.org/downloads/files/Futures-Debate-Compassion.pdf

Reflecting on the Concept of Compassion Fatigue

Brenda Sabo

A review of the literature on the health of nurses leaves little doubt that their work may take a toll on their psychosocial and physical health and well-being. Nurses working in several specialty practice areas, such as intensive care (Bakker. Le Blanc. & Schaufeli. 2005); mental health (Jenkins & Elliott. 2004), paediatrics; (Maytum. Bielski-Heiman. & Garwick. 2004); and oncology (Bakker. Fitch. Green. Butler. & Olsen. 2006; Ekedahl & Wengstrom. 2007), have been found to be particularly vulnerable to work-related stress. Researchers exploring the nature of occupational stress among care providers, including nurses, physicians, social workers, and psychologists, have suggested that aspects of the therapeutic relationship, specifically empathy and engagement, which are fundamental components of nursing, play a role in the onset of the stress. Further, non-relationship factors may also contribute to nurses experiencing a sense of ambiguity and/or conflict about their ability to provide the care they think is needed. These factors include increased patient complexity, reliance on advancing technology to sustain or prolong life, continued emphasis on medical models supporting cure over care, and perceived lack of time (Blomberg & Sahlberg-Blom. 2007; Edwards & Burnard. 2003; Ekedahl & Wengstrom. 2007; Hertting. 2003; Hertting. Nilsson. Theorell. & Larsson. 2004). It is possible that ongoing exposure to these factors may lead nurses to experience compassion fatigue, one form of occupational stress.

In this [reading] I will provide an overview of the concepts of burnout, compassion fatigue, and vicarious traumatisation (see Table). While emphasis is placed on compassion fatigue and its underlying theory, an overview of the other two types of occupational stress, namely burnout and vicarious traumatisation, are also provided. Following this overview I will address two questions: 1) Is compassion fatigue part of a continuum of occupations stress; if so, is burnout a precondition to compassion fatigue? and 2) What are the relationships between types of occupational stress and to what extent does non-resolution of compassion fatigue increase the risk for developing vicarious traumatization? I will provide three scenarios to address these questions and enhance the discussion.

Burnout

Burnout has traditionally been rooted in an understanding of the interpersonal context of the job, specifically the relationship between caregivers and recipients of care and the values and beliefs pertaining to caring work held by care providers (Maslach. Schaufeli. & Leiter. 2001). It is most commonly defined as "a syndrome of emotional exhaustion, depersonalization, and reduced accomplishments that can occur among individuals who do 'people work' of some kind" (Maslach & Jackson. 1986. p. l). Initially conceptualized to reflect the negative effects of people work, burnout has been expanded to include the negative effects of all occupations (Leiter & Schaufeli. 1996).

Possible factors leading to burnout can be classified according to personality characteristics, work-related attitudes, and work/organizational characteristics. Researchers have hypothesized three personality traits that contribute to burnout. They include type A personalities; coping styles, such as escape-avoidance, problem solving, and confrontation; and also traits sometimes referred to as the 'big five,' namely neuroticism, extroversion, openness to experience, agreeableness, and conscientiousness. However, the individual roles of these factors have yet to be fully explicated (Schaufeli & Enzmann. 1998). The big five is considered to be an empirical-based phenomenon describing personality traits rather than a theoretical model (Goldberg. 1990). These traits tend to occur in groupings in many individuals but are not always present together. It is conceivable that certain traits may predispose individuals to increased risk for the development of stress; however further research is necessary to demonstrate whether a causal link exists.

Work-related attitudes, such as the professional's idealistic expectations, have been shown to influence the onset of burnout (Laschinger & Finegan. 2005; Leiter. 2005). For example, nurses' expectation that providing a specific level of care will ultimately lead to positive outcomes for every patient is not only unrealistic and naïve but may set nurses up for stress when they are unable to meet their expected goals. Further, incongruencies between nurses' values and beliefs, which often include their philosophy of care/caring, and their organization's vision and values (e.g., biomedical philosophy) may increase the potential for burnout.

Additional factors that may influence burnout include work-related and organizational characteristics. Examples include job-related stressors (e.g., increased patient-to-nurse ratios); client-related stressors (increased patient acuity and complexity); social support factors (amount of education and collaborative practice provided, and leader/peer support); and degree of autonomy (ability to retain control over decision making at the point of care and nurses' input into changes related to unit-based care delivery within the nurses' unit) within the work environment (Schaufeli & Enzmann, 1998). The first two factors (job-related and client-related) are associated with job demands whereas the latter two (social support and autonomy) are considered potential resources. For example, restructuring within healthcare institutions may result in nurses being moved from one service to another. The mistaken belief that a nurse is a nurse may result in the individual feeling increasing stress. When this shift takes place without adequate orientation and ongoing educational and resource support, the nurse may be at increased risk for experiencing burnout.

Although a number of theoretical frameworks have been proposed to explain burnout, including individual, interpersonal, organizational, and societal frameworks, research has suggested that the most plausible explanation is found in the workplace or organizational environment (Schaufeli & Enzmann. 1998). Increasingly, research supports the notion that burnout arises out of a mismatch between the person and the job (Leiter & Laschinger. 2006; Maslach & Leiter. 1997).

Early conceptualization and research on burnout focused on the relationship between the care provider and care recipient as a necessary element in the development of burnout. In particular, the relationship was seen to contribute to emotional exhaustion which was thought to be the root cause of burnout. As research has shifted from descriptive to inferential study designs, findings have strongly suggested that this relationship was not the key driver contributing to burnout (Lee & Ashforth, 1996; Leiter, 1993). Research now supports six work-life issues involving person-job mismatch as the most likely explanation for burnout. These issues include: work overload, lack of control, lack of reward, lack of community, lack of fairness, and value conflict (Leiter & Laschinger, 2006; Leiter & Maslach, 2004; Maslach & Leiter, 1997).

Compassion Fatigue (Secondary Traumatic Stress)

The past twenty years have seen a rise in research linking exposure to pain, suffering, and trauma with the health of professionals providing care (Abendroth & Flannery, 2006; Adams, Boscarino, & Figley, 2006; Figley, 1999; Joinson, 1992; McCann & Pearlman, 1990; Pearlman, 1998; Pearlman & Saakvitne, 1995a; Sabo, 2010; Sabo, 2006). An offshoot of burnout, the term compassion fatigue first reflected the adverse psychosocial consequences experienced by emergency room nurses in a study exploring burnout (Joinson, 1992). Compassion fatigue has been described as the "natural consequent behaviours and emotions resulting from knowing about a traumatizing event experienced by a significant other—the stress resulting from helping, or wanting to help, a traumatized or suffering person" (Figley, 1995, p. 7). Researchers have suggested that the phenomenon is connected to the therapeutic relationship between the healthcare provider and patient, in that the traumatic or suffering experience of the patient triggers a response, on multiple levels, in the provider. In particular, an individual's capacity for empathy and ability to engage, or enter into, a therapeutic relationship is considered to be central to compassion fatigue. Theorists have argued that individuals who display high levels of empathy and empathic response to a patient's pain, suffering, or traumatic experience are more vulnerable to experiencing compassion fatigue (Adams, et al., 2006; Figley, 2002b).

The dominant theoretical model postulating the emergence of compassion fatigue draws on a stress-process framework (Adams, et al., 2006; Figley, 2002a). Key elements within this model include empathic ability, empathic response, and residual compassion stress. The model is based on the assumption that empathy and emotional energy are the critical elements necessary for the formation of a therapeutic relationship and a therapeutic response. Although empathic ability has been defined as "the aptitude of the psychotherapist to notice the pain of others" (Figley, 2002a, p.1436), descriptions of these factors and of how each factor potentially interacts with another has been limited. The model is depicted as a series of cascading events beginning with exposure to a patient's pain, suffering, and/or traumatic event. Empathic concern and empathic ability on the part of care providers, such as nurses, produce an empathic response which may result in compassion stress (residue of emotional energy). The risk increases if the nurse experiences (a) ongoing exposure to suffering, (b) memories that elicit an emotional response, or (c) unexpected disruptions in her/his life. Limitations of this model include an emphasis on a linear direction, along with the binary dimension of compassion fatigue, i.e., you either have it or you don't. This binary dimension seems antithetical to human behavioral responses where individuals may express varying degrees of response. For example, an individual may not have compassion fatigue, yet may be slightly, moderately, or severely affected by a given interaction with a patient.

Figley (2002) also failed to clearly articulate the interaction(s) among the various influencing factors. The premise appears to be that if nurses care for patients who are suffering and/or traumatized, then they will inevitably experience compassion fatigue because of the use of empathy in their therapeutic or healing relationships. But not all authors view empathy in the same way. Some view empathy as the ability of an individual to enter into the world of others; to perceive other's feelings/emotions and meaning associated with an experience (Walker & Alligood, 2001); and to correctly convey that understanding back to the individual, who in turn acknowledges and understands the other's perceived understanding (La Monica, 1981). La Monica (1981) identified the nurse's ability to pick up on an individual's feelings/ emotions as 'helper perception,' 'helper communication,' and 'client perception' (2001). Empathy has also been conceptualized as (a) a human trait, innate rather than taught; (b) a professional state (learned communication skill comprised of behavioral and cognitive elements); (c) caring (an understanding and need to act because of that understanding); and (d) a special relationship (reciprocity) (Kunyk & Olson, 2000). Figley's (2002) model fails to clearly articulate the conceptualization of empathy on which his model is based, making it difficult to determine if one conceptualization may be antithetical to, or have more relevance than another in an understanding of compassion fatigue.

Another limitation of Figley's (2002) model lies in its failure to address the ability 'to get off the run-away train' or to halt compassion fatigue's progress. It also fails to adequately account for the benefits that nurses may derive from their relationships with patients or for how the therapeutic relationship may potentially serve to protect the nurse from experiencing compassion fatigue (Sabo, 2009, 2010). If the relationship is an empathic one, then it seems contradictory to suggest that empathy would lead to adverse effects. Rather, the contrary seems a more likely outcome; that is, when empathy is present the relationship would be more fulfilling.

Given the lack of consideration regarding the benefits derived from the relationship, other factors may need to be explored beyond empathy. These factors may include resilience and hope, which may thwart the development of compassion fatigue allowing the nurse to experience positive effects from caring work. For example, hope may influence actions that individuals take, as well as foster and support relationships (Simpson, 2004). Building on this idea, a shared meaning of hope between nurse and patient may not only enhance the quality of the relationship but also satisfaction with the caring work. Resilience, defined as the capacity to move forward in a positive way from negative, traumatic, or stressful experiences (Walsh, 2006), has been shown to enhance relationships, facilitate emotional insight, and decrease vulnerability to adverse effects from the work environment (Jackson, Firtko, & Edenborough, 2007). Research into the role of personal characteristics, such as resilience and hope, as well as the nature of the relationship among families, patients, and nurses, and also the fit within Figley's (2002) model of compassion fatigue, may help to add clarity and depth to a one-dimensional model.

In contrast to Figley's (2002) explanatory model of compassion fatigue, Valent (2002) has hypothesized that compassion fatigue may emerge as the result of unsuccessful or maladaptive survival strategies. In particular, he attributed the development of compassion fatigue to the "unsuccessful, maladaptive psychological and social stress responses of Rescue-Caretaking. [The responses] are a sense of burden, depletion and self-concern; and resentment, neglect and rejection, respectively" (Valent, 2002, p.26) rather than as resulting from empathy. The description by Valent is somewhat reminiscent of an early label, 'savior syndrome,' used to describe the effect of the needs of nurses in providing care and also their affect responses (NiCathy, Merriam, & Coffman, 1984). Rather than nurses depicted as exemplary and selfless caregivers, they may be perceived as self-absorbed, using the therapeutic relationship for their own needs, instead of facilitating patients' ability to fulfill their own needs. Taking this perspective into consideration, it would appear that a different concept may be at work in influencing compassion fatigue, a concept separate from empathy.

In one study that focused on the prevalence and risk for compassion fatigue among 216 hospice nurses, Abendroth and Flannery (2006) found that survey respondents in the moderate to high-risk category for compassion fatigue (N =170) had 'self-sacrificing behaviors' as the major contributing factor for risk. Approximately 34% (N=47) of the 170 nurses who exhibited this behavior were in the high-risk category for compassion fatigue. This group of nurses cared more for their patients than for themselves; their experiences increased life demands, post-traumatic stress, and a lack of emotional support within the work environment. While the findings supported the notion that hospice care nursing was stressful, what remained unclear was the nature of the relationship among nurses, patients, and families and the role of relationships in either increasing or decreasing the risk for compassion fatigue. Additionally, individual characteristics (such as resilience) and organizational factors (such as management support, workload, values, and beliefs) were not considered. Research is needed to fully explore the role of self-sacrificing behavior as a contributing factor for increased risk of compassion fatigue, as well as the role of individual characteristics and organizational factors. To date, there have been few, if any studies exploring self-sacrificing behavior and the possible effects it may have on the psychosocial health of nurses. Further, there is a need to understand what effect self-sacrificing behavior may have on the ability of nurses' skills, such as empathy and health-promoting personality traits, to self-select high demand areas, such as oncology, critical care, or mental health.

Exposure to traumatic stressors does not guarantee that an individual will manifest symptoms of compassion fatigue (Valent, 2002). Nor does targeting the negative aspects and/or symptoms provide answers to what, why, and how it is that some healthcare providers achieve satisfaction/rewards from the very same work that contributes to compassion fatigue in others (Abendroth & Flannery, 2006; Sabo, 2010). In light of this fact, more energy should be focused on exploring both the nature and roles of the relationship (nurse-patient-family) and empathy versus other related concepts, including the savior syndrome and engagement, in the psychosocial health and well-being of nurses, and whether the risk changes for nurses working in different specialties.

To date, much of the research has been quantitative in nature. A variety of instruments exist to assess for the presence of secondary traumatic stress, including the Professional Quality of Life Scale-R-IV (Stamm, 2009), the Secondary Trauma Scale (Motta, Kefer, Hertz, & Hafeez, 1999), and the Secondary Traumatic Stress Scale (Bride, Robinson, Yegidis, & Figley, 2004).

While the use of instruments is helpful to highlight the incidence and prevalence of various types of occupational stress and to develop models highlighting influencing factors, it is also limiting. For example, nurses may respond to questions on one of several instruments used to indicate the presence or absence of occupational stress, yet the responses do little to explain how nurses perceive the nature of their work and what factors affect compassion fatigue or other types of occupational stress. The use of qualitative study designs may enhance an understanding of whether empathy and engagement have a role in the development of occupational stress or, perhaps more importantly, whether they serve as protective mechanisms against occupational stress by affording nurses the opportunity to share their stories and experiences in a way that goes beyond the objective and quantifiable (Sabo, 2010).

Vicarious Traumatization

Evidence within trauma research has supported the notion that psychological distress affects more than just those who have been personally traumatized (Collins & Long, 2003; Figley, 1999; Pearlman & Saakvitne, 1995a). The psychological distress experienced by healthcare professionals in their work with patients who are suffering or who have been traumatized has been labelled vicarious traumatization (Pearlman & Macian, 1995). Defined as the "[negative] transformation in the therapist's (or other trauma worker's) inner experience resulting from empathic engagement with clients' trauma material" (Pearlmann & Saakvitne, 1995b. p.151), vicarious traumatization results in the permanent disruption of the individual's cognitive schema. Researchers have suggested that ongoing exposure to graphic accounts of human cruelty, trauma, and suffering, as well as the healing work within the therapeutic relationship that is facilitated through 'empathic openness' (as is the case in compassion fatigue), may leave healthcare providers, including nurses, vulnerable to emotional and spiritual consequences (Dunkley & Whelan, 2006).

Additional factors beyond empathy have been identified as contributing to the development of vicarious traumatization. One factor considers the characteristics of healthcare professionals, including their previous personal history of abuse and/or personal life stressors, personal expectations, need to fulfill all patient needs, and inadequate training/inexperience. Another factor involves the characteristics of the treatment, such as invasiveness, life-threatening nature, and long-term effects, as well as its context, such as the type of patient and the political, social, and cultural context within which the treatment occurred and the traumatic event took place (Pearlman & Macian, 1995; Pearlman & Saakvitne, 1995b). For example, ongoing advances in medical technology are now able to keep patients alive for longer periods of time, yet the eventual outcome is not altered. By this I mean that the patient still succumbs to the disease or injury; death has only been delayed. When a healthcare system places greater value on curative intent than on supportive care, situations, such as futility of care, may occur. For nurses involved in providing such futile care, the lasting imprint may be vicarious traumatization.

McCann and Pearlman (1990), and later Pearlman and Saakvitne (1995), used constructivist self-development theory (CSDT) to explain the "progressive development of a sense of self and world view in response to life experiences" (Pearlman & Saakvitne, 1995b, p.151). In other words, one's unique history of life experiences shapes how one will experience, interpret, and adapt to traumatic or highly stressful events. This CSDT interactive model attempts to take into account the variability of life experiences, suggesting that vicarious traumatization is unique to the individual (McCann & Pearlman, 1990; Pearlman & Saakvitne, 1995b). For example, if the nurse grew up in a home environment where one coped by dealing with stressful situations through escape/avoidance behaviour (a negative coping strategy), one would likely employ the same coping strategy in other stressful situations, such as that of witnessing ongoing patient suffering. If negative coping strategies are coupled with other contributing factors, for example lack of emotional support and/or unrealistic expectations of self in one's role as care provider, the risk for vicarious traumatization may be increased (Saakvitne, Tennen, & Affleck, 1998).

This theory argues that exposure to trauma, whether direct or indirect, disrupts one's frame of reference in one of five core areas of need, namely safety, trust, esteem, control, and intimacy (McCann & Pearlman, 1990). For example, disruption may occur whether the nurse witnesses the devastation of war firsthand while serving in a MASH unit in Afghanistan or whether the nurse listens to her/his patient's eyewitness accounts of the devastation of war while providing care in a healthcare facility. As a result of either exposure the nurse may experience the following: (a) difficulty establishing and maintaining relationships with others; (b) loss of independence; (c) inability to tolerate extreme emotional responses to stressful situations; (d) intrusive memories of the traumatic experience (similar to post traumatic stress); and/or (e) an altered belief system.

CSDT emphasizes the importance of the individual's ability to connect with others, perceive the self as competent, cope effectively with stress over time, and interpret experiences in a meaningful way that allows the individual to draw on previous experience to manage new experiences successfully (McCann & Pearlman, 1990; Pearlman & Saakvitne, 1995b). Memory plays an important role in the development of vicarious traumatization by serving as a mental recording of life experiences and its interpretations. For example, healthcare providers may assimilate/integrate the patient's experiences of trauma and suffering as their own which, in turn, reshapes the provider's beliefs and values of self and of the world (McCann & Pearlman, 1990).

Although there is increasing evidence to support CSDT as an explanatory model for vicarious traumatization, more research is needed to demonstrate how, and in what way, the therapeutic relationship, individual core beliefs, and exposure to pain, suffering, and trauma may affect the psychosocial health and well-being of healthcare professionals working in high-demand, intense, complex environments. Limitations of this theory include an inability to recognize the positive effects of trauma work and distinguish between awareness and disturbances in cognitive schemas (Dunkley & Whelan, 2006). For example, a disturbance in cognitive schema (beliefs) may occur when a hematological cancer nurse finds her/himself believing that all patients with hematological cancer die. Alternatively, heightened awareness occurs when an experienced hematological cancer nurse recognizes certain cues triggering the belief that a particular patient will do poorly but not that all patients will do poorly. Changes in cognitive schema may interfere with the development of empathy leading to vicarious traumatization rather than empathy leading to vicarious traumatization.

It should be noted that not every individual who works with those who have been traumatized will develop vicarious traumatization. If, as researchers have suggested, empathy and engagement, as fundamental elements of the therapeutic relationship, are key factors in increasing the risk for vicarious traumatization, then one would expect to see large numbers of healthcare providers negatively affected as a result of their work. However, studies have suggested that only a small percentage of individuals will manifest symptoms consistent with vicarious traumatization (Hafkenscheid, 2005), far fewer individuals than what McCann and Pearlmann (1990) had hypothesized. What is still missing is a clearly articulated theoretical framework and evidence demonstrating a cause-effect relationship between adverse effects and empathy. Future research is needed to identify which characteristics or qualities of working with suffering/traumatized patients might protect the healthcare professional and/or decrease the risk for adverse effects such as vicarious traumatisation.

Relationship Between Compassion Fatigue and a Continuum of Occupational Stress

What becomes apparent in reviewing the literature on possible adverse effects of providing care is the level of complexity underlying the various types of occupational stress. This may be due, in part, to the relatively preliminary understanding of compassion fatigue and vicarious traumatisation, concepts that began to emerge only in the early 1990's. To date, a lack of empirical evidence exists to support a theoretical framework for these two types of occupational stress (Bride, et al., 2004; Jenkins & Baird, 2002; Sabin-Farrell & Turpin, 2003; Thomas & Wilson, 2004). In contrast, research exploring burnout has consistently supported the existence of a multidimensional model comprised of three critical elements: emotional exhaustion, depersonalization, and reduced personal accomplishment (Demerouti, Bakker, Vardakou, & Kantas, 2003; Kalliath, O'Driscoll, Gillespie, & Bluedorn, 2000; Kitaoka-Higashiguchi, et al., 2004; Langballe, Falkum, Innstrand, & Aasland, 2006; Maslach, et al., 2001; Roelofs, Verbraak, Keijsers, de bruin, & Schmidt, 2005). These elements, however, are no longer considered to be specific to provider-recipient interactions. Rather, burnout can occur in the absence of such interactions. Hence it would not appear unreasonable to suggest that burnout may be a pre-condition for the other types of occupational stress, namely compassion fatigue and vicarious traumatisation, by creating the fertile ground for these types of stress to develop.

While all three types of occupational stress share aspects of the therapeutic relationship (empathy and engagement) as influencing factors, researchers exploring factors associated with the onset of burnout have shifted their emphasis to work-life issues, such as lack of resources, leadership, and shared values (Leiter & Laschinger, 2006). Research has yet to provide clarity and understanding as to whether empathy and engagement have a role in contributing to or protecting the nurse from compassion fatigue and vicarious traumatisation. Further research may be helpful in explaining whether and how factors, such as (a) duration of the relationship; (b) level of experience; and (c) individual characteristics of the nurse (e.g., 'savior syndrome'); as well as (d) patient characteristics, increase risk for compassion fatigue and vicarious traumatization.

Factors within the work environment, such as workload and limited resources, have all been identified as influencing the potential risk of developing occupational stress. Differences appear to lie in the nature of the work. Individuals experiencing compassion fatigue and vicarious traumatization appear to work with high demand populations, such as paediatric oncology (Maytum, et al., 2004; Papadatou, Martinson, & Chung, 2001), critical care (Mobley, Rady, Verheiide, Patel, & Larson, 2007), mental health (Collins & Long, 2003) or those experiencing pain/suffering or trauma (Figley, 1995; Pearlman & Macian, 1995). In contrast, research on burnout has extended beyond the healthcare environment to include all work environments regardless of whether people-work is fundamental to the job (Maslach & Leiter, 1997) suggesting that the relationship is not central to the development of occupational stress. At this point in time, it is unclear whether or not burnout is a precondition for compassion fatigue. It is also worth noting that a clear distinction between compassion fatigue and vicarious traumatization lies in the permanency of change to the individual. Individuals experiencing vicarious traumatization have their cognitive schema permanently altered. In contrast, compassion fatigue is amenable to treatment intervention and individuals may continue to work successfully in their chosen field. With this in mind, it would seem plausible to suggest that compassion fatigue precedes vicarious traumatization if one chooses to envision a stress continuum.

Relationships Between Types of Occupational Stress

As of this writing there is no research to support a claim that any or all of these types of occupational stress are concept redundant or interrelated. Sufficient evidence exists to demonstrate the validity of each as a distinct concept. What is not known is the role each may play in the development of the other. In reflecting on the current theoretical conceptualizations for burnout, compassion fatigue, and vicarious traumatization, one can raise the following questions:

1. Does compassion fatigue exist on a continuum of occupational stress? If so, is burnout a precondition for compassion fatigue?
2. What are the relationships between the types of occupational stress? To what extent does non-resolution of compassion fatigue increase the risk for developing vicarious traumatization?

Let's consider the above questions within the context of the following scenarios.

Scenario One

You have been working on a medical/surgical unit for three years. Since you started working on this floor the unit has experienced numerous changes as a result of fiscal restructuring. The dedicated Clinical Nurse Educator and Charge Nurse positions have been eliminated and all nurses on the floor rotate through the latter position for six-month periods of time. Further, you no longer have a nurse as manager for your unit. Instead, several units have been consolidated under one manager who has had no prior experience in the acute care setting and who does not hold a professional degree in a health-related discipline. Rather, the manager holds a Master's in Business Administration degree. Over the past 10 months the nurses have had their workload doubled, found themselves working more overtime shifts, and seen the complexity of patients increase. Nurses rarely hear they have done a good job. Nor do they have appreciable input in the ongoing changes. They are feeling increasingly disenfranchised and stressed. Sick time has increased, more nurses are leaving, and the unit has had difficulty recruiting new nurses to the unit because of increasing interpersonal conflicts. The most likely outcome in this scenario is burnout if the situation is not resolved. Emphasis here would appear to be an apparent disconnect between job demand and available resources.

Scenario Two

Scenario one is allowed to continue without remediation. Over the next year the complexity of patients increases and favourable prognoses decline. There have been several difficult deaths in recent weeks, particularly among younger patients. With little time to connect with families in crisis because of time and resource issues, the nurses are finding it increasingly difficult to continue working on the unit. The level of emotional distress has increased. Nurses who had been friendly and outgoing are now more reserved and withdrawn. Some nurses have identified feeling guilty over poor patient outcomes while others have begun to perceive that all patients with a specific diagnosis will die. Management perceives the problem to be related to burnout. Strategies to address the problem have proven unsuccessful. Is this a situation of burnout or compassion fatigue? At what point does occupational stress stop being burnout and become compassion fatigue?

In this scenario, the nurses would appear to be experiencing compassion fatigue. In burnout, emotional exhaustion is considered a cornerstone element along with cynicism and decreased personal accomplishment. In contrast, nurses experiencing compassion fatigue exhibit an intensified level of emotional distress leading to interpersonal withdrawal and changes in their beliefs, expectations, and assumptions. Furthermore, the nurses experience 'witness guilt,' taking personal blame for their inability to resolve a situation, such as easing the pain and suffering of a patient. Although some signs and symptoms may overlap across all three types of occupational stress (See Table), the level of intensity as well as additional symptoms can be helpful in differentiating between types of occupational stress. It may well be that initially the lines are blurred between burnout and compassion fatigue because of overlap in the signs of both burnout and compassion fatigue. Yet as the situation continues to deteriorate, more signs of compassion fatigue may appear.

As a reader you may have recognized that some signs or characteristic of depression are present in compassion fatigue. In a recently completed study conducted by myself and colleagues (unpublished as of this writing) the researchers did observe a statistically significant correlation between the presence of clinical depression and compassion fatigue among caregivers of hematological stem cell transplant recipients. Hence there is evidence for some overlap between compassion fatigue and depression.

Scenario Three

A nurse working on the unit described in scenarios one and two makes the decision to change practice areas and shifts to working in a community health clinic in the belief that a change of work environment will support the return of physical, psychological, and emotional well-being. The community health clinic provides health services for a local shelter for abused women and children. Initially the nurse notes an improvement in overall health and well-being; however, this improvement is not sustained. During the course of working with clients accessing the clinic, the nurse hears ongoing stories of abuse. Over a period of time the nurse begins to experience intrusive images of clients' stories of abuse. As time continues, the nurse's relationship with her spouse deteriorates. A once loving, intimate relationship no longer exists. Touch, in particular evokes hostility. On occasion, the nurse has noted feelings of panic when in the presence of unknown males (e.g., while waiting for the bus). Further, the nurse's sense of trust in the compassion and caring of others has changed. Trust is no longer present. What is happening here? Is this vicarious traumatization? Can this occur without the presence of burnout or compassion fatigue?

In this situation, it is likely the nurse is experiencing symptoms associated with vicarious traumatization. The symptoms of intrusive imagery; changes in values, beliefs, and assumptions (cognitive shift); anxiety; and loss of trust form hallmark signs of vicarious traumatization. While it is possible that each form of stress may create the stage for the next to occur, behaviour and experience is not linear. Nor is the continuum on which burnout, compassion fatigue, and vicarious traumatization may exist. Rather, individuals may move back and forth, at times experiencing symptoms of all three. We do not currently have evidence to support a continuum of occupational stress ranging from burnout to compassion fatigue to vicarious traumatization. Nor can we say that one person, at a given time, can be described as being at only one point on the continuum. The nurse in scenario three could have come from a healthy work environment and yet still experience vicarious traumatization. It is also reasonable to assume that burnout can exist concurrently with either compassion fatigue or vicarious traumatization. What and how each form of occupational stress influences the other requires further research.

Conclusion

Research clearly demonstrates that working with patients who are in pain, suffering, or at end of life may take a toll on the psychosocial health and well being of nurses. Over the past ten years compassion fatigue has received considerable attention as a potential form of occupational stress experienced by nurses. At the same time, the lack of theoretical clarity underlying compassion fatigue has led to a number of questions ranging from the role of empathy and empathic response in the development of compassion fatigue to the possibility of a continuum of stress. More research is needed to articulate clearly not only what factors may mitigate and/or mediate the onset of compassion fatigue but also to clarify its theoretical underpinnings if we hope to develop and implement sustainable interventions to support positive psychosocial health and well being among all nurses caring for patients who are in pain, suffering, or at the end of life.

Burnout	Compassion Fatigue	Vicarious Traumatization
Hallmark Signs • Anger & frustration • Fatigue • Negative reactions towards others • Cynicism • Negativity • Withdrawal	**Hallmark Signs** • Sadness & grief • Nightmares • Avoidance • Addiction • Somatic complaints • Increased psychological arousal • Changes in beliefs, expectations, assumptions • 'witness guilt' • Detachment • Decreased intimacy	**Hallmark Signs** • Anxiety, sadness, confusion, apathy • Intrusive imagery • Somatic complaints • Loss of control, trust & independence • Decreased capacity for intimacy • Relational disturbances (crossover to personal life)
Symptoms • Physical • Psychological • Cognitive • Relational disturbances	**Symptoms (mirror PTSD)** • Physical • Psychological distress • Cognitive shifts • Relational disturbances	**Symptoms (mirror PTSD)** • Physical • Psychological distress • Cognitive shifts • Relational disturbances • Permanent alteration in individual's cognitive schema
Key Triggers • Personal characteristics • Work-related attributes • Work/ organizational characteristics	**Key Triggers** • Personal characteristics • Previous exposure to trauma • Empathy & emotional energy • Prolonged exposure to trauma material of clients • Response to stressor • Work environment • Work-related attributes	**Key Triggers** • Personal characteristics • Previous exposure to trauma • Type of therapy • Organizational context • Healthcare structure • Resources • Re-enactment

References

Abendroth, M., & Flannery, J. (2006). Predicting the risk of compassion fatigue: A study of hospice nurses. *Journal of Hospice and Palliative Nursing, 8*(6), 346–356.

Adams, R., Boscarino, J., & Figley, C. (2006). Compassion fatigue and psychological distress among social workers: A validation study. *American Journal of Orthopsychiatry, 76*(1), 103–108.

Bakker, A., Le Blanc, P., & Schaufeli, W. (2005). Burnout contagion among intensive care nurses. *Journal of Advanced Nursing, 51*(3), 276–287.

Bakker, D., Fitch, M., Green, E., Butler, L., & Olsen, K. (2006). Oncology nursing: Finding the balance in a changing health care system. *Canadian Oncology Nursing Journal, 16*(2), 79–98.

Blomberg, K., & Sahlberg-Blom, E. (2007). Closeness and distance: A way of handling difficult situations in daily care. *Journal of Clinical Nursing, 16*, 244–254.

Bride, B. E., Robinson, M. M., Yegidis, B., & Figley, C. (2004). Development and validation of the secondary traumatic stress scale. *Research on Social Work Practice, 14*(1), 27–35.

Collins, S., & Long, A. (2003). Too tired to care? The psychological effects of working with trauma. *Journal of Psychiatric and Mental Health Nursing, 10,* 17–27.

Demerouti, E., Bakker, A., Vardakou, I., & Kantas, A. (2003). The convergent validity of two burnout instruments: A multitrait-multimethod analysis *European Journal of Psychological Assessment* 19(1), 12–23.

Dunkley, J., & Whelan, T. (2006). Vicarious traumatization: Current status and future directions. *British Journal of Guidance & Counselling, 34*(1), 107–116.

Edwards, D., & Burnard, P. (2003). A systematic review of stress and stress management interventions for mental health nurses. *Journal of Advanced Nursing, 42*(2), 169–200.

Ekedahl, M., & Wengstrom, Y. (2007). Nurses in cancer care-stress when encountering existential issues. *European Journal of Oncology Nursing, 11,* 228–237.

Figley, C. (1995). *Compassion fatigue: Coping with secondary traumatic stress disorder in those who treat the traumatized.* New York, NY: Brunner-Routledge.

Figley, C. (1999). Compassion fatigue: Toward a new understanding of the costs of caring. In B. H. Stamm (Ed.), *Secondary traumatic stress: Self care issues for clinicians, researchers and educators* (2 ed., pp. 3–28). Lutherville: Sidran.

Figley, C. (2002a). Compassion fatigue: Psychotherapists' chronic lack of self care. *Psychotherapy in Practice, 58* (11), 1433–1441.

Figley, C. (2002b). *Treating compassion fatigue.* New York, NY: Brunner-Routledge.

Goldberg, L. (1990). An alternative "Description of personality": The Big-Five factor structure. *Journal of Personality and Social Psychology, 59,* 1216–1229.

Hafkenscheid, A. (2005). Event countertransference and vicarious traumatization: Theoretically valid and clinically useful concepts? *European Journal of Psychotherapy, Counselling and Health, 7*(3), 159–168.

Hertting, A. (2003). *The healthcare sector: A challenging or draining work environment. Psychosocial work experiences and health among hospital employees during the Swedish 1990's.* PhD, Karolinska Institutet, Stockholm.

Hertting, A., Nilsson, K., Theorell, T., & Larsson, U. (2004). Downsizing and reorganization: demands, challenges and ambiguity for registered nurses. *Journal of Advanced Nursing, 45*(2), 145–154.

Jackson, D., Firtko, A., & Edenborough, M. (2007). Personal resilience as a strategy for surviving and thriving in the face of workplace adversity: A literature review. *Journal of Advanced Nursing, 60*(1), 1–9.

Jenkins, R., & Elliott, P. (2004). Stressors, burnout and social support: Nurses in acute mental health settings. *Journal of Advanced Nursing, 48(6),* 622–631.

Jenkins, S. R., & Baird, S. (2002). Secondary traumatic stress and vicarious traumatization: a validational study. *Journal of Traumatic Stress, 15*(5), 423–432.

Joinson, C. (1992). Coping with compassion fatigue. *Nursing, 22*(4), 116–122.

Kalliath, T., O'Driscoll, M., Gillespie, D., & Bluedorn, A. (2000). A test of the Maslach Burnout Inventory in three samples of healthcare professionals. *Work & Stress, 14*(1), 35–50.

Kitaoka-Higashiguchi, K., Nakagawa, H., Ishizaki, M., Miura, K., Naruse, Y., Kida, T., et al. (2004). Construct validity of the Maslach Burnout Inventory-General Survey. *Stress & Health, 20,* 255–260.

Kunyk, D., & Olson, J. (2000). Clarification of conceptualizations of empathy. *Journal of Advanced Nursing, 35*(3), 317–325.

La Monica, E. (1981). Construct validity of an empathy instrument. *Research in Nursing and Health, 4,* 389–400.

Langballe, E., Falkum, E., Innstrand, S., & Aasland, 0. (2006). The factorial validity of the Maslach Burnout Inventory-General Survey in representative samples of eight different occupational groups. *Journal of Career Assessment, 14(3),* 370–384.

Laschinger, H., & Finegan, J. (2005). Empowering nurses for work engagement and health in hospital settings. *JONA, 35*(10), 439–449.

Lee, R. T., & Ashforth, B. E. (1996). A meta-analytic examination of the correlates of the three dimensions of burnout. *Journal of Applied Psychology, 81(2),* 123–133.

Leiter, M. (1993). Burnout as a developmental process: consideration of models. In W. Schaufeli, C. Maslach & T. Marek (Eds.), *Professional Burnout: Recent developments in theory and research* (pp. 237–250). London: Taylor & Francis.

Leiter, M. (2005). Perception of risk: An organizational model of occupational risk, burnout, and physical symptoms. *Anxiety, Stress and Coping, 18(2),* 131–144.

Leiter, M., & Laschinger, H. (2006). Relationships of work and practice environment to professional burnout: testing a causal model. *Nursing Research, 55*(2), 137–146.

Leiter, M., & Maslach, C. (2004). Areas of worklife: A structural approach to organizational predictors of job burnout. In P. Perrewe & D. Ganster (Eds.), *Research in occupational stress and well being: Vol 3. Emotional and physiological processes and positive intervention strategies* (pp. 91–134). Oxford: JAI Press/Elsevier.

Leiters, M., & Schaufeli, W. (1996). Consistency of the burnout construct across occupations. *Anxiety, Stress and Coping, 9,* 229–243.

Maslach, C., & Jackson, S. (1986). *Maslach Burnout Inventory Manual* (2 ed.). Palo Alto: Consulting Psychologists Press.

Maslach, C., & Leiter, M. (1997). *The Truth About Burnout: How organizations cause personal stress and what to do about it.* San Francisco, CA: Jossey-Boss.

Maslach, C., Schaufeli, W., & Leiter, M. (2001). Job burnout. *Annual Reviews in Psychology, 52,* 397–422.

Maytum, J., Bielski-Heiman, M., & Garwick, A. (2004). Compassion fatigue and burnout in nurses who work with children with chronic conditions and their families. *Journal of Pediatric Health Care, 18,* 171–179.

McCann, L., & Pearlman, L. (1990). Vicarious traumatization: A framework for understanding the psychological effects of working with victims. *Journal of Traumatic Stress, 3*(1), 131–149.

Mobley, M., Rady, M., Verheiide, J., Patel, B., & Larson, J. (2007). The relationship between moral distress and perceptions of futile care in a critical care unit *Intensive and Critical Care Nursing, 23,* 256–263.

Motta, R. W., Kefer, J. M., Hertz, M. D., & Hafeez, S. (1999). Initial evaluation of the Secondary Trauma Questionnaire. *Psychological Reports, 85,* 997–1002.

NiCathy, G., Merriam, K., & Coffman, S. (1984). *Talking it out: A guide to groups for abused women.* Seattle: Seal Press.

Papadatou, D., Martinson, I., & Chung, P. (2001). Caring for dying children: A comparative study of nurses' experience in Greece and Hong Kong. *Cancer Nursing,* 24(5), 402–412.

Pearlman, L. (1998). Trauma and the self: A theoretical and clinical perspective. *Journal of Emotional Abuse, 1,* 7–25.

Pearlman, L., & Macian, P. (1995). Vicarious traumatization: An empirical study of the effects of trauma work on trauma therapists. *Professional Psychology, Research and Practice,* 26(6), 558–565.

Pearlman, L., & Saakvitne, K. (1995a). *Trauma and the Therapist: Countertransference and vicarious traumatization in psychotherapy with incest survivors.* London: W.W. Norton.

Pearlman, L., & Saakvitne, K. (1995b). Treating therapists with vicarious traumatization and secondary traumatic stress disorders. In C. R. Figley (Ed.), *Compassion Fatigue: Coping with secondary traumatic stress disorder in those who treat the traumatized.* New York: Brunner-Routledge.

Roelofs, J., Verbraak, M., Keijsers, G., de bruin, M., & Schmidt, A. (2005). Psychometric properties of a Dutch version of the Maslach Burnout Inventory General survey (MBI-DV) in individuals with and without clinical burnout. *Stress & Health, 21,* 17–25.

Saakvitne, K., Tennen, H., & Affleck, G. (1998). Exploring thriving in the context of clinical trauma theory: constructivit self development theory. *Journal of Social Issues,* 54(2), 279–299.

Sabin-Farrell, R., & Turpin, G. (2003). Vicarious traumatization: Implications for the mental health of health workers? *clinical Psychology Review, 23,* 449–480.

Sabo, B. (2009). *Nursing from the heart: An exploration of caring work among hematology/blood and marrow transplant nurses in three Canadian tertiary care centres* PhD, Dalhousie University, Halifax.

Sabo, B. (2010). Compassionate presence: The meaning of hematopoietic stem cell transplant nursing. *European Journal of Oncology Nursing, doi:10.1016/j.ejon.2010.06.006.*

Sabo, B. M. (2006). Compassion fatigue and nursing work: Can we accurately capture the consequences of caring work? *International Journal of Nursing Practice, 12,* 136–142.

Schaufeli, W., & Enzmann, D. (1998). *The Burnout Companion to Study and Practice: A critical analysis.* London: Taylor & Francis.

Simpson, C. (2004). When hope makes us vulnerable: A discussion of patient-healthcare provider interactions in the context of hope. *Bioethics,* 18(5), 428–447.

Stamm, B. (2009). *The concise manual for the Professional Quality of Life Scale: The ProQOL.* Pocatello, ID: ProQOL.org.

Thomas, R., & Wilson, J. (2004). Issues and controversies in the understanding and diagnosis of compassion fatigue, vicarious traumatization and secondary traumatic stress disorder. *International Journal of Emergency Mental Health,* 6(2), 81–92.

Valent, P. (2002). Diagnosis and treatment of helper stresses, traumas, and illnesses. In C. Figley (Ed.), *Treating Compassion Fatigue* (pp. 17–37). New York: Brunner—Routledge.

Walker, K., & Alligood, M. (2001). Empathy from a nursing perspective: Moving beyond borrowed theory. *Archives of Psychiatric Nursing,* 15(3), 140–147.

Walsh, F. (2006). *Strengthening Family Resilience.* New York: Guilford Press.

Unit III

Moral Issues

Inventing Genetic Engineering

Hallam Stevens

Introduction: Brave New World

In 1932, the English writer Aldous Huxley (1894–1963) imagined a world in which human beings were manufactured rather than born. Huxley describes how "Podsnap's technique"—which speeds up the maturation of eggs within an ovary—is combined with "Bokanovsky's process"—that causes fertilized eggs to divide into identical copies—to produce large numbers of identical humans in a "Hatchery and Conditioning Centre." Of course, Huxley made up all of this. But it was not just wild speculation: Huxley was well versed in the latest biology of the 1930s. Aldous' brother Julian was a well-known evolutionary biologist who had taught at King's College London in the 1920s. Given Julian's enthusiasm for eugenics, it is likely that the brothers had discussed the biological possibilities of manipulating life through the application of chemicals, heat, hormones, and selective breeding.

Brave New World is most widely known as a satirical critique of totalitarian society. With the Soviet Union consolidating its power in the wake of the Russian Revolution and fascism on the rise in Italy and Germany, Huxley's book was a warning about where centralized planning of society and the economy could lead. In this *Brave New World*, planning and control extends even to reproduction. Huxley's vision shocks us because it depicts the government reaching even into the most intimate aspects of our lives. Humans have become automata, to be programmed and reprogrammed according to the needs of those in charge. But they have also become commodities, mass-produced in factories according to the principles of Fordist efficiency.

Genetic engineering still conjures up Huxley-inspired visions of mad scientists creating babies inside test tubes. It is variously understood as a triumph of biomedical progress, as a symbol of scientific hubris, and as scientists "playing God." As we try to understand the social, political, and economic significance of genetic engineering, it is worthwhile to keep Huxley's vision in mind. This scientific imaginary—in which manipulating life is associated with the totalitarian manipulation of society—influences the way society thinks about biotechnology and its consequences.

This [reading] provides a background for understanding the so-called revolution that took place in biology in the 1970s. The term *genetic engineering* is now often used in a loose way to refer to many techniques in biotechnology. But in the 1970s, genetic engineering came to be associated with a specific technique for making copies of DNA that was invented in 1972.[1] Why was this discovery so important?

Life as Code

The idea that life depends on molecules is relatively new. The sub-discipline of *molecular* biology coalesced only after World War II as biologists developed the tools to investigate life on the smallest scale. One of the factors that caused this development was the influx of physicists into biology right around this time. Physics had enjoyed enormous success by examining smaller and smaller bits of the world: atoms, electrons, protons, neutrons, and photons. Some physicists imagined they would have equal success by applying the same techniques to biology—that is, by trying to understand the very smallest constituents of a system.

An influential figure in this respect was Erwin Schrödinger. In 1925, Schrödinger had played a major role in the formulation of quantum mechanics, the key theory that underpinned physicists' understanding of matter on the subatomic level. In 1944, Schrödinger wrote a short book called *What is Life?* based on some lectures he had given the previous year in Dublin. His premise—provocative to physicists and biologists of the 1940s—was that life should be understood at the level of physics and chemistry. Schrödinger speculated on ways in which similarities between parents and offspring (heredity) could be explained in molecular terms:

> It has often been asked how this tiny speck of material, nucleus of the fertilized egg, could contain an elaborate code-script involving all the future development of the organism ... For illustration, think of the Morse code. The two different signs of dot and dash in well-ordered groups of not more than four allow thirty different specifications. Now, if you allowed yourself the use of a third sign, in addition to dot and dash, and used groups of not more than ten, you could form 88,572 different "letters."[2]

Schrödinger was suggesting that the fertilized egg contained a set of molecular symbols, like Morse

---

1. . This technique is also known as *molecular cloning* since it is used to make many copies (clones) of a DNA molecule. This is not be confused with the popular use of *cloning*, which now usually refers to reproductive cloning or therapeutic cloning[...].
2. Erwin Schrödinger, *What Is Life?* (Cambridge: Cambridge University Press, 1967 [original publication 1944]). Quotation p. 61.

code, that could specify how to build an organism. Schrödinger didn't know about DNA so he just called this an "aperiodic crystal."

Schrödinger's book did not announce any new discoveries or new theories about biology. But it was important for a different reason. As other scientists began to do experiments on the molecules in cell nuclei (proteins, DNA, and RNA) they began to adopt Schrödinger's code-script idea. They began to talk about molecules containing codes and passing information from one to another. In 1953, James Watson and Francis Crick discovered the structure of DNA. This achievement was widely celebrated because the structure immediately suggested the means by which a molecule might carry a code (see figure 3.1.1 and box 1).

All this was happening at the same time that information and communication sciences were making their first appearance. The first electronic computers were developed during World War II and were soon being put to use in a range of scientific fields. The mathematician Claude Shannon published "A Mathematical Theory of Communication" in 1948, laying the groundwork for a new discipline called information theory.

Historians have documented how "information" and "code" came to be powerful metaphors in molecular biology in the 1950s and 1960s. Biologists thought of DNA as acting like a computer program: it contained a code that was read out by the machinery of the cell in order to build proteins. Of course, DNA was not literally a piece of software and the cell did not literally act like a computer. But the language of "codes" and "information" played a crucial role in shaping how biologists thought about molecules and organisms.

For one thing, the metaphor meant that the most urgent problem for molecular biology was "cracking the code"—that is, discovering exactly how DNA built the proteins that made up living things. A single strand of DNA comprises a chemical "backbone" plus a chain of "nucleotides" or "bases"—adenine (A), guanine (G), cytosine (C), and thymine (T). This is why a DNA molecule is often represented by just a string of letters: AAGGATGCC, for example. The nucleotides can be strung along the backbone in any order: thymine-thymine-cytosine (TTC); adenine-cytosine-guanine-guanine (ACGG); and so on (see box 1). Molecular biologists suspected that particular strings of As, Gs, Ts, and Cs made up a code that provided instructions for building a protein molecule. But how did this work? Between 1961 and 1965 the painstaking laboratory work of Marshall Nirenberg, Heinrich Matthaei, and Har Ghobind Khorana eventually solved this problem. This made it possible to read the "code of life" (see table 1). This only encouraged biologists to take their metaphors more seriously. If DNA was a code, then it also represented a kind of "text" and if it was a text then the whole collection of DNA was a "book of life." Some biologists even imagined DNA as a script or a language that had biblical resonances.

DNA Replication

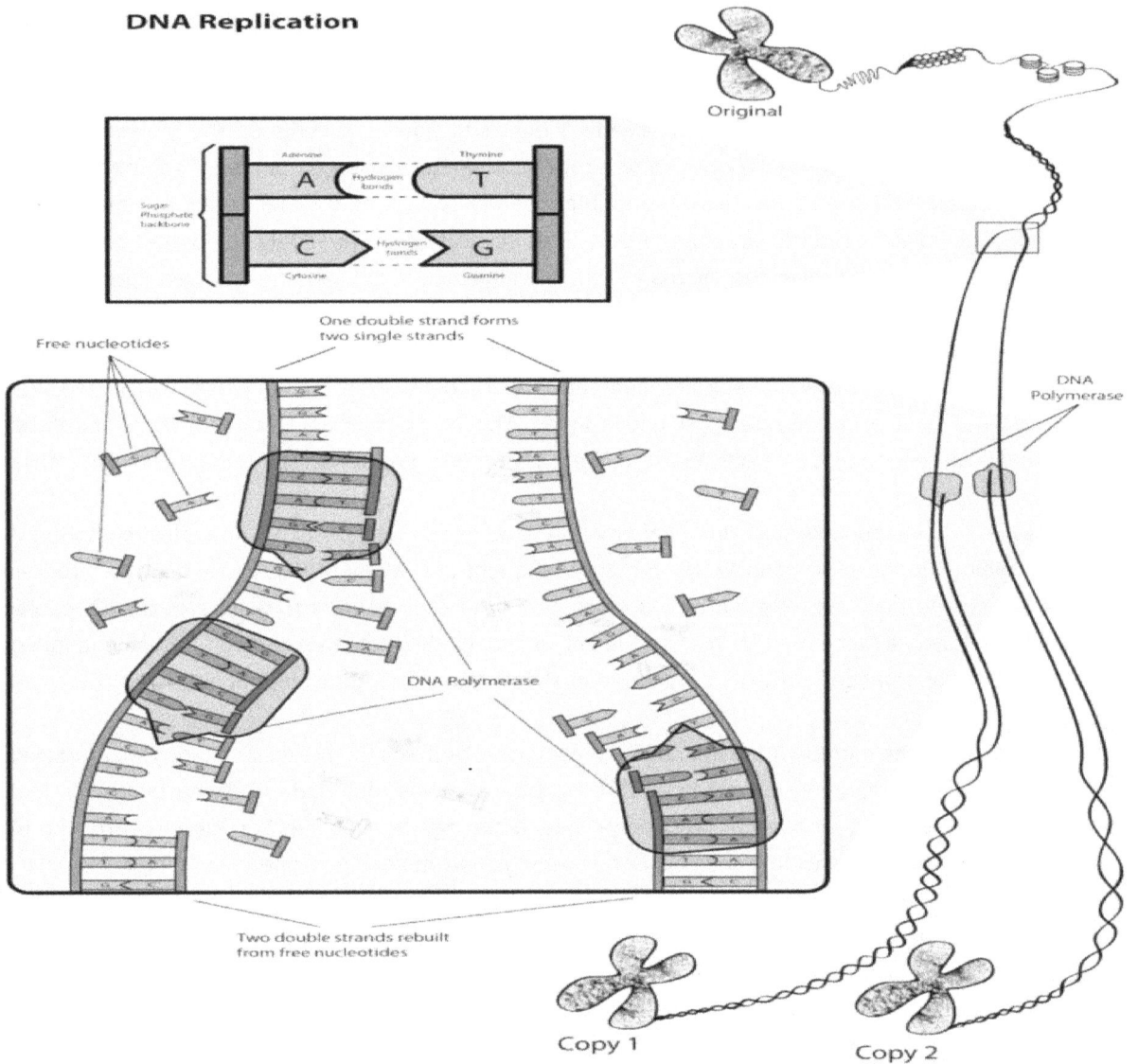

Figure 3.1.1   DNA replication. Refer to box 1. DNA is a complex double-stranded molecule twisted into a double helix shape. The order of the nucleotide bases forms a "code" that can be used to make proteins. The separation of the two strands allows each strand to be used as a template for copying the entire DNA molecule. Source: Illustration by Jerry Teo.

Box 3.1.1 A DNA Primer

Deoxyribonucleic acid is a very large molecule that consist of millions or even tens of millions of atoms (carbon, hydrogen, oxygen, nitrogen, and phosphorus). The molecule consists of two strands—the strands are each twirled into a helix and so the molecule overall is shaped like a double helix with the two strands twisting together in parallel.

Each strand has a "backbone" that is made of a kind of sugar (this is deoxyribose) and stretches along the entire length of the molecule. At regular intervals along the backbone, another kind of molecule (called *nucleotide* or *base*) is attached. These nucleotides can be one of four types: adenine, guanine, cytosine, and thymine (usually abbreviated A, G, C, and T). These are complex molecules in and of themselves, made up of one or two rings of carbon atoms. The nucleotides can be attached along the backbone in any order, forming a distinct pattern—AAGGATCCA, for instance. DNA molecules are very long, so in fact there can even be millions of nucleotides in a row.

This sequence of letters is referred to as the DNA sequence. Some parts of the DNA sequence are genes. This means that they can act as a template for building proteins. Within a gene, each triplet of nucleotides corresponds to an amino acid. For example, AAG corresponds to the amino acid called lysine; and GAT corresponds to aspartic acid (see table 3.1.1). When a gene is "expressed" this means that the DNA is being "read out" by the cellular machinery and made into a chain of amino acids. This chain of amino acids folds into a protein.

The nucleotides from each strand are also arranged to stick out towards each other so that they almost touch in the middle. If we were to flatten the double helix out onto a two-dimensional surface, it would look something like a ladder, with each rung made up of two nucleotides, one from each strand. But only specific combinations of nucleotides will join together to form rungs. As will only join with Ts and Gs will only join with Cs. So if the nucleotides on one strand are AAGGATCCA (from bottom to top), then the nucleotides on the other strand must be TTCCTGGT. If the nucleotides don't match up in this way, the rungs will not join and the two strands will split apart.

This double-strand system provides the means of copying DNA molecules. When DNA is to be copied inside the cell, the two strands are pulled apart and separated by a special enzyme. Since the nucleotides on one strand must match the nucleotides on the other (A with T and G with C), it is possible to rebuild two double strands from two single strands (figure 1). This is the job of a molecule called DNA polymerase. DNA polymerase moves along each single strand and rebuilds a double strand: where it senses an A on one strand, it places a matching T on the other strand; where it senses a G, it builds a C, etc. Eventually two complete and identical DNA strands can be reconstructed.

Table 3.1.1 The Genetic Code

	Second Nucleotide					
	T	C	A	G		

Table 3.1.1 The Genetic Code

First Nucleotide						Third Nucleotide
T	TTT—Phe TTC—Phe TTA—Leu TTG—Leu	TCT—Ser TCC—Ser TCA—Ser TCG—Ser	TAT—Tyr TAC—Tyr TAA-STOP TAG—STOP	TGT—Cys TGC—Cys TGA—STOP TGG—Trp	T C A G	
C	CTT—Leu CTC—Leu CTA—Leu CTG—Leu	CCT—Pro CCC—Pro CCA—Pro CCG—Pro	CAT—His CAC—His CAA—Gln CAG—Gln	CGT—Arg CGC—Arg CGA—Arg CGG—Arg	T C A G	
A	ATT—Ile ATC—Ile ATA—Ile ATG—Met	ACT—Thr ACC—Thr ACA—Thr ACG—Thr	AAT—Asn AAC—Asn AAA—Lys AAG—Lys	AGT—Ser AGC—Ser AGA—Arg AGG—Arg	T C A G	
G	GTT—Val GTC—Val GTA—Val GTG—Val	GCT—Ala GCC—Ala GCA—Ala GCG—Ala	GAT—Asp GAC—Asp GAA—Glu GAG—Glu	GGT—Gly GGC—Gly GGA—Gly GGG—Gly	T C A G	

3-letter code	Amino acid name
Ala	Alanine
Arg	Argenine
Asn	Aspargine
Asp	Aspartic acid
Cys	Cysteine
Gln	Glutamine
Glu	Glutamic Acid
Gly	Glycine

His	Histidine
Ile	Isoleucine
Leu	Leucine
Lys	Lysine
Met	Methionine
Phe	Phenylalanine
Pro	Proline
Ser	Serine
Thr	Threonine
Trp	Tryptophan
Tyr	Tyrosine
Val	Valine

Molecular biologists still describe biology in terms of information and codes. This is the way it is taught in classrooms and textbooks. It is hard to imagine it any other way. Can you describe the relationship between DNA and protein without using the words *code* or *information*? This suggests the deep influence this has had on our way of understanding life. But we should not make the mistake of thinking that code and information are the *only* way of describing genetics. After all, the As, Gs, Ts, and Cs are not like English or Japanese—they are not really a language. Nor are they really a code. Morse code, for instance, takes an alphabetic language and represents it as a series of dots and dashes. But the DNA code doesn't represent any other underlying language.

With enough thought it might be possible to imagine describing biology using different metaphors: templates or molecules acting as locks and keys, perhaps. In any case, it is important to remember that information and code are *metaphors* rather than literal descriptions of how biology works on a molecular level.

What is Genetic Engineering?

What does all this code talk have to do with genetic engineering? It is only really possible to understand why genetic engineering was considered to be so important if we understand that molecular biologists saw DNA as a piece of *text*. To be fluent in a language, you need not only to be able to *read* it, but also to be able to *write* it. By cracking the code molecular biologists had figured out how to read DNA, but they had not yet figured out how to write in this language, or even how to edit it. This is what genetic engineering is all about.

In 1972, Herbert Boyer was a thirty-six-year-old biochemist and molecular biologist working at the

University of California in San Francisco. Relaxed and gregarious, he usually wore jeans, running shoes, and a leather vest. He ran his lab in a casual style too, often gambling on new ideas that emerged from brainstorming sessions over a beer. Boyer's subject of research was restriction enzymes—special proteins that occur naturally within organisms and which are used to cut or cleave DNA at particular sites. These enzymes are designed to recognize specific sequences of DNA—AAGGAT, for instance—and make a cut only at this site (for instance, it could cut between the two Gs in this example).

Significantly, Boyer found that these molecular scissors did not make a straight cut across a double-stranded piece of DNA. Figure 3.1.2 shows how the restriction enzyme could cut at an angle across the double strand, leaving overhanging pieces of single-stranded DNA on both sides of the cut. These overhangs were called "sticky ends" since they could be used to re-stick pieces of DNA back together. In imagining how this works it is useful to think of a carpenter trying to join together two long pieces of wood end-to-end. Just sticking the pieces together would not make a very effective join (or it would require some very strong glue). A stronger join would be formed by removing half the thickness of each piece of wood and then overlapping them.[3]

---

3. In carpentry this is known as a half-lap joint. Just sticking the pieces end to end is known as a butt joint and is the weakest of all joints.

Recombinant DNA with Sticky Ends

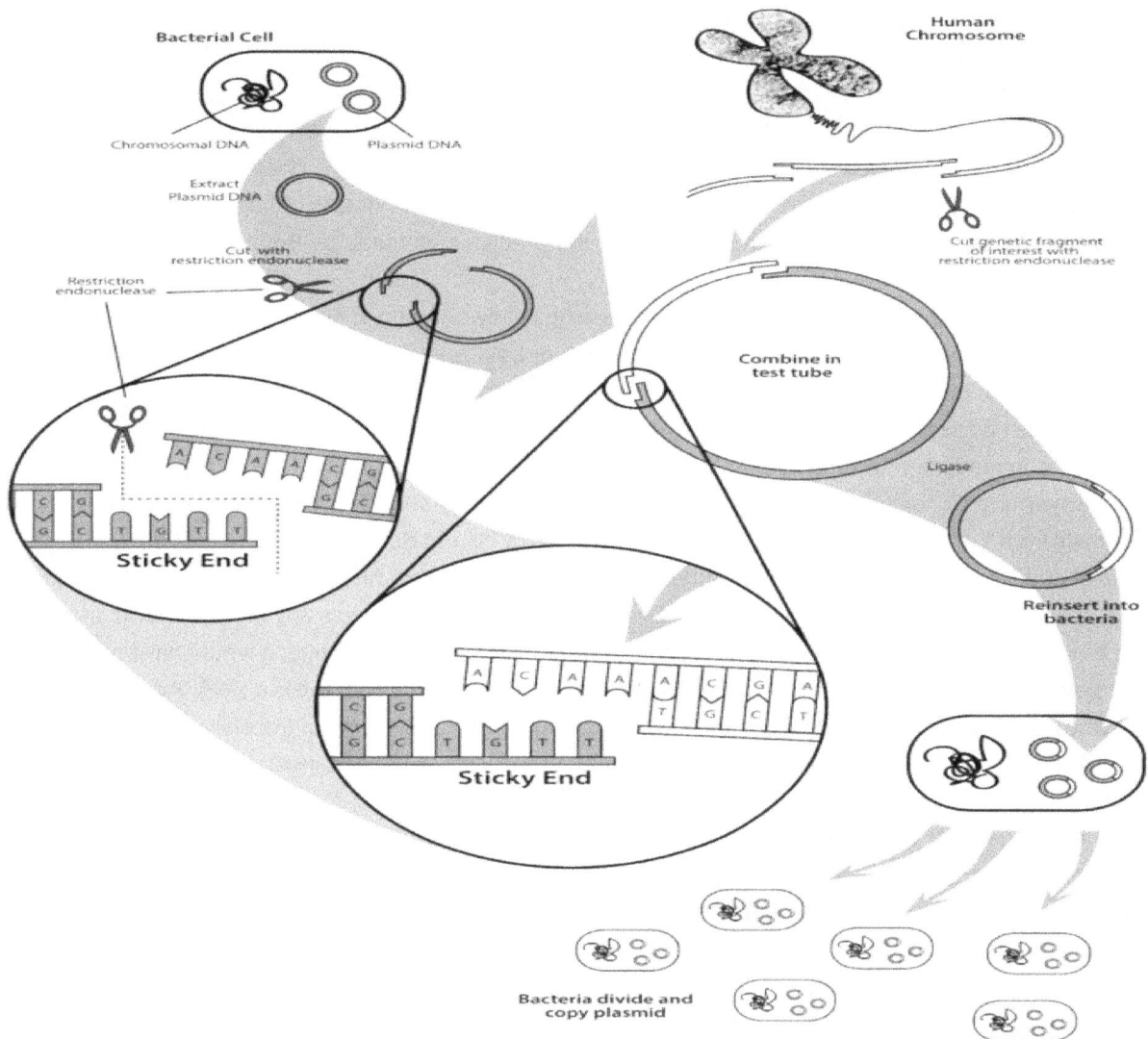

Figure 3.1.2 Recombinant DNA with sticky ends. A vector or plasmid ring is spliced open with restriction endonucleases to form an open ring. The donor DNA to be inserted into the ring is spliced with the same endonucleases. Mixing the open rings and the donor DNA and adding the enzyme ligase allows the rings to incorporate the foreign DNA. The now complete rings are reinserted into bacterial cells. The bacterial cells divide and copy, making millions of copies of the donor DNA. This DNA can then be extracted from the bacterial cells. The bacterial cells can also be used to make the protein associated with the donor DNA.

Illustration by Jerry Teo.

Stanley Cohen, a geneticist at nearby Stanford University, had little in common with Boyer. Although they were almost the same age, Cohen was meticulous, private, and circumspect. He was the consummate professor: beard, baldness, glasses, sports jacket, and serious demeanor. Cohen's interest too, was not particularly similar to Boyer's: he studied little rings of double-stranded DNA that existed inside bacteria. These plasmids, as they were called, were separate from the bacteria's main DNA chromosomes and seemed to provide the organisms resistance against antibiotics. Cohen wanted to understand how this worked. In order to study the plasmids effectively Cohen often needed to break the DNA up into small pieces. He could do this in a blender, but this left him with random fragments that were difficult to study. He wanted a more systematic approach.

In November 1972, Cohen planned a conference in Honolulu on the topic of plasmid research. Happening to have just heard about Boyer's work on restriction enzymes, Cohen invited him, almost as an afterthought. The two men had never met and knew nothing of the details of each other's work. But as Boyer presented his research, Cohen realized that the precise cuts made by Boyer's restriction enzymes were exactly what he needed.

A walk along the beach after the day's proceedings allowed them to share their ideas in more detail. The stroll ended up at a deli near Waikiki Beach and over beer and sandwiches Boyer and Cohen realized that—more than just solving Cohen's problems—they might have hit upon a way to copy or clone pieces of DNA. Not just bacterial plasmid DNA, but *any* piece of DNA. They became "jazzed" with the idea, as Boyer later put it, immediately sensing its possible importance.

Boyer and Cohen's insight can be explained in five steps (figure 3.1.1). First, you needed to remove plasmids from their bacterial cells. Cohen's lab already knew how to do this. Second, you could use Boyer's special cutting enzyme to cut open the rings at a specific point. This would leave open rings with sticky ends. Third, you could take another piece of DNA (this could be more or less any piece of DNA) and again cut it with Boyer's restriction enzyme. Because it was cut with the same enzyme, it would have sticky ends that paired with those in the rings. Fourth, mix the open-ring plasmids with the cut DNA. Adding a special enzyme called ligase (which promotes the joining of DNA) would cause some of the plasmids to incorporate the foreign DNA, re-forming a ring, but now including an extra piece. Fifth, reinsert these plasmids into the bacteria (again, Cohen's lab knew how to do this).

These bacteria containing the specially modified plasmids could then be grown in the lab. As they reproduced, not only would they copy their own DNA, but they would also make copies of the foreign DNA. One copy could be amplified into millions as the bacteria quickly divided.

At least, that was the plan. In Hawaii, Boyer and Cohen made an agreement to give the experiments a try. Beginning in January 1973, Cohen's lab isolated plasmids and Boyer's team began working with the enzymes. At first, the results were ambiguous, but by March it became clear that the "recombination" (between plasmid DNA and some foreign DNA) had worked. The plasmids had taken up the foreign DNA and copied it accurately. In just a couple of months—remarkably fast by the standard of most scientific work—they had succeeded in cloning DNA. Boyer was stunned:

> The [DNA] bands were lined up [on the gel] and you could just look at them and you knew ... [that DNA recombination and cloning] had been successful ... I was just ecstatic ... I remember going home and showing a photograph [of the gel] to my wife ... You know, I looked at that thing until early in the morning ... When I saw it ... I knew that you could do just about anything ... I was really moved by it.[4]

4. Herbert Boyer quoted in Sally Smith Hughes, *Genentech: The Beginnings of Biotech* (Chicago: University of Chicago Press, 2011), 16.

Suddenly Boyer and Cohen had in their hands a straightforward technique for taking any piece of DNA and copying it. They knew they could do "just about anything" [...].

It wasn't quite as simple as this, of course. Boyer and Cohen's initial experiments had in fact used DNA from the same bacteria as the plasmid (a common laboratory organism, *Escherichia coli*). It still remained to be shown that the system would work for DNA from a different species of bacteria (let alone from a higher organism like a frog or a human). Ultimately, the answer was a resounding "yes," but it took Boyer and Cohen a year's more work to show it. Until this point in 1973, studying the DNA of higher organisms had hardly been possible—only the tiniest amounts, just one or two copies of a gene, could be extracted from a cell. But Boyer and Cohen's method provided a way to produce millions of copies—this opened up a wealth of new possibilities for research.

A small but growing group of researchers—biochemists and molecular biologists—quickly became aware of Boyer and Cohen's work. A handful of biologists and biochemists began to use and improve the recombinant techniques. Some suspected that the bacterial cells might even be able to *express* the foreign DNA that was inserted inside it—that is, the bacteria might be able to make the protein corresponding to a foreign gene inserted into it. Insert the gene for human insulin in the bacteria and it would produce human insulin. If that possibility could be realized, it would really seem that biologists had gained the ability to build and control organisms, to write in the language of DNA.

The Multiple Meanings of Genetic Engineering

I want to interrupt this history of genetic engineering at this point to take stock of some of the long-term consequences of recombinant DNA. Why is this particular idea so important? I have already described some of the reasons for its *scientific* importance, but it also has a *symbolic* importance that needs to be explored. This symbolic importance can be divided into three kinds of meanings we might attribute to recombinant DNA: social meanings, political meanings, and economic meanings.

Social Meanings

We usually think of the world as neatly divided into two categories: natural things and social things. Natural things include inanimate objects like rocks and water, as well as living things like bacteria, trees, and human bodies. Social things include things made by us: bridges, schools, microscopes, synthetic rubber molecules, and even institutions like "science" or "government." If we take this as a reasonable description of our world, then recombinant DNA poses a big problem. Does it fit into the first category or the second? Is it "natural" or "social"? It is made up of things that we would usually think of as natural: bacteria, DNA, enzymes. It is also made using these same things as tools. But it is also constructed by humans—it is engineered like a bridge. It can even be used for human ends like making technologies or medicines.

Recombinant DNA appears to be neither entirely "natural" nor "social." It is perhaps both: a kind of *hybrid*. Why does this matter? First, it requires us to rethink justifications based on "naturalness." We hear these all the time: in arguments about everything from homosexuality to climate change one side or the other often invokes the idea that something is "natural" or "unnatural" to support their point. Such arguments certainly wouldn't make sense for a genetically engineered bacterium—they are neither natural nor unnatural. More generally, their very existence suggests that these categories are problematic—that what is natural versus what is social depends on your point of view. So recombinant DNA might call into question *all* arguments that rely on such categories.

Consequently, recombinant DNA is provocative or even disruptive. Its hybridity calls into question the kinds of categories and reasons that we use to make sense of the world around us and justify our beliefs.

Political Meanings

Genetic engineering also raises possibilities for radically altering ourselves. It may lead not only to cures for diseases, but also towards the capability to enhance our physical and mental characteristics. So far, these ideas have mostly remained in the realm of science fiction [...].

As biologists began to extend and explore the ways in which they could manipulate and recombine DNA, some social scientists became concerned about the *political* implications that such changes might bring. If the possibility of remaking one's body or mind did become a reality, it was likely to be available only to a select few. The high cost of health care meant that it was likely to be available only to the wealthy; more likely still, it would be limited to North America and Europe, leaving poorer countries behind.

Disparities in wealth would lead not only to inequities in opportunities for education and employment, but now to unequal bodies and minds. Those with access to biotechnologies could be built better, faster, stronger, and smarter. The ultimate result would be an even more divided society, or an even more divided world.

The political scientist Francis Fukuyama has predicted even graver results. Many of our political institutions—especially in a democracy—are based on the idea that all humans are "created equal." This is the basis of liberal thought and the cornerstone of human rights. If biotechnological enhancements are available for some and not others, humans may become literally unequal (some people may have better eyesight, or be able to think faster, or to live longer). This fact would undermine our democracies and our human rights, Fukuyama argues.

It is possible that we will never face these problems in the dramatic way suggested here. Nevertheless, genetic engineering's promise to reconstruct humans makes it fundamentally challenging to ideas of human equality.

Economic Meanings

Genetic engineering quickly became an economic phenomenon. Cohen and Boyer's discovery formed the basis for what became the biotech industry. Globally, the combined revenue of this industry was over $250 billion in 2013.[5] To put this in perspective, this is comparable to (but smaller than) the size of the global software industry and more than half the size of the global market for seafood. But the industry continues to grow rapidly: it includes not only the sale of drugs and therapeutics, but also genetic tests, personalized medicine, the sale of technologies such as DNA chips and sequencing machines, trade in patents, the running of global clinical trials, and the use of biotechnologies in agriculture.

5. Based on a 2013 report from Transparency Market Research. See http://www.prweb.com/releases/2013/6/prweb10848846.htm.

And all of this seems to play a more and more important role in our everyday lives. The anthropologist Kaushik Sunder Rajan has even argued that "the life sciences represent a new face, and a new phase, of capitalism."[6] There is no doubt that biotech is now immensely important for many national economies. But Rajan and others are also saying that biotechnologies have made living matter inextricably bound up with capitalism. Boyer and Cohen's discovery became a workable technology only through the workings of capitalism. This is true of most other biotechnology—it depends on capitalism. To understand our economy we need to pay attention to biotech and to understand biotech we need to pay attention to the economy. We have entered the era of "biocapital." Capitalism is no longer just about making and selling goods, but about harnessing living stuff (cells, proteins, DNA) in order to make money.

Conclusions

Genetic engineering has not created Huxley's *Brave New World*. But the issues that Huxley chose to explore in his fiction are exactly those that generate concerns around biotechnology. Huxley imagined a world of stark inequality between Alphas, Betas, Gammas, Deltas, and Epsilons—each social rank engineered to suit its appointed tasks. Genetic engineering of humans remains figuratively connected to concerns about a living in a radically unequal and divided society. Moreover, Huxley's book examines the consequences of the manufacture of human beings—in *Brave New World* humans are made on a production line, not born. Society today worries about the devaluation and commodification of life that accompanies biocapital. At the heart of both these issues—equality and commodification—is the problem of control. Ultimately, Huxley's society was intolerable because it enabled the exercise of total power. This too is perhaps what we fear most about genetic engineering: that it provides a means for a few to gain social, political, or economic power over others.

Huxley should receive some credit for his accurate depiction of the biotech future. But these convergences also suggests how our understanding of technology is influenced by imagination. Boyer and Cohen may never have read *Brave New World*, but the meanings we attach to the technology they invented are shaped by that book.

6. Kaushik Sunder Rajan, *Biocapital: The Constitution of Postgenomic Life* (Durham, NC: Duke University Press, 2006), 3.

Selections from "When Abortion Suddenly Stopped Making Sense"

Frederica Mathewes-Green

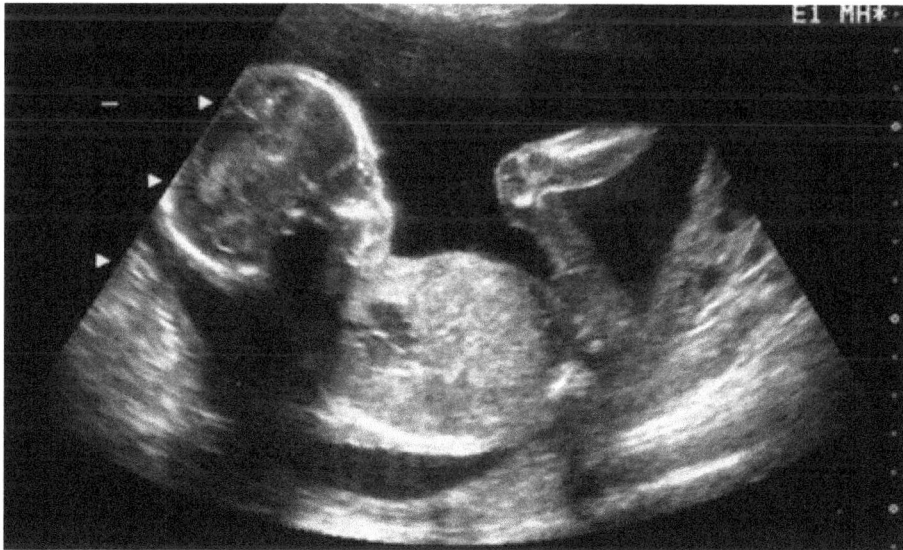

Figure 3.2.1   Abortion won the day, but sooner or later that day will end.

Suzanne Tucker/Dreamstime

At the time of the *Roe v. Wade* decision, I was a college student — an anti-war, mother-earth, feminist, hippie college student. That particular January I was taking a semester off, living in the D.C. area and volunteering at the feminist "underground newspaper" *Off Our Backs*. As you'd guess, I was strongly in favor of legalizing abortion. The bumper sticker on my car read, "Don't labor under a misconception; legalize abortion."

The first issue of *Off Our Backs* after the *Roe* decision included one of my movie reviews, and also an essay by another member of the collective criticizing the decision. It didn't go far enough, she said, because it allowed states to restrict abortion in the third trimester. The Supreme Court should not meddle in what should be decided between the woman and her doctor. She should be able to choose abortion through all nine months of pregnancy.

But, at the time, we didn't have much understanding of what abortion *was*. We knew nothing of fetal development. We consistently termed the fetus "a blob of tissue," and that's just how we pictured it — an undifferentiated mucous-like blob, not recognizable as human or even as alive. It would be another 15 years of so before pregnant couples could show off sonograms of their unborn babies, shocking us with the obvious humanity of the unborn.

We also thought, back then, that few abortions would ever be done. It's a grim experience, going through an abortion, and we assumed a woman would choose one only as a last resort. We were fighting for that "last resort." We had no idea how common the procedure would become; today, one in every five pregnancies ends in abortion.

Nor could we have imagined how high abortion numbers would climb. In the 43 years since *Roe v. Wade*, there have been 59 million abortions. It's hard even to grasp a number that big. Twenty years ago, someone told me that, if the names of all those lost babies were inscribed on a wall, like the Vietnam Veterans Memorial, the wall would have to stretch for 50 miles. It's 20 years later now, and that wall would have to stretch twice as far. But no names could be written on it; those babies had no names.

We expected that abortion would be rare. What we didn't realize was that, once abortion becomes available, it becomes the most attractive option for everyone *around* the pregnant woman. If she has an abortion, it's like the pregnancy never existed. No one is inconvenienced. It doesn't cause trouble for the father of the baby, or her boss, or the person in charge of her college scholarship. It won't embarrass her mom and dad.

Abortion is like a funnel; it promises to solve all the problems at once. So there is significant pressure on a woman to choose abortion, rather than adoption or parenting.

A woman who had had an abortion told me, "Everyone around me was saying they would 'be there for me' if I had the abortion, but no one said they'd 'be there for me' if I had the baby." For everyone around the pregnant woman, abortion looks like the sensible choice. A woman who determines instead to continue an unplanned pregnancy looks like she's being foolishly stubborn. It's like she's taken up some unreasonable hobby. People think, If she would only go off and do this one thing, everything would be fine.

But that's an illusion. Abortion can't really "turn back the clock." It can't push the rewind button on life and make it so she was never pregnant. It can make it easy for everyone *around* the woman to forget the pregnancy, but the woman herself may struggle. When she first sees the positive pregnancy test she may feel, in a panicky way, that she has to get rid of it as fast as possible. But life stretches on after abortion, for months and years — for many long nights — and all her life long she may ponder the irreversible choice she made.

This issue gets presented as if it's a tug of war between the woman and the baby. We see them as mortal enemies, locked in a fight to the death. But that's a strange idea, isn't it? It must be the first time in history when mothers and their own children have been assumed to be at war. We're supposed to picture the child attacking her, trying to destroy her hopes and plans, and picture the woman grateful for the abortion, since it rescued her from the clutches of her child.

If you were in charge of a nature preserve and you noticed that the pregnant female mammals were trying to miscarry their pregnancies, eating poisonous plants or injuring themselves, what would you do? Would you think of it as a battle between the pregnant female and her unborn and find ways to help those pregnant animals miscarry? No, of course not. You would immediately think, "Something must be really wrong in this environment." Something is creating intolerable stress, so much so that animals would rather destroy their own offspring than bring them into the world. You would strive to identify and correct whatever factors were causing this stress in the animals.

The same thing goes for the human animal. Abortion gets presented to us as if it's something women want; both pro-choice and pro-life rhetoric can reinforce that idea. But women do this only if all their other options look worse. It's supposed to be "her choice," yet so many women say, "I really didn't have a choice."

I changed my opinion on abortion after I read an article in *Esquire* magazine, way back in 1976. I was home from grad school, flipping through my dad's copy, and came across an article titled "What I Saw at the Abortion." The author, Richard Selzer, was a surgeon, and he was in favor of abortion, but he'd never seen one. So he asked a colleague whether, next time, he could go along.

Selzer described seeing the patient, 19 weeks pregnant, lying on her back on the table. (That is unusually late; most abortions are done by the tenth or twelfth week.) The doctor performing the procedure inserted a syringe into the woman's abdomen and injected her womb with a prostaglandin solution, which would bring on contractions and cause a miscarriage. (This method isn't used anymore, because too often the baby survived the procedure — chemically burned and disfigured, but clinging to life. Newer methods, including those called "partial birth abortion" and "dismemberment abortion," more reliably ensure death.)

After injecting the hormone into the patient's womb, the doctor left the syringe standing upright on her belly. Then, Selzer wrote, "I see something other than what I expected here. . . . It is the hub of the needle that is in the woman's belly that has jerked. First to one side. Then to the other side. Once more it wobbles, is tugged, like a fishing line nibbled by a sunfish."

He realized he was seeing the fetus's desperate fight for life. And as he watched, he saw the movement of the syringe slow down and then stop. The child was dead. Whatever else an unborn child does not have, he has one thing: a will to live. He will fight to defend his life.

The last words in Selzer's essay are, "Whatever else is said in abortion's defense, the vision of that other defense [i.e., of the child defending its life] will not vanish from my eyes. And it has happened that you cannot reason with me now. For what can language do against the truth of what I saw?"

The truth of what he saw disturbed me deeply. There I was, anti-war, anti–capital punishment, even vegetarian, and a firm believer that social justice cannot be won at the cost of violence. Well, this sure looked like violence. How had I agreed to make this hideous act the centerpiece of my feminism? How could I think it was wrong to execute homicidal criminals, wrong to shoot enemies in wartime, but all right to kill our own sons and daughters?

For that was another disturbing thought: Abortion means killing not strangers but our own children, our own flesh and blood. No matter who the father, every child aborted is that woman's own son or daughter, just as much as any child she will ever bear.

We had somehow bought the idea that abortion was necessary if women were going to rise in their professions and compete in the marketplace with men. But how had we come to agree that we will sacrifice our children, as the price of getting ahead? When does a man ever have to choose between his career and the life of his child?

Once I recognized the inherent violence of abortion, none of the feminist arguments made sense. Like the claim that a fetus is not really a person because it is so *small*. Well, I'm only 5 foot 1. Women, in general, are smaller than men. Do we really want to advance a principle that big people have more value than small people? That if you catch them before they've reached a certain size, it's all right to kill them?

What about the child who is "unwanted"? It was a basic premise of early feminism that women should not base their sense of worth on whether or not a man "wants" them. We are valuable simply because we are members of the human race, regardless of any other person's approval. Do we really want to say that "unwanted" people might as well be dead? What about a woman who is "wanted" when she's young and sexy but less so as she gets older? At what point is it all right to terminate her?

The usual justification for abortion is that the unborn is not a "person." It's said that "Nobody knows when life begins." But that's not true; everybody knows when life — a new individual human life — gets started. It's when the sperm dissolves in the egg. That new single cell has a brand-new DNA, never before seen in the world. If you examined through a microscope three cells lined up — the newly fertilized ovum, a cell from the father, and a cell from the mother — you would say that, judging from the DNA, the cells came from three different people.

When people say the unborn is "not a person" or "not a life" they mean that it has not yet grown or gained abilities that arrive later in life. But there's no agreement about which abilities should be determinative. Pro-choice people don't even agree with each other. Obviously, law cannot be based on such subjective criteria. If it's a case where the question is "Can I kill this?" the answer must be based on objective medical and scientific data. And the fact is, an unborn child, from the very first moment, is a new human individual. It has the three essential characteristics that make it "a human life": It's alive and growing, it is composed entirely of human cells, and it has unique DNA. It's a person, just like the rest of us.

Abortion indisputably ends a human life. But this loss is usually set against the woman's need to have an abortion in order to freely direct her own life. It is a particular cruelty to present abortion as something women want, something they demand, they find liberating. Because *nobody* wants this. The procedure itself is painful, humiliating, expensive — no woman "wants" to go through it. But once it's available, it appears to be the logical, reasonable choice. All the complexities can be shoved down that funnel. Yes, abortion solves all the problems; but it solves them inside the woman's body. And she is expected to keep that pain inside for a lifetime, and be grateful for the gift of abortion.

Many years ago I wrote something in an essay about abortion, and I was surprised that the line got picked up and frequently quoted. I've seen it in both pro-life and pro-choice contexts, so it appears to be something both sides agree on.

I wrote, "No one wants an abortion as she wants an ice cream cone or a Porsche. She wants an abortion as an animal, caught in a trap, wants to gnaw off its own leg."

Strange, isn't it, that both pro-choice and pro-life people agree that is true? Abortion is a horrible and harrowing experience. That women choose it so frequently shows how much worse continuing a pregnancy can be. Essentially, we've agreed to surgically alter women so that they can get along in a man's world. And then expect them to be grateful for it.

Nobody wants to have an abortion. And if nobody wants to have an abortion, why are women doing it, 2800 times a day? If women doing something 2,800 times daily that they don't want to do, this is not liberation we've won. We are colluding in a strange new form of oppression. [...]

Selections from "Rethinking the Abortion Debate"

Anthony Weston

Abortion may not be the most fortunate of ethical problems to take up at the start. We might do better to turn first to general questions of lifestyle or social welfare or the human relation to nature. Even with respect to abortion "the" issue may be far broader than it usually seems, which perhaps is why it has stayed alive so long. But we will come to these other questions in time. Now, however, abortion is one of the most salient problems that confronts us. If it is an unfortunate place-holder for so central a place, that too is part of the problem. [...]

Social Reconstruction and the Abortion Debate

So far this [reading] has considered "the" problem of abortion more or less in the way that philosophical ethics presently takes it. A woman unwillingly becomes pregnant; she needs to decide what to do about it; society as a whole must decide what range of options will be socially supported. I have suggested a rough set of methods for addressing these questions that I hope shows some of pragmatism's virtues: inclusiveness, flexibility, ongoing engagement. Now we must remember that pragmatism suggests a much longer term and more social point of view as well. Another major turn—indeed perhaps the most significant turn of all—remains to be taken with the abortion issue.

Remember that pragmatism challenges us to rethink the "givens" of problematic situations themselves. Rather than taking problems as fixed and inevitable, inviting only "solution," we must consider changing our practices and institutions so that such problems do not arise in so intractable a way. Following Dewey, let us call this kind of change "social reconstruction." [...]

Making Abortion Less Necessary

The need for abortion arises most directly from the problem of unintended and burdensome pregnancies and, if they are carried to term, children. The burden is both economic and personal. Eighty-two percent of all American women getting abortions in 1987 were unmarried, and nearly all were either working or attending school. Most were under twenty-five; two-thirds had family incomes under $25,000 a year.[1] A simple and direct kind of social reconstruction therefore ought to address the contemporary conditions that make pregnancy and children unacceptably burdensome for women under these conditions.

A full-scale proposal is of course beyond our means here, and is premature anyway. These are matters for extended experiment with a variety of responses. But some of the necessary steps are easy to recognize. Parts of the women's movement have cast the problem in reconstructive terms from the beginning, and major parts of the feminist agenda—creating the possibility of economic independence for women, securing pregnancy leaves from work without penalty, keeping contraception legal and expanding its availability—bear upon it. A few reorientations of policy have begun to follow these lines. In 1984 a Wisconsin state legislator, impatient with the perpetual deadlock over abortion legislation, organized a committee of legislators and activists from the opposed sides with the aim of working together, as far as possible, to identify shared goals and to draft legislation to achieve them. The resulting bill passed the legislature-unanimously-and is now law. Among other things, it provides money for sex education and pregnancy counseling, with the hope of reducing unintended pregnancies, and for a state adoption center and adoption hotline, to encourage adoption as an alternative. It begins to make the grandparents on both sides co-responsible for raising a child born of their minor children. It also makes protestors guilty of criminal trespass if they enter an abortion or family planning clinic with the intent to harass.[2]

This sort of approach is rare enough that we hardly even know how to understand it, even though it is also, perfectly obviously, far more intelligent than fighting one more bout of the contemporary debate about whether fetuses are or aren't persons. In a sense it is a compromise, but it is really more as if both sides made an end run, shifting what seemed to be the problem in order to avoid the areas where disagreement is too deep-seated. It is a good example of "lateral thinking." Of course, the two sides also *did* compromise, but we might understand that compromise not as the initial and central aim so much as a natural product of each side's attempt to address the other's real concerns without abandoning what is most essential in

1. Rosalind Petchesky, "Abortion Politics in the 90s," *Nation* 250:21 (May 28, 1990): 732.
2. See Beth Maschinot, "Compromising Positions," *In These Times* 10:3 (November 20–26, 1985): 4. Since when has any abortion legislation been *unanimous?* And since when has any such legislation been *experimental?* This bill's sponsor himself calls it a "social experiment," and certain of its provisions have built-in limits. If they don't work, they expire.

its own. It turned out that common ground was not hard to find once "the" question was put in a broader social context.[3]

There are many further possibilities. We might concentrate on making still other alternatives to abortion workable: speaking to the needs of working and professional women, for instance, by trying to reduce the practical tensions between career and family and by expanding day care, child support, and pregnancy-leave programs for both parents, and so on. It is high time that career expectations designed for and by men were challenged and revised—and for men's sake too, if we are ever to hope for the equal involvement of both genders in child rearing.

The need for abortion, then—the absolute desperation with which some women today must seek it—is not a given, not a necessary fact of life, but a social fact open to change. Indeed, it might well be seen as a social fact that is a disgrace to society. In any case, having children, or having children at the "wrong time," needn't be made such a burden for a woman in every other region of her life. The very idea of a wrong time itself might be rendered largely moot by the right kinds of social support and the sort of restructuring of single-track work and education that is overdue anyway.

None of this implies, of course, that abortion should not also be an option. Rather, the suggestion is that it is partly our lack of attention and imagination—and lack of willingness to tackle some of the structural problems of our society—that keeps it the *only* option. That pregnant women and fetuses are made to bear the cost instead, and indeed that the two should be put at odds with each other in the first place, should seem morally indefensible to both sides in the debate as it stands.

Sex and Motherhood

A step deeper into the social background of the abortion debate and larger tensions begin to emerge. According to Kristin Luker, what in the nineteenth century was mainly a debate about medicine's right to make life and death decisions has now become nothing less than "a debate about women's contrasting obligations to themselves and to others."

> New technologies and the changing nature of work have opened up possibilities for women outside of the home undreamed-of in the 19th Century; together, these changes give women—for the first time in history—the option of deciding exactly how and when their family roles will fit into the larger context of their lives. In essence, therefore, this round of the abortion debate is so passionate and hard-fought because it is a referendum on the place and meaning of motherhood.[4]

Legalized abortion is felt by its opponents to threaten not just the sanctity of life but the family, and

3. One game used to train people in conflict resolution sets up two individuals or teams to compete for the same supply of a given good, say oranges. So focused is each side on beating out the other that they may never notice that they actually need different parts of the oranges, so that by sharing the oranges they both can achieve their goals. The situation seems "zero-sum," to use the game-theoretic term (i.e., it seems as though what one side gains, the other must lose), simply because we are not in the habit of looking for other ways out.

4. Luker, *Abortion and the Politics of Motherhood,* p. 193.

indeed the social valuation of motherhood itself In particular, legalized abortion lies at the core of a larger pattern of social change that demotes motherhood, in Luker's words, "from a sacred calling to a job," and not the only job women might aspire to; in fact a particularly low paid and without the sanctity—socially disvalued job as well. It also reflects the intrusion of technological control into the family, eliminating the element of "surprise" in favor of what may seem to be a kind of arrogant intervention. This accounts for the pro-life movement's tendency to oppose not only abortion but also many forms of contraception, genetic engineering, fetal sex selection, and so on. Even people who favor legalized abortion may agree with their opponents on some of these other points.

For the "other side," meanwhile, sexual freedom is at stake, again as part of a larger pattern of values. On the traditional conception of sex and motherhood, says Luker, sexual relations are located solidly within traditional marriage, where female dependence is not only accepted but affirmed, and sex gains its primary meaning as a means of reproduction. At worst, pregnancy becomes, as it were, the "price" for sex, a kind of punishment. For the prochoice side, however, sexual relations primarily promote intimacy and pleasure, and are authentic and proper only when the partners are independent, even if they happen to be married. Thus the invocation of the right to control what happens in and with one's own body is not restricted to the right to choose abortion. For many women, the fundamental issue is the very possibility of an autonomous lifestyle and an inclusive and socially affirmed sense of self, whatever a woman's actual relation to men or her intentions about having children may be.

Here social divisions lie very deep.[5] But these still only define problematic situations, not ultimate and inevitable conditions. One fundamental problem we might take to be this: how and in what form social support for and affirmation of families can and should be continued, maybe even strengthened, without restricting the freedom of people who want something else, and without perpetuating the forms of female subordination that the traditional family undeniably involves. Certainly, as Luker points out, many people have enormous investments in the traditional patterns. On the other hand, many of those patterns are now only shells of what they once were. Only about 10 percent of American households fit the stereotypical pattern of the traditional family (working husband, "homemaker" wife, children)—down from 60 percent in 1955.[6] Thus, it is not as though change is merely an option, a future possibility. It is an already-present reality that we need to learn to live with.

Forms of Sexual Coercion

At this level a still more fundamental aspect of "the" problem of abortion emerges. The familiar problem of abortion focuses exclusively on what to do *after* a woman unintentionally or unwillingly becomes pregnant. We must also—in fact, surely, primarily—ask how it is that women become pregnant under such conditions in the first place, and what can be done, systematically and seriously, about *that*.

5. The last point, for instance, suggests one source of profound tension: the autonomy of women, and in particular the sexual autonomy of women, is deeply threatening to some people. There are also racial divisions cutting across the usual pro-choice/pro-life divisions. People of color have not notably supported either side. Rosalind Petchesky analyzes this phenomenon in some intriguing ways in her *Abortion and Women's Choice* (Boston: Northeastern University Press, 1990), especially chap. 4.
6. Ron Harris, "Experts Say Childhood Enduring Deep Change," *Raleigh News and Observer*, 13 May 1991, p. 5A.

One reason, already glancingly mentioned, is the difficulty even now of obtaining adequate contraception or information about its use, not just for teenagers but for anyone disadvantaged in this society, and even for many of the supposedly advantaged. Half of all women seeking abortions in 1987 used no birth control.[7] Some chose not to use it, no doubt, but we may be equally sure that lack of access is part of the problem. Even "choosing" not to use contraception has to be understood against a background of meager social support for contraception and resistance from male lovers ranging from noncooperation to active force.

Some of this could be changed by redesigning social policies. Schools, clinics, and even the media can much more effectively teach people about contraceptives and promote their use. Of course there are formidable barriers: sexual freedom is at stake here too, and the same interests that oppose abortion also often array themselves against sex education in the schools and public discussion of contraception.[8] So we have the bizarre spectacle of media full of graphic sexual scenes and sexual incitements with no corresponding education about even the most basic aspects of sexuality or its consequences. On the other hand, some of the resistance can evaporate very fast. The past few years have seen condom advertisements on national television, unthinkable only a few years before. AIDS was the motivator then, but there is no reason why a systematic attempt to link contraception education with a partial "resolution" of the abortion issue could not make as powerful a case.

I do not want to underestimate the obstacles to these kinds of policies. Still, *one* of those very obstacles is our failure to even pose the question in these terms. Powerful interests collaborate to keep such alternatives obscured. But there is no reason that ethics, following what I am arguing are its own most basic dynamics, cannot speak out, cannot even—in the Wisconsin spirit—propose some social experiments.

Other and less noticed kinds of sexual coercion are involved too. One is the very pressure to have sex itself, especially as concentrated on very young and therefore especially vulnerable women and reinforced and intensified in multiple ways by, for example, certain kinds of advertising. But this is not a given either. Historically, after all, the pressures have been almost overpowering in the other direction. Limiting certain kinds of advertising is not out of the question. More creatively, we should also begin to think about how we could affirm rather than repress the sexuality of the young, and in particular how we might affirm its polymorphousness, decentering the furtive and male-centered genital intercourse that now counts as sex for many young people and that also, of course, produces large numbers of pregnancies. Again I certainly do not mean that such a change is likely anytime soon, given the prevailing hysteria about anything sexual, let alone polymorphic, and again I certainly do not claim to know how things should go instead. But at the very least we might begin to see that hysteria itself as part of the problem. Certainly it is possible to argue, for instance, that by adopting a basically repressive attitude toward adolescent sexuality, mainstream society has ceded the shaping of that sexuality to commercial and even pornographic interests that are

---

7. According to a study by the Alan Guttmacher Institute as reported in *U.S. News and World Report* 105:15 (October 17, 1988): 15. That the other half did use birth control and still got pregnant also underlines the pressing need for better contraception.

8. Karen Gustafson ("The New Politics of Abortion," *Utne Reader*, [March/April 1989]: 20) reports that fewer than half of Minnesota's high schools offer any form of sex education because school officials fear the wrath of pro-lifers. See also Kristin Luker, *Taking Chances: Abortion and the Decision Not to Contracept* (Berkeley: University of California Press, 1975).

ultimately far more destructive, sexist, and restrictive than even the mainstream itself might offer were it more explicit.

Other forms of sexual coercion lie even deeper and seem still more intractable. Too often the philosophical discussion sounds as though abortion becomes an issue only when contraception unexpectedly fails.[9] But Catharine MacKinnon has stressed that any discussion of the abortion issue must be framed against the background of pervasive male violence against women. We must think about abortion not only in the context of rape but also of wife battering and marital rape, and in the context of male attitudes about sexuality in general and contraception in particular such that, as MacKinnon puts it, many women come to feel that it is less costly "to risk an undesired, often painful, traumatic, dangerous, sometimes illegal, and potentially life-threatening procedure [abortion] than to protect themselves in advance."[10] The fact is that pregnancy is often, in one way or another, forced on women. And when even the most rudimentary kinds of respect are routinely denied women, social hypersensitivity to the much more problematic rights of the fetus may seem only a vicious joke. Abortion in this context becomes one small means of empowerment, partial and full of risks but still sometimes crucial.

The question raised here is ultimately the question of misogyny itself. As a society we are only beginning to confront the pervasiveness of "domestic violence"—itself a euphemism for the wife beating and child abuse that, depending on one's, definition, occur in well over half of all households in America. Abortion itself has been cast by some: pro-life feminists as a subtly misogynist tool. Abortion, they say, allows male lovers to avoid the consequences of their own sexuality by pressuring their lovers into abortions. Abortion "allows women to become 'unpregnant' at will, so that they can be accepted in a. man's world, while men can go on ignoring the need to accept and accommodate women, their pregnancies included."[11] In any case, none of the constant reminders of physical insecurity and the multiple forms of objectification that force themselves upon women from city billboards and everyday slang would be changed even if abor1tion became every woman's ironclad right tomorrow. The underlying issue is clearly a much broader one. Feminist theory has begun to explore some of the reasons that misogyny is so deep-seated, but it is certainly no easy question. All of this may indeed make fundamental change in 'the near future seem unlikely. Nonetheless, the connection must at least be named. Even these very general and long-term projects, rethinking and resisting misogyny itself, are vital to any finally livable resolution of "the" abortion issue.

Of course everything I have said here represents only the barest beginning toward the rethinking and reconstruction that are necessary. But we have perhaps taken the first step: breaking free of the givens that frame and circumscribe "the" debate as it is presently offered to us, both by philosophers and by the

9. Recall for example the discussion of Judith Thompson's apartment analogy in n. 18 above.
10. MacKinnon, *Feminism Unmodified,* p. 95. This is why Thompson's analogies are in a way deeply insulting, even though she means them to vindicate a woman's right to abortion. For one thing, they are markedly class-relative. Poor women have few socially enforced rights either over their own bodies or over apartments or houses, and are systematically denied the means to protect themselves or their homes even when they supposedly are granted the right. Living in a culture in which, for whole classes of women, sex *is* rape-as MacKinnon would put it-is not like once or twice having your jewelry stolen by burglars who break in when you're gone.
11. Kay Castonguay, president of Feminists for Life of Minnesota, quoted in Gustafson, "New Politics of Abortion," p. 21.

familiar popular movements. That debate is but one strand in a much larger fabric. It is time to pay attention to the whole pattern.

Truth Telling

Disclosure, Privacy, and Confidentiality

Linda Farber Post and Jeffrey Blustein

Linda Farber Post and Jeffrey Blustein, "Truth Telling: Disclosure, Privacy, and Confidentiality," *Handbook for Health Care Ethics Committees*, pp. 46-66. Copyright © 2015 by Johns Hopkins University Press. Reprinted with permission.

Arguably, the most valuable health care resource is information. Clinicians depend on its accuracy in making their diagnoses and prognoses. Patients rely on its adequacy in evaluating their options and arriving at their decisions about care. Families wait for news of their loved ones' changing conditions. But beyond lab data and examination findings, how clinical information is elicited, protected, and shared is bound up with the very nature of the therapeutic relationship. It is, therefore, a matter of ethical concern for professionals and patients alike.

The idea that care professionals should tell their patients the truth seems self-evident and uncontroversial. [...]Like most other aspects of the clinical interaction, however, obligations of truth telling are complex. How do we determine the "truth"? To whom is the truth owed? When does withholding the truth, or massaging information, shade into deliberate deception? The ethics of truth telling is also complicated when patient autonomy, beneficence, nonmaleficence, and justice collide.

Mr. Nunez is a 46-year-old Hispanic man suffering from terminal esophageal cancer. He speaks no English, but his wife, who is bilingual and constantly at his bedside, translates for the care providers. This way of relating to Mr. Nunez—through his wife—is not recent. For the nine months that Mr. Nunez has been coming to the hospital for treatment, Mrs. Nunez has essentially directed his care and determined what he is to be told. Believing that she is acting in his best interest, his care providers have honored her wishes, but they are increasingly uncomfortable.

It has become clear that Mrs. Nunez is not translating everything that she is being told. In particu- lar, she seems to be censoring information about the seriousness of Mr. Nunez's condition. When asked about this, Mrs. Nunez has made it very clear that she does not want her husband told that he is dying of cancer. He knows that he has a "growth" on his esophagus but not that he has cancer. Indeed, according to her, he does not even understand what cancer is. Mr. Nunez has also recently been enrolled in a phase I/II cancer research protocol, consent for which has been given by his wife.

Mrs. Nunez is adamant that her husband not be told about his diagnosis or prognosis. She seems to believe sincerely that, if he were to find out the truth, he would do violence to himself and possibly to her. When asked why she thinks this, she cites an incident in which the patient threatened to harm himself if his condition were found to be more serious than he thought. Although she has been assured that patients usually benefit from understanding their conditions, she insists that nothing can be gained for Mr. Nunez by telling him the truth. She concedes that he occasionally asks questions, but claims that she has been able to satisfy him with evasive or deceitful answers. When asked whether she would agree to have Mr. Nunez told the truth when he is finally too weak to harm himself, she emphatically replied, "No! Never! I can't imagine what it would be like for him to know that he is dying. I won't have this!" Although she describes her husband as "like a baby," there is no reason to believe that the patient could not comprehend the nature and seriousness of his condition. His cognitive status cannot be confirmed, however, because Mrs. Nunez has forbidden a psychiatric evaluation.

Members of the care team are conflicted about the limits on their ability to interact with Mr. Nunez. Several strongly believe that he is being deprived of his rights to information, while others suggest that his wife knows him better than they do. The oncology fellow notes that "in certain countries, such as Japan, patients are not routinely told the truth about their diagnoses as a way of protecting them from stress, but at least they are not tortured by being enrolled in research that is not likely to benefit them."

How and by whom should this patient's best interests be defined? Do Mr. Nunez's rights conflict with his best interest? What arguments support disclosure or nondisclosure in this case?

Justifications

Truthfulness is a core interpersonal value in social life generally and it has particular significance in the clinician-patient relationship. Three justifications have been advanced to support the obligation of veracity in the clinical setting. They are "respect owed to persons ... fidelity, promise-keeping, and contract ... [and] the role of trust in relationships between health professionals and patients and subjects" (Beauchamp and Childress 2013, p. 303):

1. Respect for others is reflected in the ethical principle of autonomy. The capable individual's right to be self-determining imposes on clinicians the obligation to provide adequate information for informed health care decision making.
2. Fidelity and the keeping of promises are central elements in the trust-based relationship between patient and clinician. This fiduciary bond creates an implicit contract that both parties will be honest and will honor their commitments.

3. Productive therapeutic interactions rely on the truthful management of information. The effective clinician-patient relationship depends on the exchange of accurate and complete information about symptoms, diagnoses, prognoses, and treatment options, as well as confidence that care plans will be followed and patient wishes will be honored.

In this context, the uneasiness of the professionals caring for Mr. Nunez is understandable if they believe that withholding information undercuts his autonomy, erodes their trusting relationship, and inhibits effective clinical management. Only the strong likelihood that disclosure would be genuinely *harmful* to the patient can justify withholding information about his condition. This very rare therapeutic exception to the disclosure obligation is discussed below.

Disclosure

Ethical Obligation

Collaborative decision making and informed consent depend on the reasonable disclosure of necessary or material information. Capable patients or their authorized surrogates are ethically and legally entitled to information that enables them to understand the likely course of the medical condition, evaluate the therapeutic options, and make choices consistent with patient goals and values.

Disclosure invokes respect for the patient's right to information that promotes effective decision making and the ethical imperatives to maximize benefits and minimize harms. Yet, as the case of Mr. Nunez illustrates, these same principles create tension between and among professionals' obligations. The analysis weighs the benefits of disclosing information that enhances patient understanding and self-determination against the potential harms of anxiety and stress that disclosure may cause.

Because laboratory and examination findings are controlled by the care team, particularly the medical staff, disclosure of clinical information is at the discretion of the physician. Access to medical information is thus an inherently unequal process that places the patient at a potential disadvantage in decision making, although this is changing somewhat with the wide availability of the Internet and the marketing of direct-to-consumer tests. This imbalance confers on doctors the disclosure obligation.

Arguments for Disclosing Information

Ms. Kim, a 23-year-old woman, presents with an isolated case of first-bout optic neuritis. The ophthalmologist, Dr. Frank, is concerned about whether to inform her that multiple sclerosis (MS) may develop in the future. His dilemma arises because, at the time the optic neuritis presents, the likelihood of subsequent development of MS is uncertain. At one time, it was thought that the degree of association between optic neuritis and MS was around 11%. Increasing evidence, however, suggests that the association may be as high as 50% (Brodsky et al. 2008). In light of current evidence, what should Dr. Frank disclose to her? How does the degree of association between optic neuritis and MS affect Dr. Frank's disclosure obligation?

The arguments in favor of disclosure are both ethical and practical. To know the truth about one's current and future medical condition is, for many patients, essential to a sense of self-mastery, especially as that condition evolves and possibly deteriorates. In addition, the therapeutic value of patients maintaining a sense of control in such circumstances is promoted by information disclosure. Even when treatment options are limited, life plans may need to be altered, and knowing what to expect allows patients to understand and prepare for what lies ahead.

Dr. Frank's concern is that disclosing the possibility of MS could cause Ms. Kim needless anxiety about an illness that she may never develop. Moreover, because MS cannot be prevented or cured, the information will not afford her any protection against developing the disease. On the other hand, it can be argued that she has the right to prepare herself for the heightened likelihood that she may experience a debilitating condition that would inevitably affect her ability to function independently. This knowledge may be an important influence in making decisions about lifestyle, career, family, and finances, as well planning treatment that might potentially delay the onset or mitigate symptoms of MS. Finally, if Ms. Kim discovers this information independently, her trust in Dr. Frank may be damaged by the belief that he was not honest about her risks.

Evan Barry was 17 years old when he was diagnosed last year with renal cell carcinoma. His right kidney was removed and he began several rounds of chemotherapy. Earlier this year, he came to the emergency department (ED) complaining of shortness of breath and chest pain. He seemed to be unaware of his diagnosis and could not explain the scar from the kidney surgery. A chest x-ray showed metastases to his lungs.

Evan was transferred from the ED to the adolescent unit and given gamma interferon. The physicians on the adolescent floor were puzzled by his apparent ignorance of his condition. When they approached his mother, Mrs. Barry was equivocal about what her son had been told. She said that she had been candid with Evan when he was first diagnosed but, when the physicians encouraged further discussions during the current admission, she adamantly refused to allow anyone to talk with him about his diagnosis and treatment. She expressed fear that he would be devastated and become suicidal, although she acknowledged that he had never attempted or threatened to harm himself.

Staff on the adolescent unit believed that Evan was frightened and isolated by the lack of information and communication. One of the residents carefully asked questions to probe the extent of his knowledge about his cancer. Evan said tearfully that he did not know what was wrong with him and that the doctors always spoke with his mother, not with him. He also said, "My mom is very worried about me but it makes her sad to talk about my problems and I don't want to upset her even more."

The team agreed that, while the lack of information was probably very frightening for Evan, he seemed to be protecting his mother by not asking questions. Concern was expressed that, even though he was not yet an adult with legal rights to information, as a bright adolescent who appeared to want and need information and support, he should be told the truth.

What are the care providers' obligations in this situation and, if they conflict, how can they be resolved? What benefits and risks should be considered? Who should determine what Evan is told?

The assumption that truth will normally be told goes to the heart of trust-based relationships of all sorts, including relations among family members and between patients and care professionals. Shielding patients from the truth is generally an imperfect enterprise in any case, requiring the collusion of others, including staff, family, and friends, in a conspiracy of silence. Uncertainty about what the patient knows and discomfort with the deception often result in caregivers and even family avoiding contact with the patient. It is not unusual to hear, "I was so sure that I would give it away that I just didn't want to be around him."

Yet, patients—even children and adults with a history of not wanting to know—sense when things are being kept from them and may avoid discussion as a way of accommodating those protecting them. Evan, for example, is reluctant to ask questions about his condition because he knows that talking about it upsets his mother. The result is a cycle of increasingly difficult efforts for mother and son to protect each other from acknowledging their sadness and fear. The burden of the deception itself, thus, can be a barrier to communication. Paradoxically, withholding information from the patient in order to protect him ends up isolating the patient at precisely the time when close and supportive relationships are critical. In short, although the obligation of truth telling, like other obligations, is not an absolute, it is something that requires a compelling reason to disregard.

Conflicting Obligations

Tension arises when clinicians feel that their obligations require them to either disclose information that the patient may not want or withhold potentially problematic information, all in the name of promoting the patient's well-being. The challenge is determining what the patient should know about his care without causing him harm and without violating his right to make autonomous decisions.

As you might suspect at this point, disclosure is not simply a matter of rattling off the results of lab tests or physical examinations. Effective disclosure is a clinical skill that depends on physician judgment and communication, as well as knowledge. Too much information can be as harmful as too little. The difference between truth telling and truth dumping is the difference between providing specific material information that facilitates decision making and indiscriminately overloading the patient with facts in the interests of completeness. An unbroken monologue of clinical data can be counterproductive, leaving the patient with glazed eyes and little recollection of what was said. Far more useful is breaking up the explanation every few sentences with, "Does that make sense?" or "What else can I tell you that would be helpful?" or "Can you tell me what you have understood so far?" Patients often indicate what they want to know and perceptive clinicians can be guided by their spoken or unspoken signals.

Truth telling is also counterproductive when information is disclosed without the accompanying explanations or guidance that frame the decisions patients or surrogates must make. More helpful is something like, "Let me tell you what all this means and then we can figure out the reasonable choices you might consider." Finally, patients need to be reassured that they are not expected to absorb everything all at once. "I know that this is a lot to take in right now and we will talk again. When you think of questions, it might be a good idea to write them down so that we can address them next time."

Arguments for Not Disclosing Information

Patients have both the right to receive information and the right *not* to receive it. Some people, especially those who are elderly, anxious, easily confused, or from cultures that do not place a high premium on individual autonomy, find it burdensome and even frightening to learn about their conditions and be asked to make treatment decisions. For example, while persons from European American backgrounds typically value full disclosure of medical information, those from Asian and Middle Eastern cultures tend to protect patients from knowing about illness or impending death. For them, authentic decision making in the clinical setting is expressed in the capacitated request *not* to be informed and the voluntary delegation of decision-making authority to trusted others (Zahedi 2011). Implicit is a long-standing or culture-based comfort with the practice of decision making by surrogates. In that sense, Mr. and Mrs. Nunez may exemplify families that have their own decision-making patterns, which may be effective and comfortable, rather than paternalistic or coercive. Decision making, like other interpersonal dynamics, comes in assorted shapes and sizes entitled to respectful attention. [... A]waiver of informed consent is something that must be explicitly confirmed, not inferred, to demonstrate respect for the patient and protect his autonomy.

The more common disclosure dilemmas concern withholding information from patients who have not waived their right to information, usually justified by notions of shielding them from harm (invoking the principle of nonmaleficence) and sometimes by notions of promoting their interests (invoking the principle of beneficence). Disclosure, especially of bad news, is one of the most difficult clinical tasks, and evasion or awkwardness is often the result of efforts to avoid inflicting pain. Physicians frequently protect themselves and—they think—their patients by softening the message and resorting to euphemism. "The patient has a grim prognosis" becomes "The patient is not doing well." "The patient is dying" becomes "The patient is failing." Sometimes it sounds as though, if only the patient and care team tried harder, she would not be dying.

Rather than comfort, however, deliberate vagueness creates confusion, anxiety, mistrust, and unrealistic expectations. It is not uncommon for a family to react with frustration and seemingly unreasonable demands when told that, although the patient is *not doing well*, aggressive cure-directed treatments should be limited. The family argues that she could be doing *better* if only the care team were doing *more* rather than *less*. [...]

Sometimes, discomfort in discussing bad news with the patient persuades care professionals that disclosure would be *harmful*, when in fact it might only be *distressing*. The risk is that the therapeutic exception[...] may be expanded beyond its strict definition (exception to the disclosure obligation when the information itself would cause *imminent, direct, and significant harm* to the patient) and applied to situations in which the information would be upsetting, but not dangerous. The principle of nonmaleficence is formulated in terms of *harm* and does not require physicians to shield their patients from upset or distress. Whenever clinicians consider withholding information, especially from capable patients, they need to question who is being protected, whether the protection is truly warranted, and what the cost will be to the trust between doctor and patient. This dilemma, which requires balancing the ethical obligations of respect for autonomy, beneficence, nonmaleficence, and justice, often triggers a clinical ethics consultation to explore the benefits and risks of disclosure to the patient.

Pressure also comes from families—parents of young children, grown children of aging parents, or concerned spouses like Mrs. Nunez—not to share information with the patient. These are typically concerned family members who want to protect their loved one, although sometimes their motives are less creditable. In other words, "If we can't prevent Papa from having cancer, at least we can keep him from feeling anxious or scared." The reasons given are usually "The news will kill him" or "You will take away all hope." The first objection indicates the need to reassure anxious relatives that disclosure is part of clinicians' skill set and the patient will not be burdened with information that he does not want or cannot safely assimilate.

The second objection speaks to expectations and the importance of hope. Bad news or even a terminal diagnosis need not signal a future so bleak that deception is justified. Depriving patients and families of hope is never justified. It is frequently necessary, however, to redefine what can be hoped for—perhaps not long life or unlimited function, but rather increased comfort, attendance at a special celebration, or a peaceful death surrounded by loved ones. Helping patients and families adjust their goals to be achievable is an essential part of care professionals' responsibilities.

Let us consider how these issues relate to Mr. Nunez. His caregivers are faced with conflicting obligations in determining what he should be told about his condition. Because they have been prevented from interacting with him directly, they have no independent assessment of his capacity, emotional stability, or desire for information. All communications have been filtered through his wife, whose motives may be well meaning but overprotective, or possibly not in his best interest. For precisely this reason, the policies of most hospitals, as well as Joint Commission standards, require that trained and certified interpreters, rather than family, manage communications between the care team and patients who prefer to use a language other than English. Not only is this requirement a safeguard against deliberately distorted messages, it also relieves family members of the burden of trying to digest unfamiliar medical terms and clinical concepts and then translating them into another language in a way that is understandable to the patient. The care professionals need to clarify with Mrs. Nunez that providing her husband with good care requires that they interact with him directly. She should be reassured that harmful or unwanted information will not be forced on him but that his perceptions and wishes will be skillfully assessed as part of his clinical evaluation.

In addition to helping protective families appreciate the reasons supporting disclosure, it is also important to explain the risks of withholding or distorting information. They must understand that the care team will not lie to patients, that direct questions will require truthful answers. They must also realize that, given the number of people involved in patients' care and the ease with which information can be accessed from the Internet and other available sources, it will be difficult if not impossible to guarantee that they will not learn what is being kept from them. Potential damage to family relationships is another compelling argument for disclosure. "If your husband learns about his condition independently, he might begin to wonder what other things you've kept from him. Let's work together to figure out how to give him the information he needs in a way that is controlled and comfortable for both him and you."

When withholding information is suggested, it is necessary to determine the patient's capacity, understanding of the clinical situation, desire for information, and the degree to which he wants to be involved in care planning and decision making. Using the patient's preferred language, one approach might be, "Mr. Nunez, the examinations and tests will give us information about your condition and then some decisions will have to be made about your treatment. Some patients want to know all the information and others don't. What would make you comfortable? Do you want us to discuss these things with you or with someone else?" Capable patients can then elect to participate in the process or voluntarily delegate that responsibility to another person. Even if Mr. Nunez explicitly says, "I don't want to know and I want my wife to make decisions for me," he should be kept in the communication loop by being asked periodically, "Do you have any questions? Is there anything we can tell you?" A wish not to be burdened with information or decision making should not deprive patients of attention in other ways.

Disclosure of Adverse Outcomes and Medical Error

Mrs. Allen, a pregnant woman with diabetes, had been encouraged to undergo amniocentesis to determine the fetus's lung development in order to plan induction of her delivery. Because there is a window of safety in delivering diabetic patients, this procedure is considered standard of care. During the amnio, the umbilical cord was nicked, resulting in bleeding and requiring an immediate caesarean section.

The neonatology house staff has requested an ethics consult to discuss whether the parents should be told the reason for the emergency delivery and, if so, whether the information should come from the obstetric team or the neonatologists.

Adverse Outcomes and Medical Error

Disclosure of bad news is difficult under any circumstances. Disclosure of bad news when things go wrong is a clinician's worst nightmare, but it is one that must be confronted for the sake of patients and professionals. We begin with some important definitions. *Adverse outcomes* are undesired and unintended negative results of medical care that create actual or potential harm to the patient. These untoward occurrences may be the result of carelessness or ineptitude, or they may reflect foreseen but unavoidable risk even when standard of care was practiced. The former—*medical errors*—are considered avoidable, while the latter are generally seen as unavoidable, an inherent part of the imperfect art of medicine. Distinguishing between these types of adverse outcomes may be problematic, but standard of care is routinely used as an important criterion. The distinction is crucial in recognizing that unintended outcomes do not always mean that someone is to blame.

Other analyses distinguish between *system* and *individual or human errors*, attributing some adverse outcomes to problems in the health care delivery system and others to the actions of individual providers. This approach reflects the notion that "no one person [is] responsible, because it is virtually impossible for one mistake to kill a patient in the highly mechanized and backstopped world of a modern hospital" (Belkin 1997, p. 28). The 2000 Institute of Medicine report, *To Err is Human: Building a Safer Health System*, generated considerable interest in disclosure of information as a key to managing and preventing adverse outcomes. As a result, oversight and accrediting bodies, clinicians, and institutions are adopting the concept of health care delivery as a system-wide interlocking dynamic that can either allow or prevent error. In analyzing adverse events, this perspective focuses on *organizational processes* rather than *individual performance*, searching for systemic solutions rather than assigning blame.

Scope of Disclosure

Disclosure includes but is not limited to the requirements of informed consent that concern *prospective* analysis of proposed interventions. Armed with adequate information, the patient can proceed to make decisions about future care. Full disclosure that promotes patient self-determination and protection also includes *retrospective* analysis of unintended consequences, which involves informing patients that an adverse outcome has occurred and providing an explanation of why it happened. This aspect of disclosure recognizes that, in addition to patients' need for information to enhance care planning and decision making, they have a desire and a right to understand what did or will happen to them. Taken together, the *preview* and *review* aspects of the disclosure obligation can be grounded in the patient's need to *know* and *act* on the basis of adequate information.

Obligation of Disclosure

The obligation to disclose adverse outcomes rests on both ethical and legal foundations. Recognizing the need to ensure the provision of adequate information, courts have imposed fiduciary obligations of disclosure on physicians. Judicial reasoning is that these obligations exist when "one party is dependent on another for information or knowledge that only the first party possesses" (Vogel and Delgado 1980, pp. 66–67). In the clinical setting, the physician is the person most likely to have and control information about an untoward event or medical error, heightening the professional obligation of disclosure. The patient who has suffered an undisclosed adverse event is not only likely to be unaware of what happened and the actual or potential harm she faces, but she is also unable to prevent or mitigate the harm or to seek fair compensation for it. Her reliance on the physician for information that will minimize harm and help her cope with the consequences creates an ethical imperative for timely and full disclosure of the adverse event. This obligation has received explicit attention in the various codes and opinions that provide ethical guidance and analysis for physicians. In the name of transparency, health care organizations also have an obligation to promote disclosure of anticipated outcomes by their medical practitioners, and they should include this in their organizational codes of ethics.

A related basis for the disclosure obligation can be found in the values underlying informed consent. This analysis views informed consent as a compact entered into by physician and patient. The doctor says, in effect, "Here is the information you need, including the possible risks." The patient says, in effect, "I understand what you have said and I consent to the test or treatment *because I trust that you have told me everything I need to know* in order to make a decision." Implicit in the patient's response is, "I trust that you will exercise all due care in treating me. *I further trust that, if any foreseen or unforeseen harms should occur, you will disclose that information so that I can understand and manage the negative consequences.*" The informed patient is able to balance the benefits, burdens, and risks in advance of treatment and, if an untoward event occurs, mitigate any harm, protect herself from further harms, and seek appropriate compensation. Rather than a passive recipient of treatment, the patient becomes an active partner in planning for and managing the outcomes of care.

Barriers to Disclosure

Given the ethical and legal justifications, it seems hard to argue with the notion that information about untoward occurrences should be made available to patients or their surrogates. It will not be surprising, however, that physicians are very reluctant to discuss negative outcomes with patients and families. Reasons for avoiding disclosure include the difficulty of determining whether the event was medical error, the belief that the information will be needlessly upsetting, and the omnipresent fear of legal action. Additional barriers include the ideal of physician infallibility shared by patients as well as physicians, and the shame and guilt that physicians experience when admitting an untoward outcome, especially when it is a result of medical error.

Liability to medical malpractice suits is cited by physicians as the chief barrier to disclosure of unintended occurrences. Doctors' understandable risk aversion makes them uneasy about admitting error or other behavior that might have contributed to patient harm. Concerns about who assumes the duty of disclosure and bears responsibility are especially difficult in an academic medical center, with its multiple levels of interdisciplinary staff and different authority structures. That said, you should know and reinforce with physicians that legal action does not inevitably follow adverse events, including those caused by negligence. Instead, some evidence suggests that the pursuit of litigation by patients and families is related to how physicians handle discussions with them about untoward outcomes, including disclosure of information about actual or potential harm (Mastroianni et al. 2010; Liebman and Hyman 2004; Gallagher et al. 2003; Goldberg et al. 2002).

In an effort to encourage provider-patient communication about unanticipated clinical events, many states have passed "disclosure" or "apology" laws. These statutes are designed to protect communications that provide information about the event (disclosure) and expressions of sympathy and regret (apology) from being used as evidence of liability in malpractice litigation or administrative actions. As of 2010, 34 states and the District of Columbia had enacted some type of apology law; 9 had enacted mandatory disclosure laws requiring that patients or their surrogates be notified of adverse events; 6 states had enacted both types of laws; and 13 had neither (Mastroianni et al. 2010; Dresser 2008). One response to these statutory requirements and the potential that other states may enact similar legislation was the Project on Medical Liability in Pennsylvania, which used trained mediators to strengthen physicians' skills in communicating difficult news and established mediation as an alternative to litigation (Liebman and Hyman 2004).

Institutions have also developed promising initiatives that provide guidance and support to practitioners facing the daunting task of communicating bad news. These protective laws and institutional systems are still being studied to determine their impact on malpractice litigation, practitioner behavior, and organizational strategies. Your ethics committee can play an important role in educating clinical and administrative staff about these developments, as well as participating in the development of institutional systems that promote greater transparency and trust in the provider-patient relationship.

Perhaps even more threatening to physicians than the specter of malpractice litigation is the personal devaluation that accompanies acknowledging adverse events. This may include "a loss of personal confidence and self-esteem, diminished professional authority and reputation, as well as a loss of referrals and income" (Baylis 1997, p. 338). The inability to cope with untoward outcomes appears to stem less from blatant physician callousness or dishonesty than from belief in the widespread myth of infallibility and total control that define the perfect healer. This image, born in medical schools, nurtured throughout medical careers, and sold to the public, is shared by physicians and their patients, leading to unrealistic expectations, unreasonable disappointments, and unbridgeable gaps in communication.

Privacy and Confidentiality

Mr. Miller is a 42-year-old man who came to the emergency room with iritis and whose work-up was positive for syphilis. When Dr. David discussed the diagnosis with Mr. Miller, the patient requested that Dr. David not disclose the infection to his wife or report it to the state Department of Health. He said that he must have contracted the condition during a one-time extramarital encounter on a recent business trip. He also stated that he has not had sexual contact with his wife since that time and that he will undergo treatment before doing so.

Two other aspects of information management central to the therapeutic relationship are privacy and confidentiality. Privacy refers to "a state or condition of limited access," including "an agent's control over access to himself or herself" (Beauchamp and Childress 2013, p. 312). Privacy reflects the notion that one's self, whether the physical body, personal representations or identifiers, or personal information, should be guarded and under the control of the individual. The ethical obligation to protect patients' privacy recognizes that, in the clinical interaction, patients reveal sensitive physical or informational aspects of themselves, and they should retain the right to control who has access to these personal aspects.

Protecting physical privacy entails obvious measures, such as knocking before entering a patient's room; providing appropriate gowns, robes, and covers; and, during examinations, pulling the curtain, asking visitors to step outside, and admitting only those whose presence is necessary. Protecting informational privacy requires not discussing patient information in public areas and ensuring that written or electronic patient information is accessed only by those directly involved in a patient's care.

Closely related to privacy is confidentiality. "Confidentiality is present when one person discloses information to another, whether through words or an examination, and the person to whom the information is disclosed pledges not to divulge that information to a third party without the confider's permission" (Beauchamp and Childress 2001, pp. 305–6). In that sense, confidentiality, like truth telling and privacy, invokes the patient's trust in and reliance on the health care professional's integrity. When patients provide clinicians with access to their bodies and personal information, they do so with the trust-based understanding that these private aspects of themselves will be held in confidence by the professionals.

Privacy and confidentiality are associated with distinct but related ethical obligations. Although the common perception is that confidentiality binds only the patient and physician, the professional obligation also covers other clinicians, including chiropractors, clinical social workers, dentists, nurses, podiatrists, and psychologists. Moreover, with recent changes in the delivery of health care, these obligations do not only apply to the relationship between a patient and her primary practitioner. The circle of individuals who have necessary access to private information about the patient has expanded to include multiple care providers, and patients' rights to privacy are not violated simply because these individuals have access to this information. Nor has the primary practitioner failed to protect confidentiality simply because he shares patient information with other members of the care team. Obligations to respect privacy and protect confidentiality remain, but the relationships to which they apply have changed.

Justifications for Protecting Confidentiality

Mr. Gordon, a 43-year-old man, is picked up by the police on Saturday evening and rushed to the nearest emergency department after passing out on a mid-town sidewalk. ED physicians detect a high level of alcohol in his blood and a urine toxicology screen reveals opiates. Upon regaining consciousness, Mr. Gordon provides his past medical history, which is unremarkable, and says that his occupation is city sanitation truck driver. He acknowledges that he used alcohol and cocaine earlier in the evening, and reminds the physicians that they have a duty not to disclose to others confidential patient information.

What obligations do physicians have to Mr. Gordon and others, and how can they be reconciled? What ethical principles and additional factors should be considered?

The notion that the therapeutic interaction creates a zone of protected information can be supported by the same ethical considerations discussed earlier in connection with truthfulness. Respect for persons underlies patients' privacy, namely, their right to control who has access to their health care information and the requirement that medical records and communications in the clinical setting be protected from unwarranted disclosure. If personal information can be seen as a reflection of the most intimate aspects of an individual's life, then control of that information can be seen as a form of self-determination that requires provider respect. Protecting confidentiality also prevents the harms that result from unauthorized disclosure of sensitive information, such as HIV status or psychiatric history.

Fidelity and promise keeping are reflected in the bond of trust that requires professionals to hold in confidence information learned in the clinical interaction. This justification is based on the moral imperative to honor a duty or promise regardless of the results. It holds that, without explicit patient waiver, the clinician is bound by the confidentiality inherent in the relationship. The argument also encompasses the notion of secrets, those pieces of our private selves we give in trust to others with the implicit or explicit understanding that they will be held in confidence.

The effectiveness of the clinical relationship and the resulting quality of the health care provided depend on an atmosphere of trust that promotes the candid and complete exchange of information. This justification rests on the need to encourage patients to provide all relevant facts about their medical history and symptoms, no matter how private or potentially embarrassing, to facilitate accurate diagnosis and effective treatment. This is a utilitarian rationale for protecting confidentiality since it appeals to the consequences for the patient and the practitioner-patient relationship of an obligation of nondisclosure. Without strict limits on what may be disclosed to others, patients would likely avoid seeking or fully cooperating in treatment.

Challenges to Privacy and Confidentiality

It would seem that nothing could be more ethically compelling than the promise to protect what patients reveal about themselves. Like truth telling and privacy, confidentiality seems a clear and simple duty that professionals owe their patients. But, like other ethical imperatives, the confidentiality obligation is neither absolute nor always easy to honor.

So what gets in the way of protecting patient confidences and personal health information? Medical information is generated in the health care setting as a product of the therapeutic interaction between clinician and patient; it is also generated in the pharmacy, the research lab, the autopsy room, the insurance office, the medical classroom, and the hospital elevator. It goes into reports, books, lectures, legal briefs, and computers, from which it is accessed by countless people for countless valid and not-so-valid reasons.

As noted above, the treating relationship is only one context in which medical confidentiality is raised. The dramatic change in health care delivery has altered what used to be a confidential relationship between patient and family doctor. Medical treatment has moved from the home to the institutional setting; multiple disciplines and subspecialties, legal and government bureaucracies, and third-party payers now converge on each case; and computers connect all parties to the clinical interaction. The result is that the number of people with legitimate and non-legitimate access to medical information has increased geometrically. The growing use of e-medicine to provide medical services to patients, and to store, manage, and transmit patients' health information has exacerbated the problem. The contemporary clinical setting and technological developments have greatly enhanced the efficiency and efficacy of communication among care providers, but this is not an unmixed blessing: new worries arise about the extent to which the privacy of patients' medical information can actually be respected and protected. Concerns about the security of protected health information (PHI) prompted the inclusion of stringent regulations in the 1996 federal Health Insurance Portability and Accountability Act (HIPAA).

Consent to care with a loss of some measure of privacy is either explicitly obtained, through signed releases upon entering the care-providing institution, or presumed, but the consent is never to be considered unlimited. For example, although it should be explained upon admission, it is generally understood that treatment in a teaching hospital includes having one's records, examinations, and therapies available for observation and study by students and house staff. Most patients expect that their cases will be discussed formally and even informally to obtain the benefit of other opinions and to provide teaching examples. They neither expect nor deserve to have their personal or medical information shared in public hospital areas or social situations. Likewise, patients should have control over who has access to their medical information through updates in their clinical condition. As a precaution against inadvertent unwanted disclosure, it may be helpful to say early in the patient's hospital stay, "You seem to have a lot of family and friends who are concerned about you. Please know that we will not discuss your medical condition with anyone unless you specifically request that we do so."

In addition to those who use medical information for treatment purposes, such data are routinely used by medical researchers, law enforcement agencies, attorneys (requesting their own clients' records or those of other patients in connection with medical malpractice or personal injury litigation), insurers (life, health, disability, and liability), employers, and creditors. Although these secondary users are routinely required to access information through formal requests for patient record releases, they may not always follow procedure. Finally, there are other potential users of medical information who have nothing to do with the patient's health care, including those with commercial, political, and media interests.

So, are confidentiality and privacy obsolete or decrepit, as one commentator (Siegler 1982) suggested more than 30 years ago? Given the formidable barriers and incentives in the current health care setting, is it possible or even desirable to manage the flow of information?

The management of personal health information has been a concern since Hippocrates cautioned against indiscriminate disclosure. A new challenge is storing, transmitting, and selectively disclosing protected health information (PHI) in the context of e-medicine, including electronic medical records and online- and Internet-based networks linking insurance companies, hospitals, providers, and patients (Bauer 2009). Reported incidents of intentional and unintentional breaches in security have demonstrated the real and potentially disastrous risks to individual and group medical records, provider-patient relationships, quality of care, administrative efficiency, and public confidence in the health care system. In short, e-medicine has the potential to both greatly enhance and seriously jeopardize health care.

The obligations of privacy and confidentiality are being reshaped and their boundaries are in flux. Yet, the ethical core remains intact and worth preserving. The contours may be redrawn, but the central values deserve protection through policies and regulations that respond to current clinical, ethical, and legal imperatives.

Justifications for Breaching Confidentiality

Even people with little experience in the health care setting know and rely on the sanctity of clinician-patient confidentiality. Based on well-established ethical and legal justifications, this obligation normally precludes professionals from disclosing information learned in the course of diagnosis or treatment. Precisely because this ethical mandate is so central to the clinical relationship, exceptions are justified only when disclosure of confidential information is essential to preventing significant harm to other vulnerable individuals, especially those at unsuspected risk. In these select instances, the patient's right to confidentiality is considered to be outweighed by the obligation to protect those who are not in a position to protect themselves.

The following two situations that justify breaching confidentiality illustrate that the obligation of fidelity to one's patients is not the only ethical obligation that practitioners have and that conflicts can arise as a result. In both circumstances, the needs of the non-patients are elevated because their vulnerability is heightened by their very ignorance of the risks they face.

1. Providing information that prevents harm to *identified* third parties at risk (e.g., partner notification). This exception reflects the opinion in *Tarasoff v. Regents of University of California*, a 1976 case in which the court held that a psychotherapist who had prior knowledge of a patient's intention to kill his unsuspecting girlfriend had a duty to warn her. This reasoning has been incorporated into the laws of many states in addressing the needs of those who have been unwittingly exposed to HIV/AIDS or other sexually transmitted disease (STD). When the infected patient refuses to inform sexual or needle-sharing partners, some states permit or require partner notification to enable those known to be at risk to be tested and treated. While most states recognize a duty to warn identified persons at risk of intended harm or exposure to other sexually transmitted or contagious diseases, there is no authority in most states for notifying persons exposed to HIV or AIDS (Hermann and Gagliano 1989). The *Tarasoff* ruling, which is also notable for expanding the scope of practitioner responsibility, is discussed further in part IV.

2. Providing information that prevents harm to *unidentified* others at risk (e.g., public health or public safety reporting). In some instances, the potential danger is to the general population, rather than to specified individuals. To protect the public health and safety, state laws commonly require that health care providers report certain findings, including suspected cases of child abuse and neglect; wounds that are the result of gun shots, knives, or other pointed instruments; burn injuries of specified severity; and cases of reportable communicable diseases specified in state health laws.

In the case of Mr. Miller, Dr. David is in a difficult position. He knows that confidentiality is the bedrock of the patient-physician relationship, assuring the patient that he can share accurate and sensitive information with the doctor without fear of disclosure. Not only does the assurance of confidentiality promote trust, it facilitates full and candid communication that is vital to successful diagnosis and treatment. Fear that sensitive or embarrassing information, such as a diagnosis of STD, will be disclosed may dissuade Mr. Miller from providing critical facts or even seeking necessary treatment.

Sometimes, however, withholding information poses risks to others outside the physician-patient relationship. In this case, Mr. Miller's wife is at risk of contracting syphilis and she is especially vulnerable because she has no reason to suspect that she is at risk. By taking action early through testing and, if necessary, treatment, she may be able to avoid the dire consequences of syphilis and perhaps other STDs. To protect vulnerable persons, public health has traditionally intervened by contact tracing and partner notification. Clinicians are required by law to report most STDs by patient name to public health officials so that they can trace and notify partners at risk. Public officials try to maintain the anonymity of the index case as much as possible. But if Mrs. Miller's only sexual partner has been her husband, it may be difficult or impossible to prevent her from figuring out how she was exposed.

Despite pressure from Mr. Miller, it is ethically and legally unacceptable for Dr. David to cooperate with the request to withhold information that can prevent harm to an identified person at risk. Dr. David should counsel Mr. Miller about the importance of disclosure, including the legal requirements and the risks of nondisclosure, and encourage him to tell his wife. It may be helpful if he offers support in the disclosure process.

Mr. Gordon's case raises somewhat different issues. Here, the concern is whether the physicians have a responsibility to report the fact that a person who drives a sanitation truck for the city is known to have used alcohol and illegal drugs. In this analysis, the justifications underlying the confidentiality obligation would be weighed against the possible harms to unidentified persons—the public—who have no reason to believe that they are at risk. Relevant factors would include the potential for harm, the likelihood that it could be prevented, alternatives to breaching confidentiality, and the legal requirements of the state in which the situation occurs.

While no one would encourage Mr. Gordon to abuse alcohol or drugs, it can be argued that his behavior on this occasion does not place others at immediate or inevitable risk. In this case, the patient's substance-related loss of consciousness occurred on a weekend evening, not during work hours and not while he was driving a truck or any other vehicle. It would be important to know whether his use of alcohol and drugs is substantial or minimal, and whether it occurs daily or only occasionally. This information, which is relevant to his health care as well as the safety of others, is much more likely to be revealed to his caregivers if Mr. Gordon is assured that it will be kept confidential.

In terms of state law, the patient's only illegal behavior is his use of narcotics. Health care professionals should not be expected to compromise their obligations to their patients by functioning as agents of the law enforcement or judicial systems. Accordingly, all states presume a general rule of patient confidentiality, carving out selected specific instances when that obligation must be breached to protect others from harm.

If Mr. Gordon suffered from epilepsy, he would be required by all states to report his condition to the motor vehicle bureau and, if he worked as a school bus driver, his physicians would have a heightened incentive to discourage his driving. The argument might also be made that, if Mr. Gordon did not report his epilepsy, his doctors would have an ethical obligation to do so. None of those conditions apply here, however, and his care professionals are likely to respect his confidentiality, while counseling him about responsible behaviors.

Genomic Testing and Control of Information

The increasing use of and sophistication of genetic/genomic tests raise a variety of new ethical problems related to the control of personal health information. Consider the following:

Illana, a 20-year-old Orthodox Jewish woman, has been increasingly troubled about the fact that her grandmother and her mother had breast cancer. She recently read about a test for the BRCA2 gene that can provide information about the likelihood that she, her brother, or her children will develop the disease. While Illana wants to know her risk of breast cancer, she is afraid to take the test because, if the results are positive and her prospective marriage partner finds out, he may not want to marry her.

Lawrence is a 39-year-old man who works in a large manufacturing company that employs thousands of people. Recently, the management sent out a memo alerting employees to the opportunity to participate in a program of free and confidential testing for several genetic conditions. The memo strongly encouraged employees to be tested "to enhance your knowledge of your health risks and be able to make informed decisions." Lawrence is concerned because, even though the testing is supposed to be confidential, he does not want his employer to know about his family history of heart disease.

Alex and Lauren have been reading about direct-to-consumer (DTC) personal genomic testing (PGT) and they have decided to have full genomic profiles done of their 3-year-old, Hayden, and their 6-month old, Ian. When asked by their friends and family why they are having the testing done, they reply, "We want to know as much as possible about our children's health risks so that we can work with their pediatrician to keep them healthy."

Sophia, an 18-year-old college freshman, is an avid user of Facebook, Twitter, and YouTube. Especially now that she is away at school, her social networking enables her to stay in instant and constant contact with her large circle of friends and family. Prompted by her interest in Biology 101, she has decided to access information on her genetic profile through a DTC-PGT service. When asked, she says, "It's a high-tech way of learning more about myself and my genetic history. Gene mapping is the latest thing and I can't wait to tell my family and friends what I find out."

The remarkable has become commonplace. It seems that every newspaper, journal, news program, and blog features daily bulletins about wondrous technological advances and scientific discoveries, and how they will affect our lives. We have come to expect breakthroughs and wizardry.

Perhaps once or twice in every generation, however, something so momentous occurs that even the most jaded observer pauses to contemplate how the world has shifted. Such is the potential power of the genomic revolution. We have witnessed the deciphering of the human genome, which, while not yet revealing the genetic roots of disease and generating treatments, has opened a window onto who we are, where we come from, how we are constructed, and how we might ultimately enhance the quality of our lives. And, like Adam and Eve, we have also begun to glimpse some of the potential burdens and risks that attend such potent knowledge.

Genetic/genomic testing responds to our insatiable curiosity about ourselves and offers the seductive possibility that information about our genetic makeup could enable us to predict our medical future and empower us to protect ourselves and our children from undesirable medical conditions. Yet it remains unclear exactly what and how much we want or need to know. Information about the likelihood of developing a disease that can be prevented or treated is very different from discovering the inevitability of an illness that has no cure. Possessing information about family genetics begs the question of whether to alert siblings or other relatives to their potential risks. Knowledge may be power but it can also create anxiety and, once learned, it cannot be unlearned.

Some of the ethical questions that require careful attention include the following: What is the appropriate level of protection for genetic/genomic test information? Should access to genomic information be treated differently from access to other sorts of sensitive medical information? Is genetic/genomic test information exceptional with respect to permissible use? When are the risks to others revealed by genetic/genomic testing sufficient to justify breaching confidentiality? What are the ethical concerns related to DTC gene tic tests that provide information without the explanation and counseling that are routinely part of medical testing? These are cutting-edge issues that give a very contemporary spin to some traditional bioethical problems.

For those who believe in what has been called "genetic exceptionalism," the type of information acquired by gene tic testing is unique because of its implications for other persons who are genetically related to the tested individual, and the rules concerning privacy and confidentiality have to be modified accordingly. For those who reject this view, gene tic data are not the only sort of information that has health implications for those related to the tested individual and, therefore, the normal rules concerning privacy and confidentiality apply. Widespread misconceptions about the meaning and significance of genetic information also raise concerns about its proper use and the marketing of genetic/genomic tests.

References

Ahronheim JC, Moreno JD, Zuckerman C. 2000. *Ethics in Clinical Practice*. 2nd ed. Gaithersburg, MD: Aspen Publishers.

American College of Physicians. 1993. *Ethics Manual*. 3rd ed. Philadelphia: American College of Physicians. Cited in Witman AB, Park DM, Hardin SB. 1996. How do patients want physicians to handle mistakes? *Archives of Internal Medicine* 156(22):2565–69.

American Medical Association, Council on Ethical and Judicial Affairs. 1997. Patient information: Opinion E-8.12, issued March 1981, updated June 1994. *Code of Medical Ethics*. Chicago: American Medical Association.

Bauer KA. 2009. Privacy and confidentiality in the age of e-medicine. *Journal of Health Care Law & Policy* 12:47–62.

Baylis F. 1997. Errors in medicine: Nurturing truthfulness. *Journal of Clinical Ethics* 8(4):336–40.

Beauchamp TL, Childress JF. 2001. *Principles of Biomedical Ethics*. 5th ed. New York: Oxford University Press, pp. 283–319.

Beauchamp TL, Childress JF. 2013. *Principles of Biomedical Ethics*. 7th ed. New York: Oxford University Press, pp. 302–24.

Belkin L. 1997. How can we save the next victim? *The New York Times Magazine*, June 15, pp. 28–70.

Berger JT. 1998. Culture and ethnicity in clinical care. *Archives of Internal Medicine* 158(19):2085–90.

Bok S. 1983. The limits of confidentiality. *Hastings Center Report*: 24–31.

Brodsky M, et al. 2008. Multiple sclerosis risk after optic neuritis: Final optic neuritis trial follow-up. *Archives of Neurology* 65(6):727–32.

Cullen S, Klein M. 2000. Respect for patients, physicians and the truth. In Munson R, ed. *Intervention and Reflection: Basic Issues in Medical Ethics*. 6th ed. Belmont, CA: Wadsworth, pp. 435–42.

Dresser R. 2008. The limits of apology laws. *Hastings Center Report* 38(3):6–7.

Freedman B. 2003. Offering truth: One ethical approach to the uninformed cancer patient. In Steinbock B, Arras JD, London AJ, eds. *Ethical Issues in Modern Medicine*. 6th ed. Boston: McGraw-Hill, pp. 76–82.

Gallagher TH, Waterman AD, Ebers AG, Fraser VJ, Levinson W. 2003. Patients' and physicians' attitudes regarding the disclosure of medical errors. *Journal of the American Medical Association* 289(8):1001–7.

Goldberg RM, Kuhn G, Andrew LB, Thomas HA. 2002. Coping with medical mistakes and errors in judgment. *Annals of Emergency Medicine* 39(3):287–92.

Greenberg MA. 1991. The consequences of truth telling. *Journal of the American Medical Association* 266(1):66.

Hermann DHJ, Gagliano RD. 1989. AIDS, therapeutic confidentiality, and warning third parties. *Mary land Law Review* 48(1):55–76.

Institute of Medicine, Committee on Quality of Health Care in America. 2000. *To Err Is Human: Building a Safer Health System*. Washington, DC: National Academy Press.

Jansen LA, Ross LF. 2000. Patient confidentiality and the surrogate's right to know. *Journal of Law, Medicine & Ethics* 28:137–43.

Joint Commission on Accreditation of Healthcare Organizations. 2014. Patient Rights and Organization Ethics Chapter (RI), Standard

RI.1.1.3; Intent of Standard RI.1.1.3. *Comprehensive Accreditation Manual for Hospitals*. Oakbrook, IL: Joint Commission on Accreditation of Healthcare Organizations.

Kagawa-Singer M, Blackhall LJ. 2001. Negotiating cross-cultural issues at the end of life: "You've got to go where he lives." *Journal of the American Medical Association* 286(23):2993–3001.

Kohn LT, Corrigan JM, Donaldson M, eds. 1999. *To Err Is Human: Building a Safer Health System*. A report from the Committee on Quality of Healthcare in America, Institute of Medicine, National Academy of Sciences. Washington, DC: National Academy Press.

Krumholz A, Fisher RS, Lesser RP, Hauser WA. 1991. Driving and epilepsy: A review and reappraisal. *Journal of the American Medical Association* 265(5):622–26.

Levinson W, Roter DL, Mullooly JP, et al. 1997. Physician-patient communication: The relationship with malpractice claims among primary care physicians and surgeons. *Journal of the American Medical Association* 277(7):553–59.

Liebman CB, Hyman CS. 2004. A mediation skills model to manage disclosure of errors and adverse events to patients. *Health Affairs* 23(4):22–32.

Liebman CB, Hyman CS. 2006. Prescription for improving the way health care and legal systems deal with unanticipated outcomes in medical care. Presentation, the Association of the Bar of the City of New York, May 24.

Mastroianni AC, et al. 2010. The flaws in state "apology" and "disclosure" laws dilute their intended impact on malpractice suits. *Health Affairs* 29(9):1611–19.

McDonnell WM, Guenther E. 2008. Narrative review: Do state laws make it easier to say "I'm sorry?" *Annals of Internal Medicine* 149:811–15.

McGuire AL, Fisher R, Cusenza P, Hudson K, Rothstein MA, McGraw D, Matteson S, Glasser J, Henley DE. 2008 July. Confidentiality, privacy, and security of genetic and genomic test information in electronic health records: Points to consider. *Gene tic Medicine* 10(7):495–99.

Novack DH, Detering BJ, Arnold R, et al. 1989. Physicians' attitudes toward using deception to resolve difficult ethical problems. *Journal of the American Medical Association* 261(20):2980–85.

Pellegrino ED. 1992. Is truth telling to the patient a cultural artifact? *Journal of the American Medical Association* 268(13):1734–35.

Ptacek JT, Eberhardt T. 1996. Breaking bad news: A review of the literature. *Journal of the American Medical Association* 276(6):496–502.

Quill TE, Townsend P. 1991. Bad news: Delivery, dialogue, and dilemmas. *Archives of Internal Medicine* 151(3):463–68.

Ruddick W. 1999. Hope and deception. *Bioethics* 13(3/4):343–57.

Siegler M. 1982. Confidentiality in medicine—a decrepit concept. *New En gland Journal of Medicine* 307:1518–21.

Sigman GS, Kraut J, La Puma J. 2003. Disclosure of a diagnosis to children and adolescents when parents object. In Beauchamp TL, Walters L, eds. *Contemporary Issues in Bioethics*. 6th ed. Belmont, CA: Wadsworth-Thomson Learning, pp. 133–38.

Stein J. 2000. A fragile commodity. *Journal of the American Medical Association* 283(3):305–6.

Surbonne A. 1992. Truth telling to the patient. *Journal of the American Medical Association* 268(13):1661–62.

Tarasoff v. Regents of the University of California, 551 P.2d 334 (Cal. 1976).

Thomasma DC. 2003. Telling the truth to patients: A clinical ethics exploration. In Beauchamp TL, Walters L, eds. *Contemporary Issues in Bioethics*. 6th ed. Belmont, CA: Wadsworth-Thomson Learning, pp. 128–32.

Vincent C. 2003. Understanding and responding to adverse events. *New England Journal of Medicine* 348(11):1051–56.

Vogel J, Delgado R. 1980. To tell the truth: Physicians' duty to disclose medical mistakes. *UCLA Law Review* 28:52–94.

Wu AW, Cavanaugh TA, McPhee SJ, et al. 1997. To tell the truth: Ethical and practical issues in disclosing medical mistakes to patients. *Journal of General Internal Medicine* 12(12):770–75.

Zahedi F. 2011. The challenge of truth telling across cultures: A case study. *Journal of Medical Ethics and History of Medicine* 4:11.

Introduction to the Social Roots of Health Disparities

David A. Barr

*W**hy are some people healthy and others not?* This is a question that has gained increasing attention in the United States over the last several years. It is also the title of a book published in 1994. The contributors to that book come to two basic conclusions.

First, in trying to improve health in developed societies, we have focused most of our attention in recent years on improving the quality and availability of health care.

> Modern societies devote a very large proportion of their economic resources to the production of *health care*. ... Such massive efforts reflect a widespread belief that the availability and use of health care is central to the health of both individuals and populations. (Evans and Stoddart 1994, p. 27)

Second, most of the variability in health status we find in the United States and other developed countries has little to do with health care and everything to do with one's position in the social hierarchy.

> Some of the best-kept secrets of longevity and good health are to be found in one's social, economic, and cultural circumstances. ... The largest gap lies between the richest and the poorest. But the middle classes are also

affected. The lower one is situated on the social hierarchy ... the lower one's probability of staying in good health and the lower one's life expectancy. (Renaud 1994, p. 322)

Nowhere has the emphasis on improving health through advancing the technology of health care been more evident than in the United States. As shown in Figure 3.5.1, the proportion of the U.S. economy that goes for providing health care rose from just over 10 percent in 1987 to 17.9 percent in 2011.

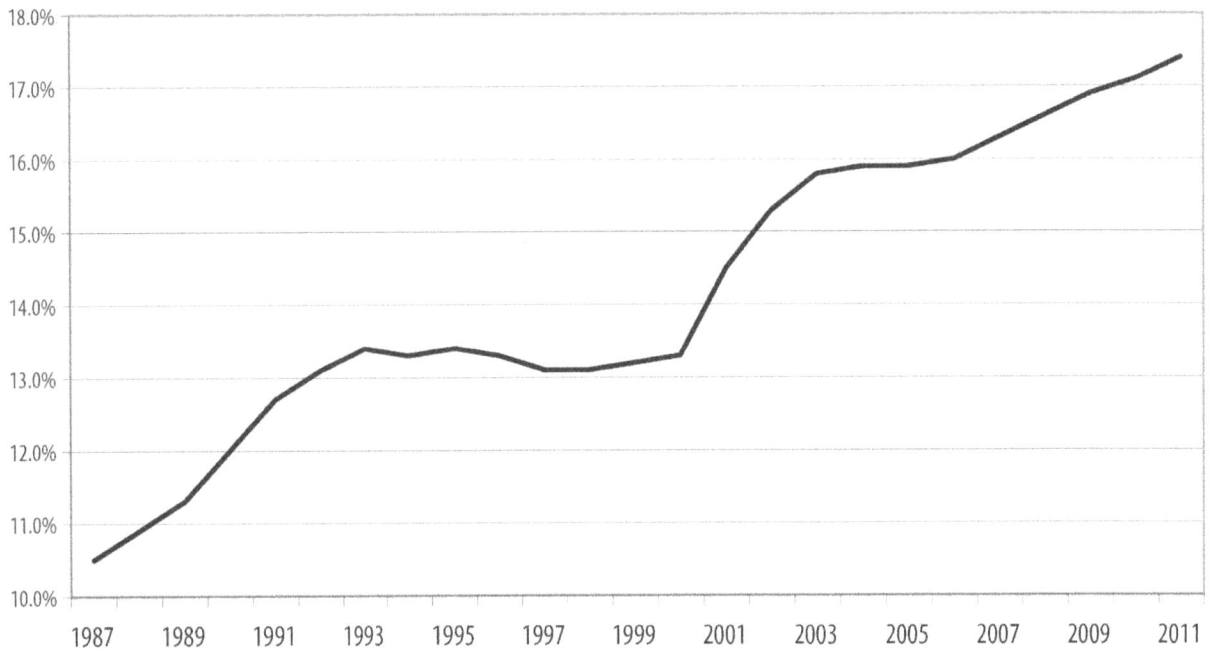

Figure 3.5.1   National health expenditures as percentage of GDP, 1987–2011.

Centers for Medicare and Medicaid Services, National Health Expenditures 1960–2011, https://www.cms.gov/Research-Statistics-Data-and-Systems/Statistics-Trends-and-Reports/NationalHealthExpendData/NationalHealthAccountsHistorical.html, accessed 5/8/13.

This heavy investment in new medications, new facilities, and the new technology of advanced procedures underscores the faith of the American public in the power of health care to improve health status. Yet, in comparing ourselves to other developed countries that have made different policy decisions about investing national resources in health care, we find a striking inconsistency. As shown in Table 3.5.1, we spend much more of our national economy on health care than any other developed country in the world. However, using two common measures of population health, our population has worse health status than the population in any of these other countries.

Life expectancy estimates how many years, on average, a baby born today can expect to live. (Given consistent difference between males and females, this figure is typically broken down by gender.) Babies born in the United States can expect to live between two and five years less than babies born in other developed countries.

Infant mortality estimates the following statistic: of a thousand babies born alive, how many will die before their first birthday? We see that the United States has the highest infant mortality rate of any of the countries listed. In fact, in 2010 the United States had a higher infant mortality rate than 30 of the 34 countries in the Organization for Economic Co-operation and Development, an association of the most developed countries in the world. The U.S. infant mortality rate was only better than those of Chile, Turkey, and Mexico.

Table 3.5.1 Health Indexes, Selected OECD Countrie010

Country	GDP Spent on Health Care (percent)	Infant Mortality Rate	Male Life Expectancy at Birth (years)	Female Life Expectancy at Birth (years)
Japan	9.5	2.3	79.6	86.4
Sweden	9.6	2.5	79.5	83.5
France	11.6	3.6	78.0	84.7
Germany	11.6	3.4	78.0	83.0
Switzerland	11.4	3.8	80.3	84.9
Greece	10.2	3.8	78.4	82.8
Canada	11.4	5.1	78.5	83.1
United Kingdom	9.6	4.2	78.6	82.6
United States	17.6	6.1	76.2	81.1

Source: Data from OECD, http://www.oecd.org/statistics/, accessed 5/8/13.

How is it that we, as a country, invest so much of our economy in providing *health care,* but we get so little in return in the form of *health*—at least health as measured by these common statistics? Perhaps our basic assumption—that more health care will lead, necessarily, to better health—is flawed. Perhaps something other than health care drives the health of a community or a society.

Economist Victor Fuchs addressed this issue in 1983 in his seminal book *Who Shall Live?* Fuchs tells us "A Tale of Two States" (pp. 52–54), comparing demographic characteristics and health status in two adjacent states in the United States, Nevada and Utah. Using data from the 1960s and 1970s, he found that the two states had similar populations using measures such as income, education, age distribution, and access to health care. However, the health of those who live in Nevada was substantially worse than that of those who live in Utah. Infant mortality was 40 percent higher in Nevada than in Utah. Death rates were consistently higher in Nevada for all age groups—a bout 40 percent higher for young adults, 50 to 70 percent higher for those ages 40 to 49. When one looks at two specific illnesses with known causes, the differences in death rates are even more striking. The combined death rate in Nevada from lung cancer (associated with cigarette smoking) and cirrhosis of the liver (associated with alcohol abuse) ranged from 100 percent higher to nearly 600 percent higher than the comparable rate in Utah, depending on the age range and gender studied.

The reader will no doubt recognize why Nevada and Utah had such strikingly different health statistics, despite having populations that were generally similar in demographic characteristics and their access to health care. The influence of the Mormon Church in Utah has led to much lower rates of smoking and alcohol abuse in that state. In addition, those in Utah experience lower rates of divorce and migration. Nevada, on the other hand, has an economy and a culture that includes higher rates of smoking and alcohol consumption, higher divorce rates, and higher rates of geographic migration. Life in Nevada is fundamentally different from life in Utah. Those lifestyle factors, and not the availability of health care, drove the differences between the two states in terms of health status. As described by Victor Fuchs (1986, pp. 274–76),

> The basic finding is the following: when the state of medical science and other health-determining variables are held constant, the marginal contribution of medical care to health is very small in modern nations. … For most of man's history, [per capita] income has been the primary determinant of health and life expectancy—the major explanation for differences in health among nations and among groups within a nation.

To illustrate the relationship between the availability of health care, the standard of living, and mortality rates, let us look at death rates from tuberculosis (TB) in England and Wales. Figure 3.5.2 shows the decline in the death rate from TB following the discovery in the late 1940s of the first drugs that were effective against TB and the development in the 1950s of the first vaccine used to prevent TB.

It appears that the advent of antituberculosis drugs and a tuberculosis vaccine—two key additions to the health care regimen available to treat TB—were effective in reducing the death rate. However, when one takes a longer time frame, the picture that emerges is quite different. Figure 3 shows the decline in the death rate from TB in England and Wales from 1840 to 1970.

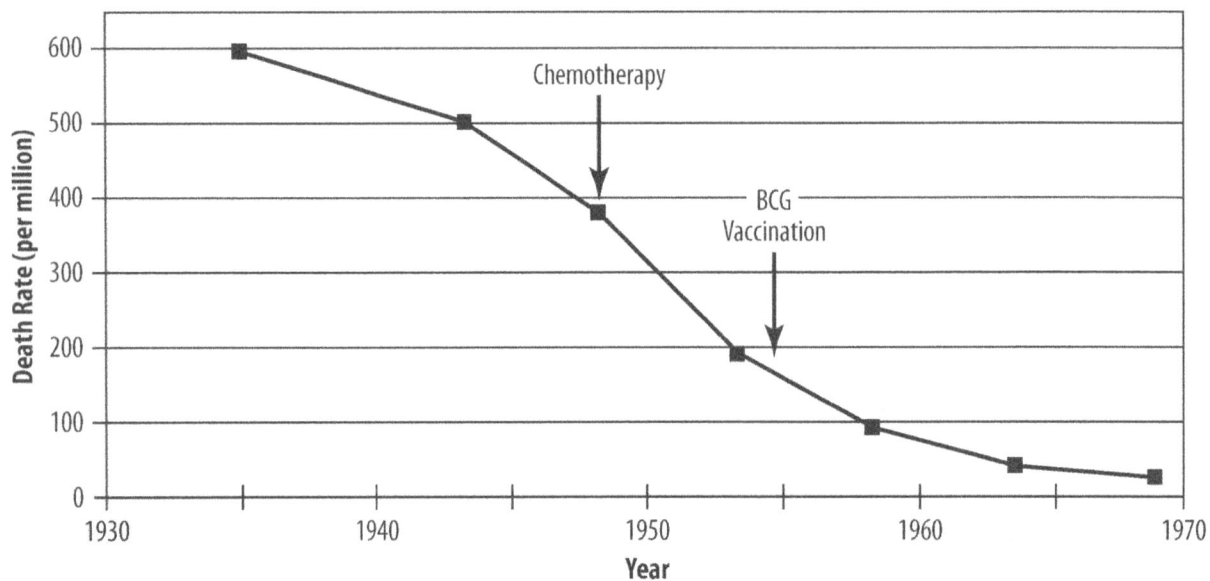

Figure 3.5.2   Mean annual death rates (standardized to 1901 population) from respiratory tuberculosis, England and Wales, 1935–70.

Evans et al. (1994); McKeown (1979).

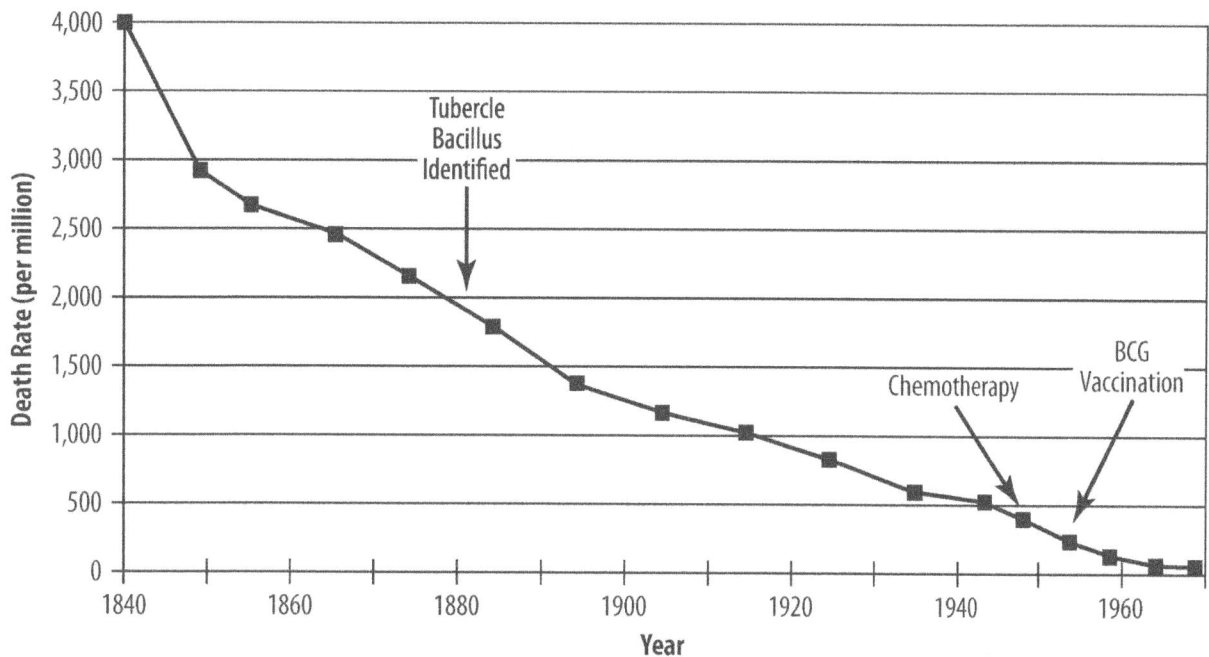

Figure 3.5.3   Mean annual death rates (standardized to 1901 population) from respiratory tuberculosis, England and Wales, 1840–1970.

Evans et al. (1994); McKeown (1979).

From the longer-range perspective, it appears that the health care developments of the mid-twentieth century had relatively little effect on the overall death rate from TB. In fact, half of the decline in the rate of death from TB took place before the tubercle bacillus responsible for TB was discovered. While the number of deaths declined by 51 percent between 1948 and 1971 following the introduction of medications and a vaccine, most of the overall decline had taken place before any effective medical treatment was available (McKeown 1979).

If health care was not responsible for the decline in death rates from TB, then what was? Consistent with Fuchs's comments above, the rising standard of living seen in England and Wales in the nineteenth and twentieth centuries can explain the falling death rates. Better nutrition, better sanitation, better housing, and less crowding, combined with public health measures to prevent the spread of TB, accounted for most of the decline in death rate over the last 200 years.

To illustrate this point, and to underscore the role income and standard of living play in reducing the chance of death from TB, let us consider two fictional persons, one from the world of music and one from the field of literature. The opera *La Boheme,* first performed in 1896, tells the story of Mimi, a poor seamstress struggling to survive in the Latin quarter of Paris. She meets and falls in love with Rodolfo, an equally poor poet who has to burn the pages of a play he was writing to stay warm. The opera tells us of the love between Rodolfo and Mimi and of Rodolfo's hesitance when he learns Mimi has TB. The lovers struggle to stay together (and to stay warm), only to have Mimi die tragically, succumbing to her disease.

Thomas Mann first began writing his novel *Magic Mountain* in 1912. It tells the story of Hans Castorp, the son of a well-to-do German family who goes to visit his cousin in a TB sanatorium high in the Swiss Alps. What was originally intended as a stay of only a few weeks extends to seven years of intensive therapy, as it turns out that Hans himself has developed TB. Seven years of sumptuous meals, fresh air, exercise, and companionship help Hans to fight off his disease, only to be drafted into the German army at the beginning of World War I (a conflict in which he is likely to be killed).

What if their roles had been reversed? If Mimi had been from a wealthy French family and Hans from a poor German family, which one would have survived TB? For more than a century, where you are on the social hierarchy has been a strong predictor of whether you live or die from a disease such as TB.

The standard of living available to those lower on the social hierarchy has been a powerful predictor of how many of them would die from the many infectious diseases that ravaged Eu rope and North America during much of the twentieth century. From 1900 through 1970, the United States experienced a steady decline in the overall death rate. As was the case in England and Wales, the rising standard of living seen in the United States during this period was associated with a steady fall in the rate of death from infectious diseases such as measles, tuberculosis, pneumonia, diphtheria, typhoid, and polio. It was also the case that the antibiotics and vaccines to treat these diseases were among the important medical discoveries of the twentieth century. However, as with the case of tuberculosis in England and Wales, most of the decline in the death rate for each of nine most feared infectious diseases occurred before the medical treatment for that disease was discovered (McKinlay and McKinlay 1997). Better health, in this case measured by reduced death rates from infectious diseases, was associated principally with rising levels of income and improvements in the standard of living. Advances in medical care played a smaller role in reducing the death rate from these illnesses.

By the end of the twentieth century, deaths from infectious diseases had declined substantially and were largely replaced by deaths from three major chronic diseases: heart disease, cancer, and stroke. With the tremendous advances in medical care seen during the last part of the twentieth century, we might expect to see death rates from these and other chronic diseases falling substantially. Yet, when we look at the actual death rates in the United States from the six leading causes of death, adjusted for changes in the age distribution of the population over this time, we see a mixed record of success (Jemal et al. 2005). The death rate from heart disease and accidents showed a sharp decline from 1970 through 2002, while the death rate from stroke declined at a slower rate. The death rate from cancer and diabetes changed relatively little during this time, and the death rate from chronic lung disease actually rose. By 2011, heart disease, cancer, chronic lung disease, and stroke accounted for 59 percent of all deaths in the United States (National Center for Health Statistics, 2013).

If measles, tuberculosis, and pneumonia have now been replaced by heart disease, cancer, and stroke as principal causes of death, will Fuchs's point—that differences in income are the principal determinant of differences in health status—still hold? An answer to this question has been provided by the Whitehall study, conducted over a period of several decades in Eng land. The study has been following employees in the British Civil Service, recording many aspects of their health status over time. It compares the health of four principal groups of employees:

1. the administrators who work at the highest ranks of the Civil Service
2. the professional and executive employees who carry out much of the work of the Civil Service, under the supervision of the administrators
3. the clerical workers who provide the staff support for their professional and executive

supervisors

4. the other workers, not in any of these employment categories, who clean the floors, take out the trash, and serve the food in the cafeteria

As one might expect, the level of education and training required to work in each of these categories is quite different. The administrators tend to have more education than the executive employees, who in turn have more education than the clerical workers, and so on down the line. Also not surprisingly, the income of each category tends to be higher than the income of the category immediately below it.

Each category of worker is fully employed, and each tends to work in similar physical surroundings. Each has access to the full level of health care provided by the British National Health Service. Will we see the same hierarchical difference in death rates in British Civil Service workers that we saw between Mimi and Hans when faced with tuberculosis? Figure 3.5.4 provides an answer to this question.

Figure 3.5.4 graphs the cumulative death rate from all causes over 10 years of observation for each of the four categories of employee described above. It seems clear that administrative employees have a substantially lower rate of death than the janitors, cafeteria workers, and "others" in this category. If Hans had been an administrator in the British Civil Service and Mimi a maid who cleans the bathrooms for the Civil Service, she would be more likely to die during this time period than he.

However, the comparison between the highest class of worker and the lowest is only part of the story. Each category of worker has a lower death rate than the category immediately below it. With each step down the employment hierarchy, health deteriorates and the chance of death goes up. Repeating Renaud's comment from the beginning of this [reading], "the lower one is situated on the social hierarchy ... the lower one's probability of staying in good health and the lower one's life expectancy" (Renaud 1994, p. 322)

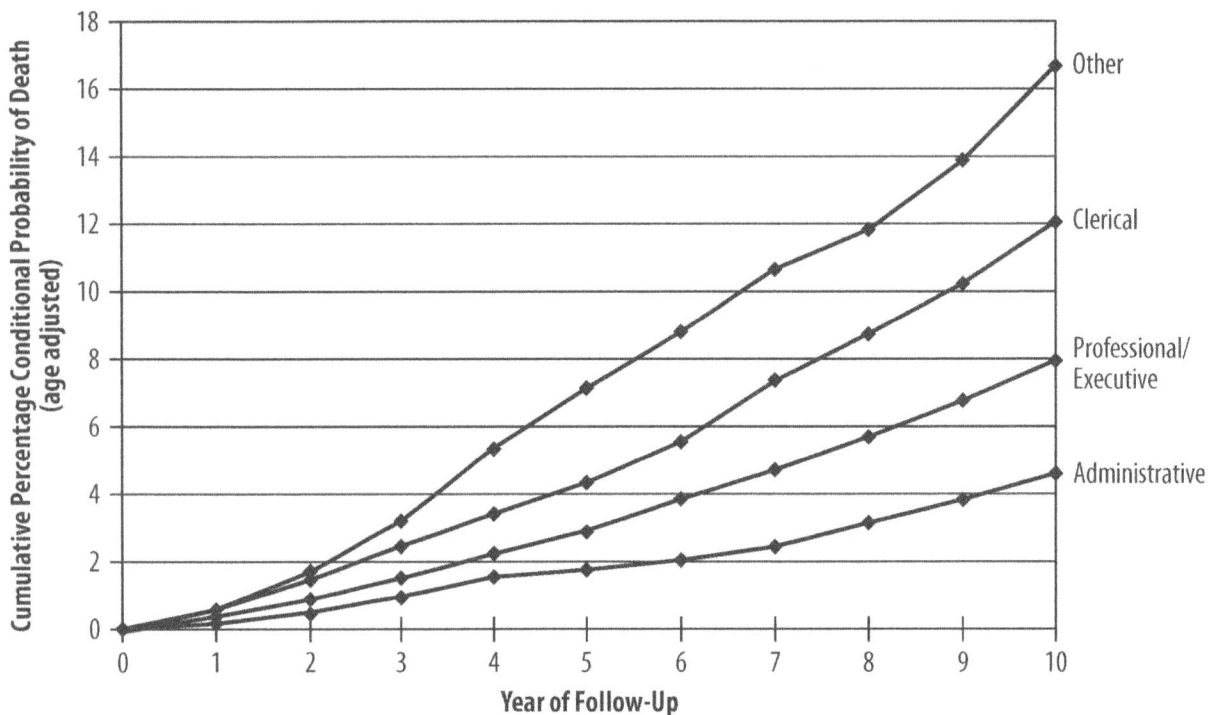

Figure 3.5.4   Cumulative probability of death based on occupational category within the British Civil Service—the Whitehall study.

Marmot et al. (1984), used by permission of Elsevier Limited.

The Whitehall study is not a study of how poverty is related to the chance of death or illness. It is a study of people who are employed and who have regular access to health care. It is important to appreciate that the relationship between income and health is not dichotomous, with only those who fall below some threshold of poverty suffering the health consequences of being at the bottom of the social hierarchy. Even though the majority of research published between 1975 and 2000 on the relationship between social class and health focused on the effects of poverty, it is clear from the Whitehall study and numerous others that the relationship between social class and health—between one's position on the social hierarchy and one's likelihood of either illness or death—is a continuous relationship that spans all levels of the social hierarchy, from the very lowest to the very highest (Adler and Ostrove 1999).

Figure 3.5.5 illustrates the two conceptual models of the relationship between income and health. The horizontal axis measures income—typically family income. The vertical axis represents the likelihood that an individual at a given income level will enjoy good health, whether measured by the rate of illness or the chance of death. In the threshold model, those who live in poverty have lower health status than those who live above the poverty line (the poverty line measured by the federal government and used to qualify those who fall below it for a variety of benefits). Once a family receives a level of income sufficient to meet its basic needs for food, clothing, and housing, there is no further health benefit to a rising standard of living.

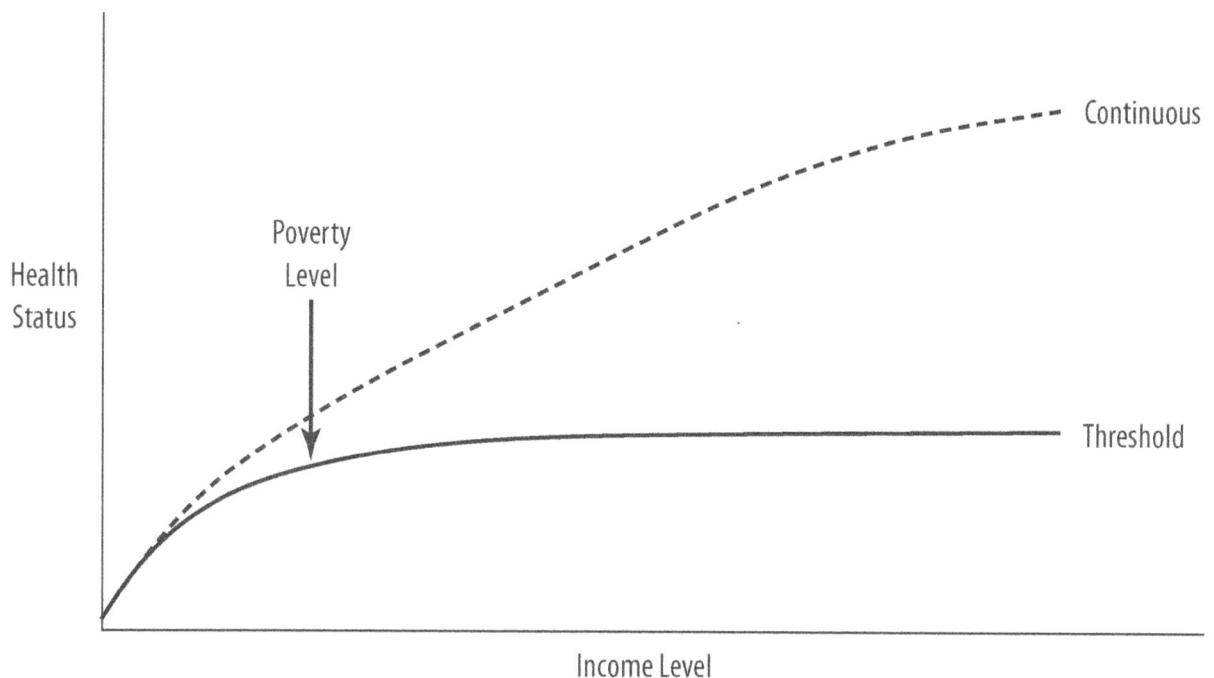

Figure 3.5.5   Two models of the association between income level and health status

By contrast, the continuous model in Figure 3.5.5 suggests that there is, indeed, a health benefit to escaping poverty. However, the farther a family gets from poverty—the higher its income and associated standard of living—the better its health becomes. Even though neither lives in poverty, an executive employee brings in more income than a clerical employee and accordingly enjoys better health. That better health status extends to the members of the executive's family as well. An administrative employee, in turn, enjoys a higher standard of living and better health than the executive employee who works under his or her direction. This is the message of the Whitehall study.

Health psychologist Nancy Adler and colleagues have looked thoroughly at the association between socioeconomic status (SES) and health status. (SES measures status within the social hierarchy according to a number of measures in addition to income. [...]) In a series of publications (Adler et al. 1994; Adler and Ostrove 1999), they summarized the research in this area that firmly supports the continuous model of this association. They analyzed the results of eight separate studies, each measuring the association between SES and the mortality rate—either the overall adult mortality rate for those at a given level of SES or the infant mortality rate. In each of these studies, with every step down the SES hierarchy, the chance of death, either adult death or infant death, goes up.

Adler and colleagues also summarized studies investigating the association between SES and health measured as the rate of certain chronic illness within a given SES group. Again, the relationship is clearly a continuous one. With every step down the SES hierarchy, the chances go up of having arthritis, high blood pressure, and other chronic diseases that reduce one's quality of life. Of course, this does not mean that every person in a lower SES category will have a higher rate of illness and an earlier death than every person in a higher SES category. The mortality rates and illness rates are statistical averages that accurately state the likelihood that an individual within the indicated category will have the outcome that is being measured. In 1900 a poor seamstress was more likely to die from tuberculosis than was the son of an affluent family. In 2000 a poor seamstress was more likely to contract high blood pressure and arthritis, to have her infant die before its first birthday, and herself to die earlier than the son of an affluent family. While the circumstances in which Mimi and Hans Castorp lived have changed dramatically over the hundred years following their fictional lives, with countless medical advances, their health status relative to each other has changed little.

This association between social status and health status holds both for the United Kingdom and for the United States. In the United Kingdom, all residents are provided health care through the British National Health Service. The United States has taken a more fragmented and incremental approach to providing health care to its residents. Rather than a right of citizenship, health care in the United States has historically been treated largely as a market commodity, available to those who are willing (and able) to pay for it. As described in 1986 by health economist Uwe Reinhardt: "Americans have ... decided to treat health care as essentially a private consumer good of which the poor might be guaranteed a basic package, but which is otherwise to be distributed more and more on the basis of ability to pay" (Reinhard and Relman 1986, p. 23).

Since the 1960s the federal and state governments have provided coverage for certain of the most vulnerable segments of our society, including the elderly and the very poor. However, in 2012, two years after the Affordable Care Act (ACA) was signed into law, 48 million people, most of them in low-to moderate-income working families, had no health insurance and as a result had little access to health care (U.S. Census Bureau 2013). Beginning in 2014, the changes enacted as part of ACA are expected to reduce the number of uninsured Americans by between 30 and 33 million people, while still leaving between 26 and 27 million people without health insurance (U.S. Congressional Bud get Office 2012).

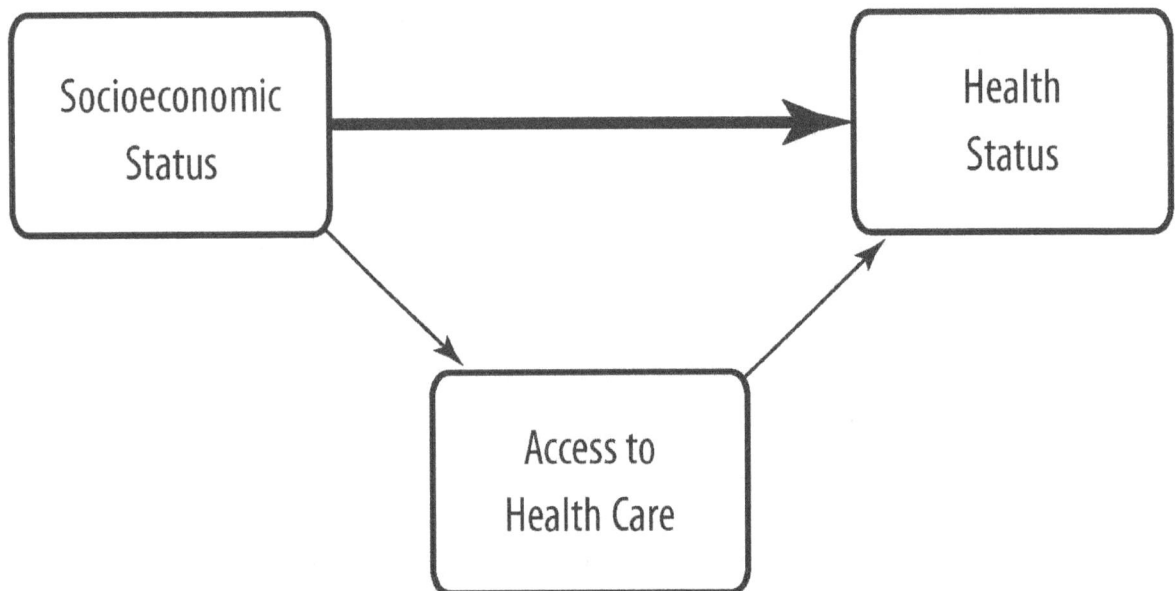

Figure 3.5.6   The association between social position, access to health care, and health status

In understanding the association between social position and health in the United States, we cannot ignore the very real economic barriers to health care that still exist. It seems clear that income and other measures of social position affect health directly, as well as affecting it indirectly through impaired access to health care. This relationship is illustrated in Figure 3.5.6, in which the width of the arrows indicates the strength of the relationship.

Before we can understand these relationships and the causal factors behind them more fully, we first need to look at the SES concept in more depth. What are the measures of SES other than income? Does it matter how long one is in a position of disadvantaged SES? [...]

Before looking at the relationship between SES and health, we must first under-stand what we mean by "health." Is there more than one way to measure health? Which is more important, health as perceived by the individual or health as measured by objective scales or the impressions of health professionals?

References

Adler, N. A., Boyce, T., Chesney, M. A., et al. 1994. Socioeconomic status and health: The challenge of the gradient. *American Psychologist* 49:15– 24.

Adler, N., and Ostrove, J. 1999. Socioeconomic status and health: What we know and what we don't. *Annals of the New York Academy of Sciences* 896:3– 15

Evans, R. G., Barer, M. L., and Marmor, T. R., eds. 1994. *Why Are Some People Healthy and Others Not?* New York: Aldine De Gruyter.

Evans, R. G., and Stoddart, G. L. 1994. Producing health, consuming health care. In Evans, R. G., Barer, M. L., and Marmor, T. R., eds., *Why Are Some People Healthy and Others Not?* 27– 54. New York: Aldine De Gruyter.

Fuchs, V. R. 1983. *Who Shall Live?* New York: Basic Books.

Fuchs, V. R. 1986. *The Health Economy*. Cambridge, MA: Harvard University Press.

Jemal, A., Ward, E., Hao, Y., and Thun, M. 2005. *Trends in the leading causes of death in the United States, 1970– 2002*. JAMA 294:1255– 59.

McKeown, T. 1979. *The Role of Medicine*. Princeton: Prince ton University Press.

McKinlay, J., McKinlay, S. 1997. Medical measures and the decline of mortality. In Conrad, P., ed. *The Sociology of Health and Illness*, 10– 23. New York: St. Martin's Press.

Reinhardt, U. E., Relman, A. S. 1986. Debating for-profit health care and the ethics of physicians. *Health Affairs* 5(2):5– 31.

Renaud, M. 1994. The future: Hygeia versus Panakeia. In Evans, R. G., Barer, M. L., Marmor, T. R., eds., *Why Are Some People Healthy and Others Not?* 317– 34. New York: Aldine De Gruyter.

U.S. Centers for Medicare and Medicaid Services. Data on national health care expenditures. Available at www.cms.hhs.gov/NationalHealthExpendData.

U.S. Congressional Bud get Office. 2012. Updated Estimates for the Insurance Coverage Provisions of the Affordable Care Act. Available at http://www.cbo.gov/sites/default/files/cbofiles/attachments/03-13-Coverage %20Estimates.pdf (accessed May 9, 2013).

Selections from "Securing Access to Health Care"

President's Commission for the Study of Ethical Problems in Medicine and Biomedical and Behavioral Research

President's Commission for the Study of Ethical Problems in Medicine and Biomedical and Behavioral Research, Selections from *Securing Access to Health Care*, pp. 1-7, 11-13, 16-47, 1983.

Introduction

The prevention of death and disability, the relief of pain and suffering, the restoration of functioning: these are the aims of health care. Beyond its tangible benefits, health care touches on countless important and in some ways mysterious aspects of personal life that invest it with significant value as a thing in itself. In recognition of these special features, the President's Commission was mandated to study the ethical and legal implications of differences in the availability of health services.[1] In this Report to the President and Congress, the Commission sets forth an ethical standard: access for all to an adequate level of care without the imposition of excessive burdens. It believes that this is the standard against which proposals for legislation and regulation in this field ought to be measured.

In fulfilling its mandate from Congress, the Commission discusses an ethical response to differences in people's access to health care. To do so, it is necessary both to examine

1. 42 U.S.C. § 300v-1(a)(1)(D)(Supp. 1981).

the extent of those differences and to try to understand how they arise. This focus on the problems of access ought not to obscure the great strengths of the American health care system. The matchless contributions made by America's biomedical scientists to medical knowledge and techniques, the high skill and compassionate devotion of countless physicians and other health professionals, the extensive financial protection against health care costs available to most people, the great generosity with time and funds of many individuals and organizations—these are the hallmarks of health care in the United States. Therefore, the objective here is not to disparage the system but merely to encourage responsible decisionmakers—in the private sector and at all levels of government—to strive to ensure that every American has a fair opportunity to benefit from it.

Health care is a field in which two important American traditions are manifested: the responsibility of each individual for his or her own welfare and the obligations of the community to its members. These two values are complementary rather than conflicting; the emphasis on one or the other varies with the facts of a particular situation. In the field of health care, personal responsibility is a corollary of personal self-determination, which the Commission discussed in its recent report on informed consent.[2] At the same time, ill health is often a matter of chance that can have devastating consequences; thus, concern has long been expressed that health care be widely available and not unfairly denied to those in need.

Since the nineteenth century, the United States has acted—through the founding of the Public Health Service and of hospitals for seamen, veterans, and native Americans, and through special health programs for mothers and infants, children, the elderly, the disabled, and the poor—to reaffirm the special place of health care in American society. With the greatly increased powers of biomedical science to cure as well as to relieve suffering, these traditional concerns about the special importance of health care have been magnified.

In both their means and their particular objectives, public programs in health care have varied over the years. Some have been aimed at assuring the productivity of the work force, others at protecting particularly vulnerable or deserving groups, still others at manifesting the country's commitment to equality of opportunity. Nonetheless, most programs have rested on a common rationale: to ensure that care be made accessible to a group whose health needs would otherwise not be adequately met.[3]

The consequence of leaving health care solely to market forces—the mechanism by which most things are allocated in American society—is not viewed as acceptable when a significant portion of the population lacks access to health services. Of course, government financing programs, such as Medicare and Medicaid as well as public programs that provide care directly to veterans and the military and through local public hospitals, have greatly improved access to health care. These efforts, coupled with the expanded availability of private health insurance, have resulted in almost 90% of Americans having some form of health insurance coverage. Yet the patchwork of government programs and the uneven availability of private health insurance through the workplace have excluded millions of people. The Surgeon General

2. President's Commission for the Study of Ethical Problems in Medicine and Biomedical and Behavioral Research, MAKING HEALTH CARE DECISIONS, U.S. Government Printing Office, Washington (1982).

3. Although public programs have generally rested on this rationale, some have been structured so as to include people who could obtain adequate care on their own without excessive burdens. Medicare, for example, covers virtually all of the elderly, not only those who cannot afford the cost of care.

has stated that "with rising unemployment, the numbers are shifting rapidly. We estimate that from 18 to 25 million Americans—8 to 11 percent of the population—have no health insurance coverage at all."[4] Many of these people lack effective access to health care, and many more who have some form of insurance are unprotected from the severe financial burdens of sickness.

Nor is this a problem only for the moment. The Secretary of Health and Human Services recently observed that despite the excellence of American medical care, "we do have this perennial problem of about 10% of the population falling through the cracks."[5] What is needed now are ethical principles that offer practical guidance so that health policymakers in Federal, state, and local governments can act responsibly in an era of fiscal belt tightening without abandoning society's commitment to fair and adequate health care.

Summary of Conclusions

In this Report, the President's Commission does not propose any new policy initiatives, for its mandate lies in ethics not in health policy development. But it has tried to provide a framework within which debates about health policy might take place, and on the basis of which policymakers can ascertain whether some proposals do a better job than others of securing health care on an equitable basis.

In 1952, the President's Commission on the Health Needs of the Nation concluded that "access to the means for the attainment and preservation of health is a basic human right."[6] Instead of speaking in terms of "rights," however, the current Commission believes its conclusions are better expressed in terms of "ethical obligations."

The Commission concludes that society has an ethical obligation to ensure equitable access to health care for all. This obligation rests on the special importance of health care: its role in relieving suffering, preventing premature death, restoring functioning, increasing opportunity, providing information about an individual's condition, and giving evidence of mutual empathy and compassion. Furthermore, although life-style and the environment can affect health status, differences in the need for health care are for the most part undeserved and not within an individual's control.

In speaking of society, the Commission uses the term in its broadest sense to mean the collective American community. The community is made up of individuals who are in turn members of many other, overlapping groups, both public and private: local, state, regional, and national units; professional and workplace organizations; religious, educational, and charitable institutions; and family, kinship, and ethnic groups. All these entities play a role in discharging societal obligations.

---

4. *Interview with Dr. C. Everett Koop, U.S. Surgeon General,* U.S. NEWS & WORLD REPORT 35, 36 (June 28, 1982). The Director of the Congressional Budget Office recently stated that almost 11 million former workers and their dependents have already lost their coverage under their employers' health insurance plan because of unemployment, and that more will lose coverage as their extended benefits expire. This is in addition, she points out, to roughly 20 million persons who are uninsured for other reasons. Alice M. Rivlin, *Health Insurance and the Unemployed,* Statement before the Subcomm. on Health and the Environment, Comm. on Energy and Commerce, U.S. House of Representatives (Jan. 24, 1983).

5. Larry Frederick, *Schweiker on Health Policy,* MEDICAL WORLD NEWS 61, 69 (July 19, 1982). 401-553 0-83-2

6. 1 PRESIDENT'S COMMISSION ON THE HEALTH NEEDS OF THE NATION, U.S. Government Printing Office, Washington (1953) at 3.

The societal obligation is balanced by individual obligations. Individuals ought to pay a fair share of the cost of their own health care and take reasonable steps to provide for such care when they can do so without excessive burdens. Nevertheless, the origins of health needs are too complex, and their manifestation too acute and severe, to permit care to be regularly denied on the grounds that individuals are solely responsible for their own health.

Equitable access to health care requires that all citizens be able to secure an adequate level of care without excessive burdens. Discussions of a right to health care have frequently been premised on offering patients access to all beneficial care, to all care that others are receiving, or to all that they need—or want. By creating impossible demands on society's resources for health care, such formulations have risked negating the entire notion of a moral obligation to secure care for those who lack it. In their place, the Commission proposes a standard of "an adequate level of care," which should be thought of as a floor below which no one ought to fall, not a ceiling above which no one may rise.

A determination of this level will take into account the value of various types of health care in relation to each other as well as the value of health care in relation to other important goods for which societal resources are needed. Consequently, changes in the availability of resources, in the effectiveness of different forms of health care, or in society's priorities may result in a revision of what is considered "adequate."

Equitable access also means that the burdens borne by individuals in obtaining adequate care (the financial impact of the cost of care, travel to the health care provider, and so forth) ought not to be excessive or to fall disproportionately on particular individuals.

When equity occurs through the operation of private forces, there is no need for government involvement, but the ultimate responsibility for ensuring that society's obligation is met, through a combination of public and private sector arrangements, rests with the Federal government. Private health care providers and insurers, charitable bodies, and local and state governments all have roles to play in the health care system in the United States. Yet the Federal government has the ultimate responsibility for seeing that health care is available to all when the market, private charity, and government efforts at the state and local level are insufficient in

The cost of achieving equitable access to health care ought to be shared fairly. The cost of securing health care for those unable to pay ought to be spread equitably at the national level and not allowed to fall more heavily on the shoulders of particular practitioners, institutions, or residents of different localities. In generating the resources needed to achieve equity of access, those with greater financial resources should shoulder a greater proportion of the costs. Also, priority in the use of public subsidies should be given to achieving equitable access for all before government resources are devoted to securing more care for people who already receive an adequate level.[7]

Efforts to contain rising health care costs are important but should not focus on limiting the attainment of equitable access for the least well served portion of the public. The achievement of equitable access is an obligation of sufficient moral urgency to warrant devoting the necessary resources

---

7. Although the Commission does not endorse devoting public resources to individuals who already receive adequate care, exceptions arise for particular groups with special ethical claims, such as soldiers injured in combat, to whom the nation owes a special debt of gratitude.

to it. However, the nature of the task means that it will not be achieved immediately. While striving to meet this ethical obligation, society may also engage in efforts to contain total health costs—efforts that themselves are likely to be difficult and time-consuming. Indeed, the Commission recognizes that efforts to rein in currently escalating health care costs have an ethical aspect because the call for adequate health care for all may not be heeded until such efforts are undertaken. If the nation concludes that too much is being spent on health care, it is appropriate to eliminate expenditures that are wasteful or that do not produce benefits comparable to those that would flow from alternate uses of these funds. But measures designed to contain health care costs that exacerbate existing inequities or impede the achievement of equity are unacceptable from a moral standpoint. Moreover, they are unlikely by themselves to be successful since they will probably lead to a shifting of costs to other entities, rather than to a reduction of total expenditures.

Overview of the Report

The Commission was instructed by Congress to study the "ethical and legal implications of differences in the availability of health services as determined by the income or residence of the person receiving the service."[8] To translate "differences in availability" into ethical terms, it is necessary to develop standards of equity of access to health care. The term "equity" means different things to different people. Does equity, for example, require that all individuals receive all potentially beneficial health care, or whatever health care is available to others, or some other level of care? Does it require only that the government ensure that people have the financial means for obtaining care, whether or not the services are available? Or does it encompass an obligation, as well to see that health services are available should the market fail to provide them? In Chapter One of this Report, the Commission attempts to respond to such questions and presents an ethical framework as a foundation for evaluating current patterns of access to health care and recommendations for change.

Chapter Two shows that differences in the ability to pay for health care and in the distribution of health care services have been reduced substantially in the past 15 years. However, inequities related to income, place of residence, race, and ethnicity still exist in the financial protection people have against the cost of care, in the availability of health professionals and facilities, in the use of services, and in the quality of care received.[9]

Chapter Three of the Report examines the impact of a range of existing government policies and programs on access to health care. Some of the improvement over the past few decades can be attributed to Federal, state, and local government policies that both directly and indirectly affect people's ability to secure health services. These actions themselves raise important—albeit sometimes

8. 42 D.S.C. § 300v-1(a)(1)(D)(Supp. 1981). Early in its deliberations, the Commission decided to include race and ethnic origin as other factors to be examined in evaluating differences in the availability of health care.

9. While the statistics in Chapter Two establish the existence of disparities based on race and ethnicity, they appear to result from many interrelated factors and not necessarily from conscious racial discrimination. Commissioner Moran believes that such disparities may perhaps exist but does not think the evidence presented here substantiates this conclusion; for the views of Commissioner Ballantine, see his dissenting statement, pp. 199–204 *infra*.

unrecognized—ethical questions. For example, public policies have subsidized the purchase of health services for some individuals but have failed to help others with comparable needs who are unable to pay for health care. The impact of government actions on the costs of health care itself has ethical implications since increased expenditures for health care mean that fewer resources can be devoted to other important social endeavors. Chapter Three also addresses a concern common to all public policy: to what extent have government efforts affected individual choice?

The final chapter examines the problems of achieving equitable access within the context of rising health care costs and expenditures. The Commission believes that efforts to improve equity need not conflict with strategies to halt the rapid escalation of health care costs and to bring the benefits derived from health care into proportion with the resources devoted to it. Indeed, such efforts offer policymakers an excellent opportunity to implement changes that could make health care not only more efficient and less costly but also more equitable.

Through an application of the Commission's analysis to several possible remedies for current problems, Chapter Four offers further refinements in the ethical framework by which policymakers in the Congress and Executive agencies can judge proposals in the health care arena. The policies discussed were chosen not because of any particular importance attached to them, but because the Commission hopes that a review of several ideas currently under consideration will demonstrate the importance of taking into account ethical implications—in addition to biomedical, economic, social, and political factors—when health policy is being framed.

An Ethical Framework for Access to Health Care

A half century ago a national Committee on the Costs of Medical Care concluded that "many persons do not receive service which is adequate either in quantity or quality, and the costs of service are inequitably distributed. The result is a tremendous amount of preventable physical pain and mental anguish, needless deaths, economic inefficiency, and social waste."[10] Although much progress has been made in the past 50 years through the advent of private health insurance and public programs, problems of access remain and are compounded by the perceived need to respond to rapidly rising health care costs and expenditures. As that earlier committee observed, "The United States has the economic resources, the organizing ability, and the technical experience to solve this problem."[11] The question now is whether the country's formidable health care resources can be applied in a way that is fair to all—be they patient, provider, or taxpayer.

Most Americans believe that because health care is special, access to it raises special ethical concerns. In part, this is because good health is by definition important to well being. Health care can relieve pain and suffering, restore functioning, and prevent death; it can enhance good health and improve an individual's opportunity to pursue a life plan; and it can provide valuable information about a person's overall health. Beyond its practical importance, the involvement of health care with the most significant

10. Committee on the Costs of Medical Care, MEDICAL CARE FOR THE AMERICAN PEOPLE (1932), Dept. of Health, Education, and Welfare, U.S. Government Printing Office, Washington (reprinted 1970) at 2.
11. Id.

and awesome events of life—birth, illness, and death—adds a symbolic aspect to health care: it is special because it signifies not only mutual empathy and caring but the mysterious aspects of curing and healing.

Furthermore, while people have some ability—through choice of life-style and through preventive measures—to influence their health status, many health problems are beyond their control and are therefore undeserved. Besides the burdens of genetics, environment, and chance, individuals become ill because of things they do or fail to do—but it is often difficult for an individual to choose to do otherwise or even to know with enough specificity and confidence what he or she ought to do to remain healthy. Finally, the incidence and severity of ill health is distributed very unevenly among people. Basic needs for housing and food are predictable, but even the most hardworking and prudent person may suddenly be faced with overwhelming needs for health care. Together, these considerations lend weight to the belief that health care is different from most other goods and services. In a society concerned not only with fairness and equality of opportunity but also with the redemptive powers of science, there is a felt obligation to ensure that some level of health services is available to all.

There are many ambiguities, however, about the nature of this societal obligation. What share of health costs should individuals be expected to bear, and what responsibility do they have to use health resources prudently? Is it society's responsibility to ensure that every person receives care or services of as high quality and as great extent as any other individual? Does it require that everyone share opportunities to receive all available care or care of any possible benefit? If not, what level of care is "enough"? And does society's obligation include a responsibility to ensure both that care is available and that its costs will not unduly burden the patient?

The resolution of such issues is made more difficult by the specter of rising health care costs and expenditures. Americans annually spend over 270 million days in hospitals,[12] make over 550 million visits to physicians' offices,[13] and receive tens of millions of X-rays.[14] Expenditures for health care in 1981 totaled $287 billion—an average of over $1225 for every American.[15] Although the finitude of national resources demands that trade-offs be made between health care and other social goods, there is little agreement about which choices are most acceptable from an ethical standpoint. In this chapter, the Commission attempts to lay an ethical foundation for evaluating both current patterns of access to health care and the policies designed to address remaining problems in the distribution of health care resources.

The sheer size and complexity of the enterprise encourages abstract thinking about large-scale issues of social policy. But every significant issue of social policy dealt with in this Report, no matter how abstract and impersonal it seems, derives its ethical and social importance from its bearing on the ability of the health care system to respond appropriately to the individual seeking care—whether it be a pregnant woman in need of prenatal and obstetrical care, a worker disabled by arthritis, or an injured motorist who requires emergency treatment.

12. National Center for Health Statistics, HEALTH UNITED STATES, 1981, Dept. of Health and Human Services, U.S. Government Printing Office, Washington (1981) at 162.
13. Unpublished data from the National Ambulatory Medical Care Survey, National Center for Health Statistics, U.S. Dept. of Health and Human Services (1982).
14. *Id.*
15. Robert M. Gibson and Daniel R. Waldo, *National Health Expenditures: 1981*, 4 HEALTH CARE FINANCING REV. 1 (Sept. 1982).

To explore "differences in the availability of health care," as required by the Commission's mandate, is to raise issues of profound ethical importance. There is no question that differences in access to health care in the United States do exist, though there is disagreement about the nature and magnitude of these differences. Describing these differences is a factual task that rests on empirical research, but to conclude that certain differences constitute inequities is to make an ethical judgment that access to health care is unfair or otherwise morally unacceptable. Plainly, then, findings of equity must be based on a standard of what constitutes equity. This chapter does not offer a policy blueprint for health care, but it seeks to provide an ethical framework for determining when differences in access to health care are inequitable and to identify who is responsible for addressing these inequities.

The Special Importance of Health Care

Although the importance of health care may, at first blush, appear obvious, this assumption is often based on instinct rather than reasoning. Yet it is possible to step back and examine those properties of health care that lead to the ethical conclusion that it ought to be distributed equitably.

Well-Being. Ethical concern about the distribution of health care derives from the special importance of health care in promoting personal well-being by preventing or relieving pain, suffering, and disability and by avoiding loss of life. The fundamental importance of the latter is obvious; pain and suffering are also experiences that people have strong desires to avoid, both because of the intrinsic quality of the experience and because of their effects on the capacity to pursue and achieve other goals and purposes. Similarly, untreated disability can prevent people from leading rewarding and fully active lives.

Health, insofar as it is the absence of pain, suffering, or serious disability, is what has been called a primary good, that is, there is no need to know what a particular person's other ends, preferences, and values are in order to know that health is good for that individual. It generally helps people carry out their life plans, whatever they may happen to be. This is not to say that everyone defines good health in the same way or assigns the same weight or importance to different aspects of being healthy, or to health in comparison with the other goods of life. Yet though people may differ over each of these matters, their disagreement takes place within a framework of basic agreement on the importance of health. Likewise, people differ in their beliefs about the value of health and medical care and their use of it as a means of achieving good health, as well as in their attitudes toward the various benefits and risks of different treatments.

Opportunity. Health care can also broaden a person's range of opportunities, that is, the array of life plans that is reasonable to pursue within the conditions obtaining in society.[16] In the United States equality of opportunity is a widely accepted value that is reflected throughout public policy. The effects that meeting (or failing to meet) people's health needs have on the distribution of opportunity in a society become apparent if diseases are thought of as adverse departures from a normal level of functioning. In this view, health care is that which people need to maintain or restore normal functioning or to compensate

16. Norman Daniels, *Health Care Needs and Distributive Justice,* 10 PHIL. & PUB. AFF. 146 (1981).

for inability to function normally. Health is thus comparable in importance to education in determining the opportunities available to people to pursue different life plans.

Information. The special importance of health care stems in part from its ability to relieve worry and to enable patients to adjust to their situation by supplying reliable information about their health. Most people do not understand the true nature of a health problem when it first develops. Health professionals can then perform the worthwhile function of informing people about their conditions and about the expected prognoses with or without various treatments. Though information sometimes creates concern, often it reassures patients either by ruling out a feared disease or by revealing the self-limiting nature of a condition and, thus, the lack of need for further treatment. Although health care in many situations may thus not be necessary for good physical health, a great deal of relief from unnecessary concern and even avoidance of pointless or potentially harmful steps is achieved by health care in the form of expert information provided to worried patients. Even when a prognosis is unfavorable and health professionals have little treatment to offer, accurate information can help patients plan how to cope with their situation.

The Interpersonal Significance of Illness, Birth, and Death. It is no accident that religious organizations have played a major role in the care of the sick and dying and in the process of birth. Since all human beings are vulnerable to disease and all die, health care has a special interpersonal significance: it expresses and nurtures bonds of empathy and compassion. The depth of a society's concern about health care can be seen as a measure of its sense of solidarity in the face of suffering and death. Moreover, health care takes on special meaning because of its role in the beginning of a human being's life as well as the end. In spite of all the advances in the scientific understanding of birth, disease, and death, these profound and universal experiences remain shared mysteries that touch the spiritual side of human nature. For these reasons a society's commitment to health care reflects some of its most basic attitudes about what it is to be a member of the human community.

The Concept of Equitable Access to Health Care

The special nature of health care helps to explain why it ought to be accessible, in a fair fashion, to all.[17] But if this ethical conclusion is to provide a basis for evaluating current patterns of access to health care and proposed health policies, the meaning of fairness or equity in this context must be clarified. The concept of equitable access needs definition in its two main aspects: the level of care that ought to be available to all and the extent to which burdens can be imposed on those who obtain these services.

Access to What? "Equitable access" could be interpreted in a number of ways: equality of access, access to whatever an individual needs or would benefit from, or access to an adequate level of care.

Equity as equality. It has been suggested that equity is achieved either when everyone is assured of receiving an equal quantity of health care dollars or when people enjoy equal health. The most common characterization of equity as equality, however, is as providing everyone with the same level of health care. In this view, it follows that if a given level of care is available to one individual it must be available to all. If the initial standard is set high, by reference to the highest level of care presently received, an enormous

---

17. For a discussion of other important factors, the uneven distribution of need, and its largely underserved nature, see pp. 23-25 *infra*.

drain would result on the resources needed to provide other goods. Alternatively, if the standard is set low in order to avoid an excessive use of resources, some beneficial services would have to be withheld from people who wished to purchase them. In other words, no one would be allowed access to more services or services of higher quality than those available to everyone else, even if he or she were willing to pay for those services from his or her personal resources.

As long as significant inequalities in income and wealth persist, inequalities in the use of health care can be expected beyond those created by differences in need. Given people with the same pattern of preferences and equal health care needs, those with greater financial resources will purchase more health care. Conversely, given equal financial resources, the different patterns of health care preferences that typically exist in any population will result in a different use of health services by people with equal health care needs. Trying to prevent such inequalities would require interfering with people's liberty to use their income to purchase an important good like health care while leaving them free to use it for frivolous or inessential ends. Prohibiting people with higher incomes or stronger preferences for health care from purchasing more care than everyone else gets would not be feasible, and would probably result in a black market for health care.

Equity as access solely according to benefit or need. Interpreting equitable access to mean that everyone must receive all health care that is of any benefit to them also has unacceptable implications. Unless health is the only good or resources are unlimited, it would be irrational for a society—as for an individual—to make a commitment to provide whatever health care might be beneficial regardless of cost. Although health care is of special importance, it is surely not all that is important to people. Pushed to an extreme, this criterion might swallow up all of society's resources, since there is virtually no end to the funds that could be devoted to possibly beneficial care for diseases and disabilities and to their prevention.

Equitable access to health care must take into account not only the benefits of care but also the cost in comparison with other goods and services to which those resources might be allocated. Society will reasonably devote some resources to health care but reserve most resources for other goals. This, in turn, will mean that some health services (even of a lifesaving sort) will not be developed or employed because they would produce too few benefits in relation to their costs and to the other ways the resources for them might be used.

It might be argued that the notion of "need" provides a way to limit access to only that care that confers especially important benefits. In this view, equity as access according to need would place less severe demands on social resources than equity according to benefit would. There are, however, difficulties with the notion of need in this context. On the one hand, medical need is often not narrowly defined but refers to any condition for which medical treatment might be effective. Thus, "equity as access according to need" collapses into "access according to whatever is of benefit."

On the other hand, "need" could be even more expansive in scope than "benefit." Philosophical and economic writings do not provide any clear distinction between "needs" and "wants" or "preferences." Since the term means different things to different people, "access according to need" could become "access to any health service a person wants." Conversely, need could be interpreted very narrowly to encompass only a very minimal level of services—for example, those "necessary to prevent death."[18]

Equity as an adequate level of health care. Although neither "everything needed" nor "everything beneficial" nor "everything that anyone else is getting" are defensible ways of understanding equitable access, the special nature of health care dictates that everyone have access to *some* level of care: enough care to achieve sufficient welfare, opportunity, information, and evidence of interpersonal concern to facilitate a reasonably full and satisfying life. That level can be termed "an adequate level of health care," The difficulty of sharpening this amorphous notion into a workable foundation for health policy is a major problem in the United States today. This concept is not new; it is implicit in the public debate over health policy and has manifested itself in the history of public policy in this country. In this chapter, the Commission attempts to demonstrate the value of the concept, to clarify its content, and to apply it to the problems facing health policymakers.

Understanding equitable access to health care to mean that everyone should be able to secure an adequate level of care has several strengths. Because an adequate level of care may be less than "all beneficial care" and because it does not require that all needs be satisfied, it acknowledges the need for setting priorities within health care and signals a clear recognition that society's resources are limited and that there are other goods besides health. Thus, interpreting equity as access to adequate care does not generate an open-ended obligation. One of the chief dangers of interpretations of equity that require virtually unlimited resources for health care is that they encourage the view that equitable access is an impossible ideal. Defining equity as an adequate level of care for all avoids an impossible commitment of resources without falling into the opposite error of abandoning the enterprise of seeking to ensure that health care is in fact available for everyone.

In addition, since providing an adequate level of care is a limited moral requirement, this definition also avoids the unacceptable restriction on individual liberty entailed by the view that equity requires equality. Provided that an adequate level is available to all, those who prefer to use their resources to obtain care that exceeds that level do not offend any ethical principle in doing so. Finally, the concept of adequacy, as the Commission understands it, is society-relative. The content of adequate care will depend upon the overall resources available in a given society, and can take into account a consensus of expectations about what is adequate in a particular society at a particular time in its historical development. This permits the definition of adequacy to be altered as societal resources and expectations change.[19]

With What Burdens? It is not enough to focus on the care that individuals receive; attention must be

18. The Federal government employed this criterion in the mid-1970s when it dropped requirements providing dental care for adult public program beneficiaries under Medicaid. It claimed that dental services were not services whose absence could be considered as "life-threatening." 401-553 0-83-3

19. There are practical as well as ethical reasons for a nation like the United States, which possesses resources to provide a high level of services, not to take a narrow view of "adequacy." A lesser level of care would make it extremely difficult to establish a desirable mix of services; narrow limits would foster intense competition among different types of care and possibly skew the adequate level toward life-threatening care to the exclusion of other very beneficial forms of care such as preventive medicine. An inadequate level, accompanied by a private market in alternative treatments, would generate inequities by encouraging the flight of resources (as is now the case with physicians who choose to serve privately insured patients to the exclusion of noninsured and publicly insured individuals).

paid to the burdens they must bear in order to obtain it—waiting and travel time, the cost and availability of transport, the financial cost of the care itself. Equity requires not only that adequate care be available to all, but also that these burdens not be excessive.

If individuals must travel unreasonably long distances, wait for unreasonably long hours, or spend most of their financial resources to obtain care, some will be deterred from obtaining adequate care, with adverse effects on their health and well-being. Others may bear the burdens, but only at the expense of their ability to meet other important needs. If one of the main reasons for providing adequate care is that health care increases welfare and opportunity, then a system that required large numbers of individuals to forego food, shelter, or educational advancement in order to obtain care would be self-defeating and irrational.

The concept of acceptable burdens in obtaining care, as opposed to excessive ones, parallels in some respects the concept of adequacy. Just as equity does not require equal access, neither must the burdens of obtaining adequate care be equal for all persons. What is crucial is that the variations in burdens fall within an acceptable range. As in determining an adequate level of care, there is no simple formula for ascertaining when the burdens of obtaining care fall within such a range. Yet some guidelines can be formulated. To illustrate, since a given financial outlay represents a greater sacrifice to a poor person than to a rich person, "excessive" must be understood in relation to income. Obviously everyone cannot live the same distance from a health care facility, and some individuals choose to locate in remote and sparsely populated areas. Concern about an inequitable burden would be appropriate, however, when identifiable groups must travel a great distance or long time to receive care—though people may appropriately be expected to travel farther to get specialized care, for example, than to obtain primary or emergency care.

Although differences in the burdens individuals must bear to obtain care do not necessarily represent inequities, they may trigger concern for two reasons. Such discrepancies may indicate that some people are, in fact, bearing excessive burdens, just as some differences in the use of care may indicate that some lack adequate care. Also, certain patterns of differences in the burdens of obtaining care across groups may indicate racial or ethnic discrimination.

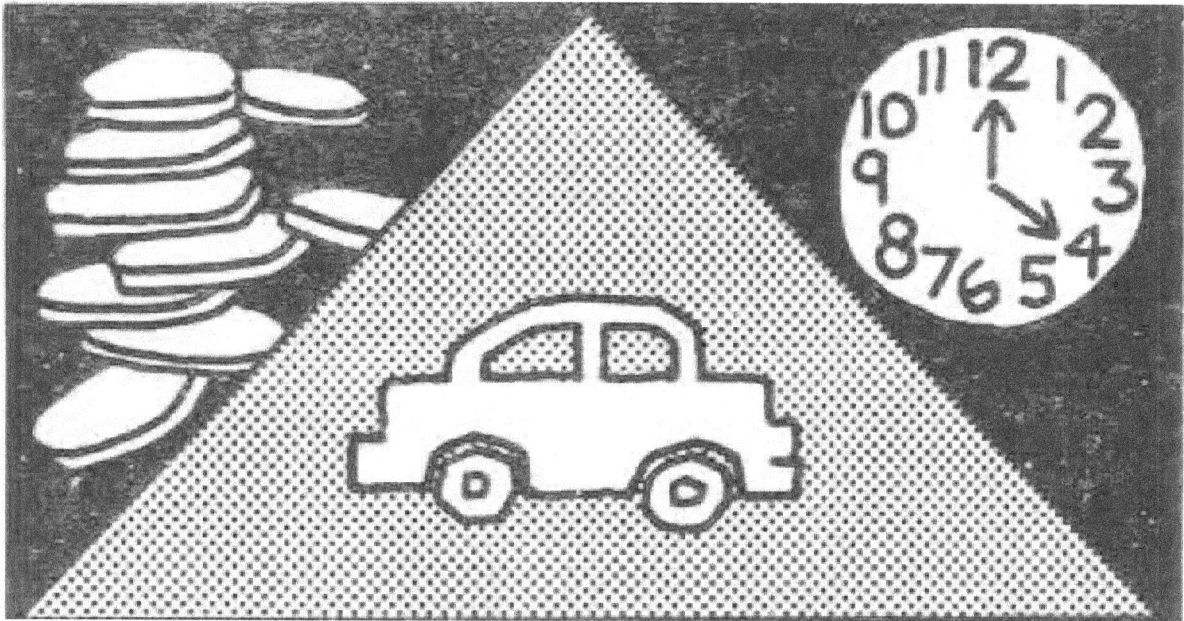

Image 3.6.1

Whether any such discrepancies actually constitute an inequitable distribution of burdens ultimately depends upon the role these differences play in the larger system under which the overall burdens of providing an adequate level of care are distributed among the citizens of this country. It may be permissible, for example, for some individuals to bear greater burdens in the form of out-of-pocket expenses for care if this is offset by a lower bill for taxes devoted to health care. Whether such differences in the distribution of burdens are acceptable cannot be determined by looking at a particular burden in isolation.

A Societal Obligation

Society has a moral obligation to ensure that everyone has access to adequate care without being subject to excessive burdens. In speaking of a societal obligation the Commission makes reference to society in the broadest sense—the collective American community. The community is made up of individuals, who are in turn members of many other, overlapping groups, both public and private, local, state, regional, and national units; professional and workplace organizations; religious, educational, and charitable organizations; and family, kinship, and ethnic groups. All these entities play a role in discharging societal obligations.

The Commission believes it is important to distinguish between society, in this inclusive sense, and government as one institution among others in society. Thus the recognition of a collective or societal obligation does not imply that government should be the only or even the primary institution involved in the complex enterprise of making health care available. It is the Commission's view that the societal obligation to ensure equitable access for everyone may best be fulfilled in this country by a pluralistic approach that relies upon the coordinated contributions of actions by both the private and public sectors.

Securing equitable access is a societal rather than a merely private or individual responsibility for several reasons. First, while health is of special importance for human beings, health care—especially scientific health care—is a social product requiring the skills and efforts of many individuals; it is not something that individuals can provide for themselves solely through their own efforts. Second, because the need for health care is both unevenly distributed among persons and highly unpredictable and because the cost of securing care may be great, few individuals could secure adequate care without relying on some social mechanism for sharing the costs. Third, if persons generally deserved their health conditions or if the need for health care were fully within the individual's control, the fact that some lack adequate care would not be viewed as an inequity. But differences in health status, and hence differences in health care needs, are largely undeserved because they are, for the most part, not within the individual's control.

Uneven and Unpredictable Health Needs. While requirements for other basic necessities, such as adequate food and shelter, vary among people within a relatively limited range, the need for health care is distributed very unevenly and its occurrence at any particular time is highly unpredictable. One study shows 50% of all hospital billings are for only 13% of the patients, the seriously chronically ill.[20]

Moreover, health care needs may be minor or overwhelming, in their personal as well as financial impact. Some people go through their entire lives seldom requiring health care, while others face medical expenses that would exceed the resources of all but the wealthiest. Moreover, because the need for care cannot be predicted, it is difficult to provide for it by personal savings from income. Under the major program that pays for care for the elderly, 40% of aged enrollees had no payments at all in 1977 and 37% fell into a low payment group (averaging only $129 per year), while 8.8% averaged $7011 in annual expenditures.[21]

Responsibility for Differences in Health Status. Were someone responsible for (and hence deserving of) his or her need for health care, then access to the necessary health care might be viewed as merely an individual concern. But the differences among people's needs for health care are for the most part not within their control, and thus are not something for which they should be held accountable. Different needs for care are largely a matter of good or bad fortune—that is, a consequence of a natural and social lottery that no one chooses to play.

In a very real sense, people pay for the consequences of the actions that cause them illness or disability—through the suffering and loss of opportunity they experience. The issue here is a narrower one: to what extent is the societal responsibility to secure health care for the sick and injured limited by personal responsibility for the need for health care? It seems reasonable for people to bear the foreseeable consequences (in terms of health care needs) of their informed and voluntary choices. Indeed, as an ethical matter, the principle of self-determination implies as a corollary the responsibility of individuals for their choices.

However, to apply the notion of personal responsibility in a fair way in setting health care policy

20. C.J. Zook and F.D. Moore, *High-Cost Users of Medical Care,* 302 NEW ENG. J. MED. 996 (1982).
21. Karen Davis, *Medicare Reconsidered,* Duke University Medical Center Private Sector Conference, Durham, N.C., March 15-16, 1982.

would be a complex and perhaps impossible task. First, identifying those people whose informed, voluntary choices have caused them foreseeable harm would be practically as well as theoretically very difficult. It is often not possible to determine the degree to which an individual's behavior is fully informed regarding the health consequences of the behavior. Efforts to educate the public about the effects of life-style on health status are desirable, but it must also be acknowledged that today people who conscientiously strive to adopt a healthy life-style find themselves inundated with an enormous amount of sometimes contradictory information about what is healthful. Voluntariness is also especially problematic regarding certain behaviors that cause some people ill health, such as smoking and alcohol abuse.[22] Moreover, there are great difficulties in determining the extent of the causal role of particular behavior on an individual's health status. For many behaviors, consequences appear only over long periods of time, during which many other elements besides the particular behavior have entered into the causal process that produces a disease or disability. For example, the largely unknown role of genetic predispositions for many diseases makes it difficult to designate particular behaviors as their "cause."

Second, even if one knew who should be held responsible for what aspects of their own ill health, policies aimed at institutionalizing financial accountability for "unhealthy behavior" or at denying the necessary health care for those who have "misbehaved" are likely to involve significant injustices and other undesirable consequences. Leaving people free to engage in health-risky behavior only if they can afford to pay for its consequences is fair only if the existing patterns of income distribution are fair, and if the payment required fully accounts for all the costs to society of the ill health and its treatment. Moreover, since some unhealthy behavior can be monitored more easily than others, problems of discrimination would inevitably arise; even when feasible, monitoring such behavior would raise serious concerns about the invasion of privacy. Finally, the ultimate sanction—turning away from the hospital door people who are responsible for their own ill health—would reverberate in unwanted and perhaps very harmful ways in the community at large. The Commission concludes that within programs to secure equitable access to health care, serious practical and ethical difficulties would follow attempts to single out the consequences of behavior and to make individuals of health-risky behavior solely responsible for those consequences.

However, even if it is inappropriate to hold people responsible for their health status, it is appropriate to hold them responsible for a fair share of the cost of their own health care. Society's moral obligation to provide equitable access for all and the individual responsibility for bearing a share of the costs of achieving equity rest on the same considerations of fairness. Individuals who—because they know that others will come to their aid—fail to take reasonable steps to provide for their own health care when they could do so without excessive burdens would be guilty of exploiting the generosity of their fellow citizens. The societal obligation is therefore balanced by corresponding individual obligations.

In light of the special importance of health care, the largely undeserved character of differences in health status, and the uneven distribution and unpredictability of health care needs, society has a moral obligation to ensure adequate care for all. Saying that the obligation is societal (rather than merely individual) stops short, however, of identifying who has the ultimate responsibility for ensuring that the obligation is successfully met.

22. Daniel Wikler, *Persuasion and Coercion for Health,* 56 MILBANK MEMORIAL FUND Q./HEALTH & SOCIETY 303 (1978).

Who Should Ensure that Society's Obligation is Met?

In this country, the chief mechanism by which the cost of health care is spread among individuals is through the purchase of insurance. Another method of distributing health care costs is to rely on acts of charity in which individuals, such as relatives and care givers, and institutions assume responsibility for absorbing some or all of a person's health care expenses. These private forces cannot be expected to achieve equitable access for all, however, States and localities have also played important roles in attempting to secure health care for those in need. To the extent that actions of the market, private charity, and lower levels of government are insufficient in achieving equity, the responsibility rests with Federal government. The actual provision of care may be through arrangements in the private sector as well as through public institutions, such as local hospitals.

Market Mechanisms in Health Care. One means societies employ for meeting needs for goods and services that individuals cannot produce by themselves is the complex legal and economic mechanism known as a market. When health care is distributed through markets, however, an acceptable distribution is not achieved; indeed, given limitations in the way markets work, this result is practically inevitable.

The inability to ensure adequate care. First, many people lack the financial resources to obtain access to adequate care. Since American society encompasses a very wide range in income and wealth, distributing goods and services through markets leads to large differences in their consumption. The variations in need for health care do not, however, match variations in ability to purchase care. The market response to variable risk is insurance. Insurance has long existed for certain calamities—such as fire damage to property—and in the past 30 years, a huge market in health insurance has developed that enables people to share some of the financial risk of ill health. The relevant question for determining equity of access thus becomes: Is everyone able to afford access to adequate care through some combination of insurance and direct payment?

Admittedly, "ability to afford" is an ambiguous concept, given different attitudes toward risk and the importance of health care, and, even more important, possibly insufficient information about the likelihood of ill health and about the possible effects of care. For example, people may want an adequate level of care and may be able to afford to pay for it, but they may lack information about the amount of coverage needed to secure adequate care. As a result, the insurance market may not do a good job of providing plans that actually do protect people adequately. And, of course, some people who can afford to pay for their health care (and who would if they knew they would have to go without it otherwise) fail to make sufficient provisions because they rely on others not being willing to let them suffer. Furthermore, the cost of basic health insurance (which does not even guarantee financial access to adequate care in all cases) is high enough to place it beyond the reach of many families by *any* reasonable standard of affordability.[23] Ironically, those who need the most care will find it most difficult to obtain it, both because their disease or disability impairs their opportunities for accumulating financial resources and because insurers will charge them higher rates.

---

23. For a detailed discussion of insurance costs, see pp. 90–100 *infra*.

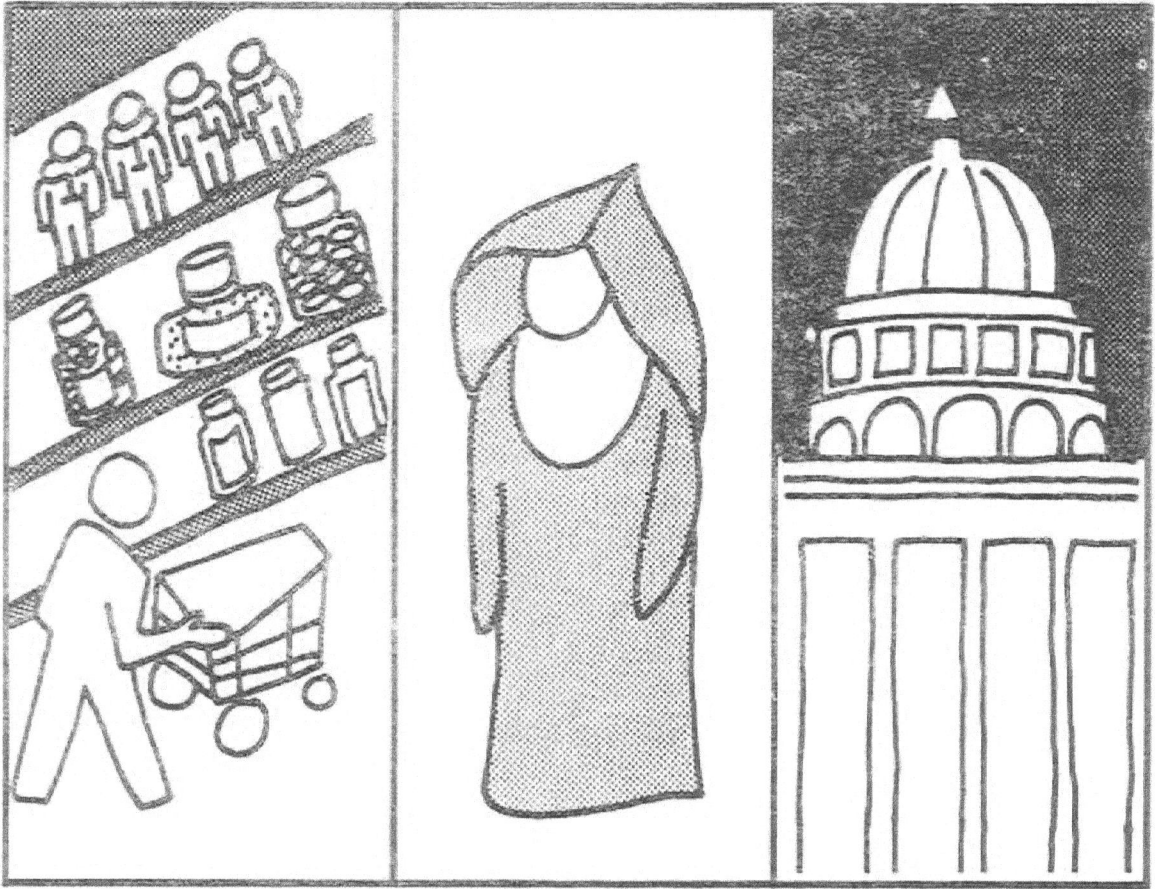

Image 3.6.2

Second, many people will be unable to obtain adequate care if the distribution of care is left exclusively to the market because services are not available in the areas in which they live. These geographical availability problems are often really financial problems: in certain areas with a high proportion of poor people, there are not enough personnel and facilities because the residents cannot afford to pay to use them. Even when people do have the ability to pay, however, they may be unable to obtain services. The area may be too sparsely populated to provide enough demand to support a practitioner or a facility; or even though the demand is sufficient, providers may not respond. In health care, decisions are often made by nonprofit institutions, whose decisions may not be keyed to market forces, or by health care professionals, who are influenced by factors other than financial incentives. Such decisions can leave some areas inadequately served. Thus in a market system, people will not necessarily obtain adequate care, and lack of access to such care will be correlated with income and place of residence.

While some people lack access to very essential care, many will receive not just an adequate level, but more than they themselves would want to have if they were well informed about the benefits of care and took its full cost into account. In deciding whether a service is worth having, an insured individual will tend to consider only what he or she must pay out-of-pocket, rather than the total costs. In the long run, additional use raises premiums, but the extra cost is spread over all policyholders, a situation known as the phenomenon of moral hazard.[24] These incentives mean that policyholders pay higher total costs for health care than they would choose to pay if they had to weigh its full costs to themselves against the benefits they receive.

The patient's lack of information and consequent reliance on professional advice for many of his or her health care decisions may make this problem more serious, depending on what practitioners consider to be their professional duty. Most believe that it is their duty to do all they can for their patients. Even uninsured patients may find it difficult to convey their preferences about trade-offs between financial costs and the benefits of care to providers who believe strongly in the value of medical care. It follows that merely giving people money (to pay their medical bills directly or to buy insurance) to assure them access to adequate care may be a very expensive proposition.

To summarize, if the distribution of health care were left solely to the market, some people would not get an adequate amount and others would get too much—not just more than an adequate level but more than they themselves really want given the costs they bear directly and through insurance premiums. The first is an ethical issue; the second, though not a moral problem, makes the solution of the first more difficult.

The inequities in costs and burdens. In the absence of insurance, a market puts the cost of goods and services on those who consume them. Normally this seems appropriate; the person who wants to see a movie or to buy an automobile must pay for it. In the case of health care, this is not so appealing: the person who suffers the largely undeserved burden of ill health also suffers the financial burdens of obtaining and paying for health care. Those who lack financial resources may suffer severely.

Private insurance markets only spread the financial risk to a limited extent. Whenever they can, insurance companies will set premiums in accord with a person's risk of experiencing ill health. At the outer limit, certain people (for example, those with preexisting disabilities) may find it nearly impossible to obtain insurance at any price—or at least to get insurance that will encompass care for their disabilities.

The private market does not adjust the financial burden of care to differences in income. Yet poverty and ill health are correlated—with the causal factors working in both directions. Therefore, the poor are in a double bind: they need more medical care but they have less money to purchase it or less insurance protection to secure it.

The market determines a geographical distribution of care that reflects providers' preferences (about where they want to live for example), the differential cost of providing services in different places, and the distribution of ill health and ability to pay. Even when it works efficiently—when the geographical distribution of services reflects the real costs of geographical location—it may result in heavy burdens on some individuals in time and cost to get to care. And, as already discussed, the process may not work efficiently, and can produce arbitrarily great differences in the burdens of obtaining care in different geographical settings. For example, in a sparsely populated state, some residents might have to travel

---

24. The classic illustration of this arises when some people dine out and agree in advance to split the check evenly. Each person has an incentive to order more expensively than that individual would if he or she were paying only for their own meal. Yet in the end each individual, as a member of the group, actually bears the cost of the collective "over-ordering."

long distances for hospital care because it is uneconomic to build a larger number of smaller hospitals and spread them evenly throughout the state. Or a state may have a small number of large hospitals because the philanthropists and hospital administrators who make the investment decisions prefer large hospitals for prestige reasons, and the market forces that would normally counteract such preferences are too weak to do so.

Private Charity as a Source of Care. There is a strong tradition of private charity in the United States, including free services by health professionals, and charitable organizations continue to play an important role in health care research and delivery. Yet, as discussed in Chapter Two, charitable efforts have not achieved equity of access.

The most obvious explanation of the inadequacy of charity is the countervailing pressure of self-interest. Especially in an acquisitive society, even the best of intentions to aid others may fall short of action. It is not necessary, however, to assume that Americans are unduly self-interested to understand why charity alone has not provided everyone with an adequate level of health care. There are two other explanations, neither of which presupposes selfishness. The first is the pervasiveness of what has been called "limited altruism." The difficulty is not that individuals are only concerned about their own interests, but rather that the focus of their concern tends to be limited to those who are near at hand, such as family and friends.

The second, less obvious factor is that effective charitable action, particularly in an area such as health care where large-scale capital investment is required, needs the coordinated efforts of many people. Unless potential contributors can be assured that a sufficient number of other people will also contribute to some appropriately identified goal, they may conclude either that they should not contribute at all or that their resources would be better used in some private act of charity, even though this will not be as effective as a coordinated action. In this sense, charity—like national defense or energy conservation—has the characteristic features of a public good in the technical sense. In general, the problems of supplying public goods illustrate the limits of private voluntary action and often provide a legitimate reason for government action.[25] Furthermore, it has often been noted that while the charitable impulses are laudable, recipients sometimes feel demeaned by their dependence on the benevolence of others. (This unfortunate feature, which is affected by the manner and setting in which aid is rendered, can be a problem not only for private but also for governmental programs, as discussed in the next section.)

A Role for Government. The extent of governmental involvement in securing equitable access to care depends on the extent to which the market and private charity achieve this objective. The limitations that have just been enumerated are not absolute barriers. Although it is clear that—even for those with adequate resources—the purchase of health care differs from other market transactions, the market (which includes private health insurance) is capable of providing many people with an adequate level of health care. However, when the market and charity do not enable individuals to obtain adequate care or cause them to endure excessive burdens in doing so, then the responsibility to ensure that these people have equitable access to health care resides with the local, state, and Federal governments.

Locating responsibility. Although it is appropriate that all levels of government be involved in seeing that equitable access to health care is achieved, the ultimate responsibility for ensuring that this obligation

25. Allen Buchanan, *Philosophical Foundations of Beneficence,* in Earl E. Shelp, ed., BENEFICENCE AND HEALTH CARE, Reidel Publishing Co., Dordrecht, Holland (1982) at 33.

is met rests with the Federal government. The Commission believes it is extremely important to distinguish between the view that the Federal government ought to provide care and the view that the Federal government is ultimately responsible for seeing that there is equitable access to care. It is the latter view that the Commission endorses. It is not the purpose of this Report to assign the precise division of labor between public and private provision of health care. Rather, the Commission has attempted here only to locate the ultimate responsibility for ensuring that equitable access is attained.

A view that has gained wide acceptance in this country is that the government has a major responsibility for making sure that certain basic social goods, such as health care and economic security for the elderly, are available to all. Over the past half-century, public policy and public opinion have increasingly reflected the belief that the Federal government is the logical mechanism for ensuring that society's obligation to make these goods available is met. In the case of health care, this stance is supported by several considerations. First, the obligation in question is society-wide, not limited to particular states or localities; it is an obligation of all to achieve equity for all. Second, government responsibility at the national level is needed to secure reliable resources. Third, only the Federal government can ultimately guarantee that the burdens of providing resources are distributed fairly across the whole of society. Fourth, meeting society's obligation to provide equitable access requires an "overview" of efforts. Unless the ultimate responsibility has been clearly fixed for determining whether the standard of equitable access is being met, there is no reason to believe it will be achieved.

The limitations of relying upon the government. Although the Commission recognizes the necessity of government involvement in ensuring equity of access, it believes that such activity must be carefully crafted and implemented in order to achieve its intended purpose. Public concern about the inability of the market and of private charity to secure access to health care for all has led to extensive government involvement in the financing and delivery of health care. This involvement has come about largely as a result of ad hoc responses to specific problems; the result has been a patchwork of public initiatives at the local, state, and Federal level. These efforts have done much to make health care more widely available to all citizens, but, as discussed in Chapters Two and Three, they have not achieved equity of access.

To a large extent, this is the result of a lack of consensus about the nature of the goal and the proper role of government in pursuing it. But to some degree, it may also be the product of the nature of government activity. In some instances, government programs (of all types, not just health-related) have not been designed well enough to achieve the purposes intended or have been subverted to serve purposes explicitly not intended.

In the case of health care, it is extremely difficult to devise public strategies that, on the one hand, do not encourage the misuse of health services and, on the other hand, are not so restrictive as to unnecessarily or arbitrarily limit available care. There is a growing concern, for example, that government assistance in the form of tax exemptions for the purchase of employment-related health insurance has led to the overuse of many services of only very marginal benefit. Similarly, government programs that pay for health care directly (such as Medicaid) have been subject to fraud and abuse by both beneficiaries and providers. Alternatively, efforts to avoid misuse and abuse have at times caused local, state, and Federal programs to suffer from excessive bureaucracy, red tape, inflexibility, and unreasonable interference in individual choice. Also, as with private charity, government programs have not always avoided the unfortunate effects on the human spirit of "discretionary benevolence," especially in those programs requiring income or means tests.

It is also possible that as the government role in health care increases, the private sector's role will decrease in unforeseen and undesired ways.[26] For example, government efforts to ensure access to nursing home care might lead to a lessening of support from family, friends, and other private sources for people who could be cared for in their homes. Although these kinds of problems do not inevitably accompany governmental involvement, they do occur and their presence provides evidence of the need for thoughtful and careful structuring of any government enterprise.

A Right to Health Care? Often the issue of equitable access to health care is framed in the language of rights. Some who view health care from the perspective of distributive justice argue that the considerations discussed in this chapter show not only that society has a moral obligation to provide equitable access, but also that every individual has a moral right to such access. The Commission has chosen not to develop the case for achieving equitable access through the assertion of a right to health care. Instead it has sought to frame the issues in terms of the special nature of health care and of society's moral obligation to achieve equity, without taking a position on whether the term "obligation" should be read as entailing a moral right. The Commission reaches this conclusion for several reasons: first, such a right is not legally or Constitutionally recognized at the present time; second, it is not a logical corollary of an ethical obligation of the type the Commission has enunciated; and third, it is not necessary as a foundation for appropriate governmental actions to secure adequate health care for all.

Legal rights. Neither the Supreme Court nor any appellate court has found a constitutional right to health or to health care.[27] However, most Federal statutes and many state statutes that fund or regulate health care have been interpreted to provide statutory rights in the form of entitlements for the intended beneficiaries of the program or for members of the group protected by the regulatory authority. As a consequence, a host of legal decisions have developed significant legal protections for program beneficiaries. These protections have prevented Federal and state agencies and private providers from withholding authorized benefits and services. They have required agencies and providers to deliver health care to eligible individuals—the poor, elderly, handicapped, children, and others.[28]

In addition, Federal statutes protecting the civil rights of all citizens and the constitutional provisions on equal protection and due process have been interpreted to apply both to governmental agencies and to private health care providers in certain circumstances. Decisions affecting beneficiaries and providers

---

26. Similarly, sometimes governmental decisions decrease the private sector's role in foreseeable ways. For example, the advent of Medicare was accompanied by a sharp alteration in the types and amount of private health insurance available to persons over 65 years of age. In 1965, 57% of this age-group had some form of private insurance. At present, 57% have private insurance but the current policies are designed to fill in the gaps in Medicare coverage and not to cover basic costs.

27. *See* Harris v. McRae, 448 U.S. 297, 318 (1980) (publicly funded abortions); Maher v. Roe, 432 U.S. 464, 469 (medical treatment).

28. The majority of the litigation has focused on the Medicare and Medicaid programs. One line of cases concerns questions of eligibility, such as Schweiker v. Gray Panthers, 453 U.S. 1 (1981) ("deeming" resources as available to the beneficiary for purposes of determining eligibility). Another line concerns limitations in services, such as White v. Beal, 413 F.Supp. 1141, *aff'd* 555 F.2d 1146 (3rd Cir. 1977) (impermissibly reducing Medicaid services by identifying mandatory services as optional). Still another line concerns the procedures that states are required to follow in administering the programs, such as Elder v. Beal, 609 F.2d 695 (3rd Cir. 1979) (requiring the state to notify beneficiaries adequately of reduction in services).

must be made through orderly and fair processes, and there can be no discrimination based on race, sex, handicap, or age in the allocation of resources and operation of the health care programs.[29] A recent study by the Institute of Medicine presents evidence showing the continuing existence of distinctive, separate, or segregated patterns in the sources of care and the amount of care received. These patterns were found to be influenced by such factors as patient income, source of payment for care, geographic location, race, and ethnicity.[30]

Moral obligations and rights. The relationship between the concept of a moral right and that of a moral obligation is complex. To say that a person has a moral right to something is always to say that it is that person's due, that is, he or she is morally entitled to it. In contrast, the term "obligation" is used in two different senses. All moral rights imply corresponding obligations, but, depending on the sense of the term that is being used, moral obligations mayor may not imply corresponding rights. In the broad sense, to say that society has a moral obligation to do something is to say that it ought morally to do that thing and that failure to do it makes society liable to serious moral criticism. This does not, however, mean that there is a corresponding right. For example, a person may have a moral obligation to help those in need, even though the needy cannot, strictly speaking, demand that person's aid as something they are due.

The government's responsibility for seeing that the obligation to achieve equity is met is independent of the existence of a corresponding moral right to health care. There are many forms of government involvement, such as enforcement of traffic rules or taxation to support national defense, to protect the environment, or to promote biomedical research, that do not presuppose corresponding moral rights but that are nonetheless legitimate and almost universally recognized as such. In a democracy, at least, the people may assign to government the responsibility for seeing that important collective obligations are met, provided that doing so does not violate important moral rights.[31]

As long as the debate over the ethical assessment of patterns of access to health care is carried on simply by the assertion and refutation of a "right to health care," the debate will be incapable of guiding policy. At the very least, the nature of the right must be made clear and competing accounts of it compared and evaluated. Moreover, if claims of rights are to guide policy they must be supported by sound ethical reasoning and the connections between various rights must be systematically developed, especially where rights are potentially in conflict with one another. At present, however, there is a great deal of dispute among competing theories of rights, with most theories being so abstract and inadequately developed that their implications for health care are not obvious. Rather than attempt to adjudicate among competing

---

29. The courts have differed, however, in their determinations of what constitutes prohibited discrimination. Thus, Cook v. Ochsner, 61 F.R.D. 354 (E.D. La. 1972), holds that HEW was obligated to require private hospitals, funded partly by Federal Hill-Burton funds, to accept Medicaid patients, regardless of conflicting hospital policies. The court in NAACP v. Wilmington Medical Center, 453 F.2d 1247 (3rd Cir. 1979), found that the plaintiffs had not proved discrimination, but also held that an inner-city hospital receiving Medicaid reimbursement could relocate its services to the suburbs only if it demonstrated that no alternatives existed that would produce less of a discriminatory impact on the hospital's minority, aged, and handicapped inner-city patients.

30. Institute of Medicine, HEALTH CARE IN A CONTEXT OF CIVIL RIGHTS, National Academy of Sciences, Washington (1981).

31. Where a basic right is concerned, such as the right to free speech, even an increase in social welfare is not a sufficient reason for stifling the exercise of that right. However, both the legal system and sound ethical tradition recognize that people have no absolute moral or legal right to use their property as they see fit. This right is limited by government's authority to tax, so long as the requirements of due process are satisfied.

theories of rights, the Commission has chosen to concentrate on what it believes to be the more important part of the question: what is the nature of the societal obligation, which exists whether or not people can claim a corresponding right to health care, and how should this societal obligation be fulfilled?[32]

Meeting the Societal Obligation

How Much Care is Enough? Before the concept of an adequate level of care can be used as a tool to evaluate patterns of access and efforts to improve equity, it must be fleshed out. Since there is no objective formula for doing this, reasonable people can disagree about whether particular patterns and policies meet the demands of adequacy. The Commission does not attempt to spell out in detail what adequate care should include. Rather it frames the terms in which those who discuss or critique health care issues can consider ethics as well as economics, medical science, and other dimensions.

Characteristics of adequacy. First, the Commission considers it clear that health care can only be judged adequate in relation to an individual's health condition. To begin with a list of techniques or procedures, for example, is not sensible: A CT scan for an accident victim with a serious head injury might be the best way to make a diagnosis essential for the appropriate treatment of that patient; a CT scan for a person with headaches might not be considered essential for adequate care. To focus only on the technique, therefore, rather than on the individual's health and the impact the procedure will have on that individual's welfare and opportunity, would lead to inappropriate policy.

Disagreement will arise about whether the care of some health conditions falls within the demands of adequacy. Most people will agree, however, that some conditions should not be included in the societal obligation to ensure access to adequate care. A relatively uncontroversial example would be changing the shape of a functioning, normal nose or retarding the normal effects of aging (through cosmetic surgery). By the same token, there are some conditions, such as pregnancy, for which care would be regarded as an important component of adequacy. In determining adequacy, it is important to consider how people's welfare, opportunities, and requirements for information and interpersonal caring are affected by their health condition.

Any assessment of adequacy must consider also the types, amounts, and quality of care necessary to respond to each health condition. It is important to emphasize that these questions are implicitly comparative: the standard of adequacy for a condition must reflect the fact that resources used for it will not be available to respond to other conditions. Consequently, the level of care deemed adequate should reflect a reasoned judgment not only about the impact of the condition on the welfare and opportunity of the individual but also about the efficacy and the cost of the care itself in relation to other conditions and the efficacy and cost of the care that is available for them. Since individual cases differ so much, the

---

32. Whether the issue of equity is framed in terms of individual rights or societal obligation, it is important to recall that society's moral imperative to achieve equitable access is not an unlimited commitment to provide whatever care, regardless of cost, individuals need or that would be of some benefit to them. Instead, society's obligation is to provide adequate care for everyone. Consequently, if there is a moral right that corresponds to this obligation, it is limited, not open-ended. 401-553 0-83-4

health care professional and patient must be flexible. Thus adequacy, even in relation to a particular health condition, generally refers to a range of options.

The relationship of costs and benefits. The level of care that is available will be determined by the level of resources devoted to producing it. Such allocation should reflect the benefits and costs of the care provided. It should be emphasized that these "benefits," as well as their "costs," should be interpreted broadly, and not restricted only to effects easily quantifiable in monetary terms. Personal benefits include improvements in individuals' functioning and in their quality of life, and the reassurance from worry and the provision of information that are a product of health care. Broader social benefits should be included as well, such as strengthening the sense of community and the belief that no one in serious need of health care will be left without it. Similarly, costs are not merely the funds spent for a treatment but include other less tangible and quantifiable adverse consequences, such as diverting funds away from other socially desirable endeavors including education, welfare, and other social services.

There is no objectively correct value that these various costs and benefits have or that can be discovered by the tools of cost/benefit analysis. Still, such an analysis, as a recent report of the Office of Technology Assessment noted, "can be very helpful to decision makers because the process of analysis gives structure to the problem, allows an open consideration of all relevant effects of a decision, and forces the explicit treatment of key assumptions."[33] But the valuation of the various effects of alternative treatments for different conditions rests on people's values and goals, about which individuals will reasonably disagree. In a democracy, the appropriate values to be assigned to the consequences of policies must ultimately be determined by people expressing their values through social and political processes as well as in the marketplace.

Approximating adequacy. The intention of the Commission is to provide a frame of reference for policymakers, not to resolve these complex questions. Nevertheless, it is possible to raise some of the specific issues that should be considered in determining what constitutes adequate care. It is important, for example, to gather accurate information about and compare the costs and effects, both favorable and unfavorable, of various treatment or management options. The options that better serve the goals that make health care of special importance should be assigned a higher value. As already noted, the assessment of costs must take two factors into account: the cost of a proposed option in relation to alternative forms of care that would achieve the same goal of enhancing the welfare and opportunities of the patient, and the cost of each proposed option in terms of foregone opportunities to apply the same resources to social goals other than that of ensuring equitable access.

Furthermore, a reasonable specification of adequate care must reflect an assessment of the relative importance of many different characteristics of a given form of care for a particular condition. Sometimes the problem is posed as: What *amounts* of care and what *quality* of care? Such a formulation reduces a complex problem to only two dimensions, implying that all care can readily be ranked as better or worse. Because two alternative forms of care may vary along a number of dimensions, there may be no consensus among reasonable and informed individuals about which form is of higher overall quality. It is worth bearing in mind that adequacy does not mean the highest possible level of quality or strictly equal quality any more

33. Office of Technology Assessment, U.S. Congress, THE IMPLICATIONS OF COST-EFFECTIVENESS ANALYSIS OF MEDICAL TECHNOLOGY, SUMMARY, U.S. Government Printing Office, Washington (1980) at 8.

than it requires equal amounts of care; of course, adequacy does require that everyone receive care that meets standards of sound medical practice.

Any combination of arrangements for achieving adequacy will presumably include some health care delivery settings that mainly serve certain groups, such as the poor or those covered by public programs. The fact that patients receive care in different settings or from different providers does not itself show that some are receiving inadequate care. The Commission believes that there is no moral objection to such a system so long as all receive care that is adequate in amount and quality and all patients are treated with concern and respect.

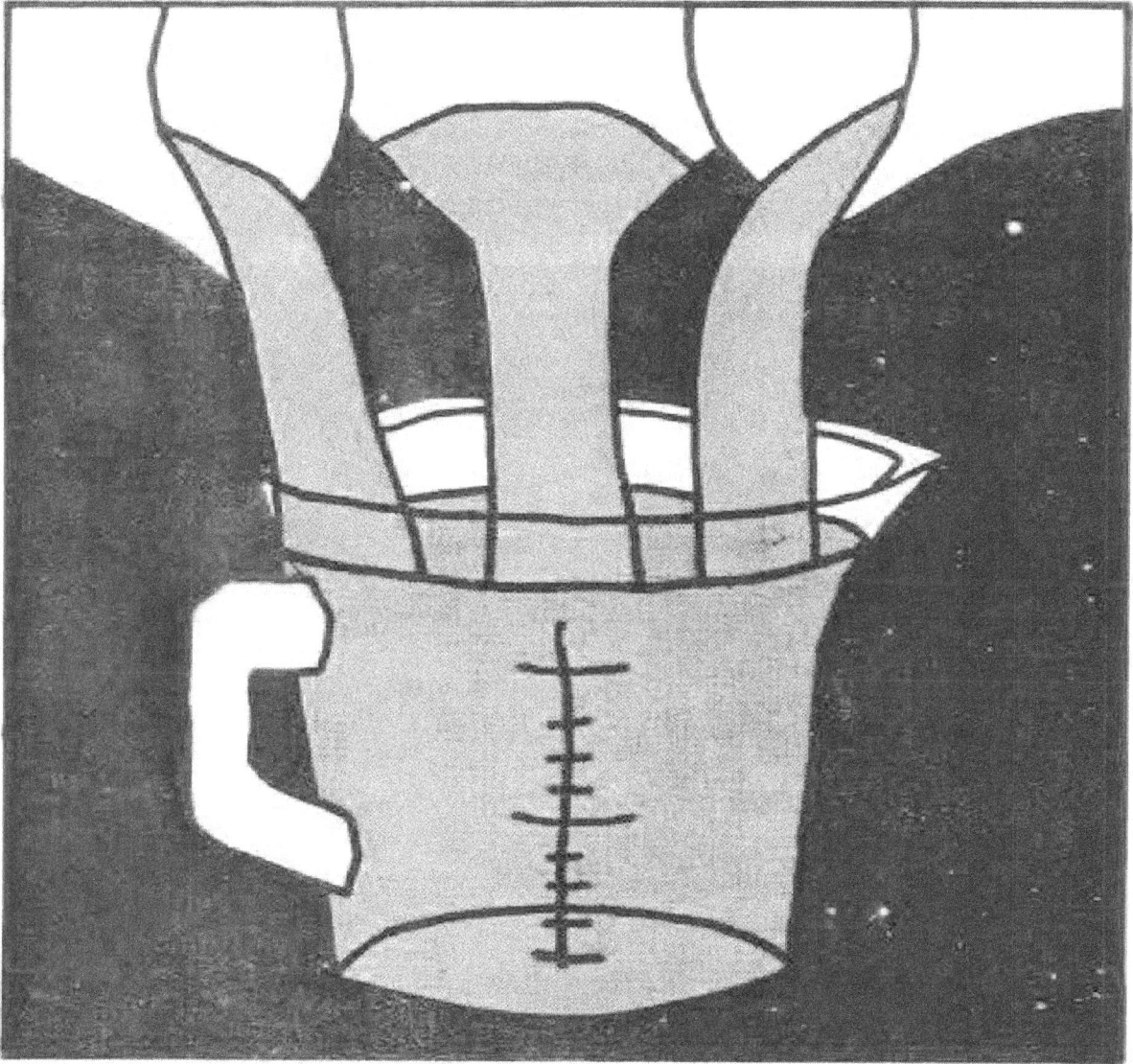

Image 3.6.3

At this point, the complexity of the problem of deciding what constitutes adequate care is apparent.

However, clear and useful conclusions can emerge even when there is no agreement on the details of adequacy. In the case of pregnant women, for example, there is a consensus in the United States that some prenatal care, the attention of a trained health professional during labor and delivery, and some continuity between the two are all essential for an adequate level of care.

A stronger consensus is required if proposals for change are to be evaluated. Some of the processes that may be used to develop a societal consensus on adequacy are already a familiar feature of the health care system, and do in fact play a role in determining the amount of care that is provided, especially to beneficiaries of public programs.[34]

Professional judgment. Physicians and other professionals who provide health care are familiar with human needs for care, so that the first means that might be employed in defining an adequate level of health care would be a reliance on individual health care practitioners' judgment of the "medical necessity" of any particular service. However, sole reliance on professional judgment in setting limits is not appropriate because of professionals' tendency to provide all possible medically beneficial care. At the very least, the extent and manner in which professionals exercise judgment to limit the use of care that is of little benefit (relative to cost) varies widely. Thus, without substantial changes in individual health care professionals' present practices, this method of defining adequate health care is likely to result in an uncertain and overly inclusive definition.

Another way that professional judgment might be used to define adequacy is to rely on the standards of medical practice as adopted by the professional community through, for example, consensus conferences. The advantage of such an approach is the specialized knowledge of the effects of care that such people have. However, there are also serious disadvantages.

Professionals have no special expertise in deciding how the effects of medical care ought to be valued, either with respect to the relative value of different dimensions of care or, particularly, the value attached to health care relative to other goods. In the last two or three decades, for example, there have been major changes in prenatal and obstetrical care, in many cases in response to the preferences of parents: changes in the use of anesthesia; the kind of contact possible between mother, father, and infant in the hospital; the information provided to the family about the birth process; support for breast-feeding as opposed to formula-feeding. These changes were never shown to be harmful or uniformly beneficial, but rather represent differences in the valuing of benefits.[35]

Professionals often have no special knowledge of the costs of different alternatives and perhaps little appreciation of the other goods foregone for the sake of health care. Studies show that practitioners are frequently unaware of the financial costs of many of the tests and procedures that they order.[36]

---

34. For a discussion of determinations of the amount and type of care under public programs, see Chapter Three *infra,* although the processes now used would not necessarily have the same role in the determinations of adequacy recommended here.

35. In many cases there is now a medical consensus that the new practices are in fact superior. Nevertheless, strong pressure from consumers was required to bring some of them about.

36. "Indeed, there is ample evidence that medical students, interns, residents, and even medical faculty are equally uninformed about the prices of the tests and treatments they order." Anthony L. Komaroff, *The Doctor, the Hospital, and the Definition of Proper Medical Practice* (1981), Appendix U, in Volume Three of this Report, at *Education,* in section five. Komaroff cites a number of studies as examples: S.P. Kelly, *Physicians' Knowledge of Hospital Costs,* 6 J. FAM. PRAC. 171 (1978); S.J. Dresnick *et al., The Physician's*

Finally, their involvement with the delivery of care may sometimes create a barrier to full consideration of all options. Many observers have noted a bias in health care in this country toward the introduction of expensive, high-technology-based procedures delivered by existing institutions and against the introduction of alternative ways to provide services at lower cost.[37]

Because of these factors, professional judgment cannot stand alone as the determinant of adequate care, but the specialized knowledge of health care professionals about the effects of health care is essential as part of any process of determining adequacy.

Average current use. The United States at present has a sophisticated health care system and there is reason to suppose that the average American obtains an adequate total amount of care. Defining adequacy in terms of the level of care presently enjoyed by the average person has the advantage of realism: it reflects the outcome of the health care system as it now operates—what actually happens as a result of patient-provider interaction, not merely what planners believe ought to happen.

Nevertheless, there are good reasons to pause before adopting "current use" as the benchmark of adequacy. Many distortions in people's true preferences for health care affect the average level of care received—for example, those whose access is now unduly limited bring down the average, while those who overspend for health care because of insurance and tax advantages (discussed in Chapter Three) inflate the average. Also, structural characteristics of the delivery system can mean that even people with good access do not necessarily receive an appropriate mix of services.

A possible variation of the concept of average use is to adopt as a point of reference the care received by people of average financial means who live in areas that are sufficiently provided with health care resources. This approach could incorporate a broader dimension of preferences, including an explicit consideration of the value of care relative to its cost. Unlike most approximations of adequacy this concept is more amenable to measurement. In fact, a modification of average use—people with similar health conditions receiving the same volume of care at a standard acceptable to middle-class Americans—is now employed by the Robert Wood Johnson Foundation in determining when adequacy is achieved.[38]

Unfortunately, this approach also has its weaknesses. Again, in making choices about health care, patients may inappropriately evaluate those costs that are covered by insurance. Moreover, recognizing their lack of knowledge, patients generally rely heavily on their practitioner's judgment, which as noted earlier may favor care that is disproportionately costly relative to its benefits. On the other hand, if a patient makes an independent choice it may be an uninformed one that rejects care that is actually of significant

---

Role in the Cost-Containment Problem, 241 J.AM.A 1606 (1979); J.K. Skipper et al., Medical Students' Unfamiliarity with the Cost of Diagnostic Tests, 50 J. MED. EDUC. 683 (1975); L.R. Kirkland, The Physician and Cost Containment, 242 J.AM.A 1032 (1979).

37. Dean David Mechanic of Rutgers University gives the following example of this: "One of the most prevalent conditions among children is sore throats, and it is routine to take a throat culture before treatment to assess whether the cause is a streptococcal infection. Typically, the mother is required to bring the child to a pediatrician for the culture, often involving inconvenience and considerable expense. As an experiment at the Columbia Medical Plan has demonstrated, mothers can be effectively instructed to take a throat culture at home, negating the need for physician and nurse care in most instances and increasing the convenience and satisfaction of the mother. The barriers to individual responsibility built in to medical care must be reviewed carefully, and efforts should be made to modify them." David Mechanic, FUTURE ISSUES IN HEALTH CARE: SOCIAL POLICY AND THE RATIONING OF MEDICAL SERVICES, The Free Press, New York (1979) at 37 (citation omitted).

38. Testimony of Robert J. Blendon, transcript of 24th meeting of the President's Commission (Sept. 10, 1982) at 21.

benefit relative to its cost. Thus, people of average means may lack some care that ought to be part of an adequate level while they receive some care that ought not to be included in it.

Nevertheless, this concept also has a role to play in determining adequacy. In particular, if some of the distorting factors could be lessened, the care sought by well-educated people of average means might be a reasonable benchmark, at least for the treatment of serious conditions.

List of services. Another alternative is to attempt to specify a list of services to be included within an adequate level of health care. An example is the list of "basic health services" in the Health Maintenance Organization (HMO) Act of 1973 (as amended), which includes physician services, inpatient and outpatient hospital services, emergency health services, short-term outpatient mental health services (up to 20 visits), treatment and referral for drug and alcohol abuse, laboratory work and X-rays, home health services, and certain preventive health services.[39]

The broad categories on this list might be broken down into more specific services. However, such a list of services is no more a specification of an adequate level of care than a list of foods is an adequate diet. What makes the HMO list into an "adequate level" specification is its combination with a delivery mechanism that relies on professional judgment to determine the appropriate amounts of services on a case-by-case basis, with organizational and financial incentives to weigh the benefits of services against cost. Other approximations in this same spirit include insurance contracts that incorporate reviews of the appropriateness of services received.

Overall evaluation. It would, of course, be possible to combine several approaches—by specifying categories of services that must be available as part of adequate care, for example, while placing limits on the overall use of services through a health insurance package valued at a specified amount. Another variation of this approach would involve an effort by the medical profession to redefine standards of practice to incorporate some assessments of the costs and benefits of acceptable alternative therapies. This might be achieved through medical education, consensus conferences, and other methods. Such determinations would, of course, take place within a process that allowed an interplay between the health care professions and political and other social factors.

The Commission cites these alternatives as examples of possible initial approaches to approximating an adequate level of health care that should be available to all Americans. There are both theoretical and practical differences between these approaches, yet each has something to offer, separately and together. For the purpose of health policy formulation, general theories as well as ordinary views of equity do not determine a unique solution to defining adequate care but rather set some broad limits within which that definition should fall. It is reasonable for a society to turn to fair, democratic political procedures to make a choice among just alternatives. Given the great imprecision in the notion of adequate health care, however, it is especially important that the procedures used to define that level be—and be perceived to be—fair.

When Are Burdens Excessive? As in the definition and assessment of adequacy, reasonable people may hold a range of views about what is an excessive or disproportionate burden in obtaining care under particular circumstances. Virtually unanimous agreement can be expected in judging some burdens to be too great, but a consensus on others will be more difficult to achieve.

---

39. Health Maintenance Organization Act of 1973 (Pub. L. No. 93-222).

It is reasonable to assume, for example, not only that adequacy includes the availability of a health care professional at the delivery of a baby, but also that women living in rural communities should generally not have to travel so far that their health or that of their infants is endangered. Obviously every rural county need not have a tertiary-care medical center. Rather, initial access to a basic range of services should be reasonably available. A referral system should be in place for more specialized services not locally available. This may require providing transportation to the more specialized provider as well as other ancillary and support services.

Some reasonable assumptions can also be made about the level at which the financial burden incurred in obtaining adequate care becomes excessive. The financial outlay for a medical procedure can be considered excessive if it drains the family's resources and precludes the purchase of other necessities such as food or shelter. Individual circumstances are also important in evaluating a financial burden: the cost of obtaining adequate care will fall differently on families of similar income, for example, if one family has six children and another has none.

Wide variations in the proportion of income devoted to securing adequate care among families of different incomes do not necessarily constitute inequities. However, such differences should trigger concern that inequities could exist and should be carefully scrutinized to determine if this is the case.

What Distribution of Cost is Fair? Equity not only requires that no one bear an excessive burden to obtain care; it also requires fairness in the distribution of the cost to achieve this situation. If an individual does not shoulder the full cost of obtaining the care that he or she uses (through out-of-pocket payments, insurance premiums, and taxes) then someone else will bear a share of the cost. Where the cost of care should fall is a political decision, but it should be guided by ethical principles that reflect the societal concern about the fair distribution of health care in the first place.

A fundamental conclusion from these principles is that the healthy should share in the cost of adequate care for those who are less healthy. In light of the importance of health care and the fact that differences in the need for care are largely undeserved, the cost of illness should be spread broadly without regard to people's actual or probable use of care. In practical terms, this means out-of-pocket payments for health care should be minimized and insurance premiums or health care taxes should be independent of a person's state of health.

This argument applies only to adequate care; it does not mean that the cost of care above the level of adequacy ought to be spread widely.[40] However, special moral arguments exist for providing extra care to certain individuals; for example, society has shown a sense of obligation to provide more extensive care to soldiers injured in combat. Each category needs to be evaluated on its merits. Outside of these special situations, the Commission believes that the moral obligation to ensure adequate care to all ought to be fulfilled before public resources are used to provide care above this level. Moreover, the Commission

---

40. Although it would not be immoral to fail to provide additional beneficial care, society might be better served if it were provided, and there may be sound practical reasons for doing so collectively rather than leaving it to private initiative. For example, there may be benefits to society as a whole as well as to the individuals who receive the care. Everyone could benefit from a healthier work force, for example, or a healthier soldiery. Moreover, individuals may wish to guarantee themselves access to these benefits through voluntary private insurance arrangements, or a collective decision could be taken to provide additional care at public expense to some or all individuals.

believes that the moral obligation to ensure equitable access to health care should take precedence over other public activities that are legitimate matters for public concern but that are of lesser moral significance.

Although spreading the cost of care broadly is desirable in that it lessens the burdens imposed on those who need health care, the disadvantages of this approach cannot be ignored. Whenever insurance is provided, individuals have little or no personal incentive to limit their consumption; therefore, this way of redistributing costs is likely to increase total expenditures on the activity. To address this difficulty, it is acceptable to take measures to limit "overuse"—including direct charges to individuals for the care they use—as long as these measures neither prevent people from receiving adequate care nor impose excessive burdens.[41]

Unfortunately, it is difficult to devise measures that can make the necessary distinctions. It is difficult to develop insurance contracts that insure people for just an adequate level of care and no more, or delivery systems that deliver just adequate care. The result is that individuals are covered for too little or too much; in fact, the combination of cost-sharing and third-party coverage (private and public) that most people have usually does both at the same time. They receive too much care for some conditions and/or bear too little of the cost; for other conditions, they receive too little care and/or bear too much of the cost. A major point of ethical evaluation of any health policy must be the way in which it distinguishes adequate from more-than-adequate care and spreads the cost of each appropriately.

People with greater financial resources should share the cost of adequate care for those with fewer financial resources. Just as those who have higher incomes can afford a greater financial outlay for their own care without excessive sacrifice, so can they bear a greater share of the cost of adequate care for the low income. A fair distribution of cost across income groups may be brought about in many different ways—through various combinations of insurance premiums, out-of-pocket payments, taxes, and publicly and privately provided free care. The issue of ethical significance is the equity of the total distribution of costs across individuals at different income levels.[42]

Direct payment of insurance premiums and of charges for care at the time of use are possible mechanisms to restrain overuse and to foster an appreciation of the cost of the care received. However, special attention must be paid to finding a level of personal payment that will be high enough to achieve the desired results but not so great as to prevent poorer patients from receiving adequate care or as to saddle such patients with excessive costs. One method is to scale premiums or out-of-pocket charges to patients' incomes.

The cost of adequate care for people of varying health status and income should be shared on a national basis. A sick person in Mississippi imposes as much of a moral obligation on a taxpayer in Connecticut as a sick person in Connecticut does. There are both practical and ethical reasons why cost should be distributed broadly among parts of the country as among individuals. People, goods, and

41. The moral implications of measures such as cost-sharing differ when they are limiting access to adequate, rather than more-than-adequate, care. The cost of securing adequate care should be spread as broadly as possible; the cost of more-than-adequate care ought normally to fall in relation to actual or probable use.

42. Although wealthy individuals can contribute more for the care of others without excessive sacrifice, people in the middle class, a far larger part of the population, are likely to be the major source of the funds required to secure equitable access because of their greater numbers.

financial resources move freely throughout the United States. The prosperity of each section of the country rests to a considerable extent on what happens in the rest of the country. Furthermore, the number of people who need help to obtain health care in a given state or locality is often partly the result of national policies. The number of unemployed auto workers in Detroit, for example, or of Cuban and Haitian refugees in Florida is influenced by national policies on interest rates and immigration. It would be unfair, therefore, for all governmental health care funds to be raised on a state or local basis, since that would force some people to face a much higher share of such costs because they live in an area that is adversely affected by national policies. It would also provide an incentive for states to set such low health care budgets for their care that some people might feel that they will be able to obtain adequate care only by moving to another state.[43]

This does not mean, however, that all the institutions designed to help bring about equitable access to care must be governmental, or, when they are governmental, that they must be Federal. What is important is who ultimately bears the cost. There are many different combinations of public and private mechanisms that could spread the cost of guaranteeing equitable access appropriately across individuals of different health statuses and financial resources without regard to place of residence. There may be excellent reasons for locating the administration of policies and programs at lower levels of government and requiring the use of local fiscal resources. Nevertheless oversight is required at the highest level of government to ensure that the resulting distribution of cost is, in fact, equitable.[44]

Limitations on Individuals' Choices. Every system for organizing an activity places some limitations on individual choice. In the existing health care system, for example, many Americans are unable to choose the source or type of health care they would prefer or are even unable to obtain care because they do not have adequate health insurance. The difficulties created by lack of care can in turn limit individuals' freedom if their ill health deprives them of opportunities. Restricted alternatives also regularly confront health care practitioners and hospital administrators—for example, whether to turn away those who cannot pay for care or to absorb the cost of treating them (sometimes by shifting the burden to their paying patients). Moreover, lack of adequate care itself greatly limits individuals' freedom of choice when illness deprives them of opportunities.

Thus, the issue is what kinds of limitations on choice are most consistent with fulfilling society's moral obligation to provide equitable access to health care for all. Certain types of restrictions appear to be acceptable. For example, the freedom of people to seek or to provide health care is limited by licensure, in order to protect against quackery. Similarly, since an adequate level is something less than all care that might be beneficial, patients' choices will be limited to that range unless they are able to pay for care that exceeds adequacy.

Any pursuit of equity entails some limitations on choice. However, limitations that occur in pursuit of

43. This is not to say that individual localities, following the usual democratic processes, are not free to choose to support the provision of care over and above an adequate level for their residents. But Federal support of the latter should not be provided until access to adequate care without excessive burdens is assured nationwide.

44. It would also be inequitable were some health care providers to be penalized financially because society has failed to fulfill its obligation to secure equitable access to care. For example, in a rural area with limited medical services, a physician may be forced to choose between leaving some poor patients without care and absorbing costs that should be spread more equitably.

equity are more ethically acceptable than those that occur when no principle of comparable importance is being advanced.

The Ethics and Reality of Rationing in Medicine

Leslie P. Scheunemann and Douglas B. White

Leslie P. Scheunemann and Douglas B. White, "The Ethics and Reality of Rationing in Medicine," *Chest*, vol. 140, no. 6, pp. 1625-1632. Copyright © 2011 by Elsevier B.V. Reprinted with permission.

Rationing is the allocation of scarce resources, which in health care necessarily entails withholding potentially beneficial treatments from some individuals. Rationing is unavoidable because need is limitless and resources are not. How rationing occurs is important because it not only affects individual lives but also expresses society's most important values. This [reading] discusses the following topics: (1) the inevitability of rationing of social goods, including medical care; (2) types of rationing; (3) ethical principles and procedures for fair allocation; and (4) whether rationing ICU care to those near the end of life would result in substantial cost savings.

CHEST 2011; 140(6):1625–1632

Abbreviations: QALY = quality-adjusted life year; UNOS = United Network for Organ Sharing

Health-care reform has remained a controversial sociopolitical issue for the last 2 decades. Part of the controversy at the policy level arises from the question of whether health-care reform will involve rationing medical care. This topic raises fears about unfair treatment of individuals,[1] which have been inflamed by assertions that rationing devalues human life.[2]

Physicians have struggled with the controversy surrounding rationing.[3,4] Some deny that rationing occurs and contend that their professional obligations require them not to participate in rationing.[5,6,7] Others admit to rationing[8,9] and see just allocation of medical care as part of physicians' ethical duties.[10] Intensivists share this ambivalence. In a recent survey, only 60% vouched that they provide "every patient all beneficial therapies without regard to costs."[11]

To be thoughtful participants in the social debate about rationing in medicine, physicians must be well informed. The purpose of this [reading] is to address the following topics: (1) the inevitability of rationing of social goods, including medical care; (2) types of rationing; (3) ethical principles and procedures for fair allocation; and (4) whether rationing ICU care to those near the end of life would result in substantial cost savings.

What Is Rationing?

Although rationing has been defined in slightly different ways by different groups, most definitions cluster around one central idea: denying a potentially beneficial treatment to a patient on the grounds of scarcity.[12] The focus on potentially beneficial treatments is appropriate because virtually no treatment in medicine offers certain benefit for an individual patient and because a central point of controversy is whether the potential benefit is large enough or likely enough to occur in order to justify the expense. In this document, we use the terms "rationing" and "resource allocation" synonymously, although we acknowledge that the emotional valence of the two terms is clearly different.

1. Holtz-Eakin D. All's not fair in health reform bills. *The Boston Globe*. December 10, 2009. http://www.boston.com/bostonglobe/editorial_opinion/oped/articles/2009/12/10/alls_not_fair_in_health_reform_bills. Accessed December 28, 2010.
2. Singer P. Why we must ration healthcare. The New York Times. July 15, 2009. www.nytimes.com/2009/07/19/magazine/19healthcare-t.html. Accessed December 28, 2010.
3. Levinsky NG. The doctor's master. N Engl J Med. 1 984; 311 (24):1573–1575.
4. Strech D, Persad G, Marckmann G, Danis M. Are physicians willing to ration health care? Conflicting findings in a systematic review of survey research. Health Policy. 2009; 90 (2–3):113–124.
5. Strech D, Synofzik M, Marckmann G. How physicians allocate scarce resources at the bedside: a systematic review of qualitative studies. J Med Philos. 2008; 33 (1):80–99.
6. Sulmasy DP. Physicians, cost control, and ethics. Ann Intern Med. 1992; 116 (11): 920–926.
7. Angell M. The doctor as double agent. Kennedy Inst Ethics J. 1993; 3(3):279–286.
8. Hurst SA, Slowther A M, Forde R, e t al. Prevalence and determinants of physician bedside rationing: data from Europe. J Gen Intern Med. 2006; 21 (11):1138–1143.
9. Sinuff T, Kahnamoui K, Cook DJ, Luce JM, Levy MM; Values Ethics and Rationing in Critical Care Task Force. Rationing critical care beds: a systematic review. Crit Care Med. 2004; 32 (7):1588–1597.
10. Cooke M. Cost consciousness in patient care–what is medical education's responsibility? N Engl J Med. 2010; 362 (14):1253–1255.
11. Ward NS, Teno JM, Curtis JR, Rubenfeld GD, Levy MM. Perceptions of cost constraints, resource limitations, and rationing in United States intensive care units: results of a national survey. Crit Care Med. 2008; 36 (2):471–476.
12. Truog RD, Brock DW, Cook DJ, et al; for the Task Force on Values, Ethics, and Rationing in Critical Care (VERICC). Rationing in the intensive care unit. Crit Care Med. 2006; 34 (4):958–963.

It is also important to note that not all efforts to control health-care costs involve rationing. For example, choosing a less expensive treatment over a more-expensive one does not entail rationing if both are equally effective, because selecting the less costly of the two does not result in the patient being denied a potentially beneficial treatment.[12] In addition, strategies focused on reducing administrative costs and waste in health care (eg, reducing duplicative testing and administrative inefficiencies) are generally not rationing because they do not entail denying patients potentially beneficial care.

Rationing Is Unavoidable

In many industrialized countries, social goods—including health care, education, defense, infrastructure, environmental protection, and public health—draw funding from a common pool. Although need for such social goods is limitless, the resources available to supply them are limited.[6,131415] Inevitably, difficult choices must be made to allocate finite resources in a way that achieves a reasonable balance across the range of important social goods. Attempting to meet all healthcare needs would likely overwhelm our capacity to supply basic elements of other social goods, such as public safety, education, and defense. Therefore, some degree of rationing of health care is necessary for the overall well-being of society.

Rationing decisions pervade daily practice in ICUs.[5,12,16] For example, it is common to transfer a patient out of an ICU when she might still derive some small degree of benefit from ongoing monitoring; such transfers accommodate the needs of sicker patients in the face of a finite number of ICU beds. Physicians in ICUs also routinely ration their time. They must decide which patients to see first and how much time to spend with each. Physicians also must balance the needs of patients against their nonprofessional obligations, such as responsibilities to their families. It is undoubtedly true that physicians cannot provide every potential benefit to every critically ill patient. Therefore, the reality of practice in ICUs is that patients are routinely denied some potential benefit—however small—through implicit rationing decisions made by physicians at the bedside.

The Appropriateness of Rationing Is Context Specific

The necessity of some rationing in medicine does not mean that all such rationing is ethically justifiable, and a justifiable rationing decision in one health-care system may not be similarly justifiable in another. One example is the rules in many health systems requiring less expensive, less beneficial drugs to be first-line choices over more expensive, more beneficial drugs. This type of rationing is relatively easy to justify in single-payer systems (eg, the government-sponsored health-care plans in Canada and many

13. Veatch RM. Physicians and cost containment: the ethical conflict. Jurimetrics. 1990; 30 (4):461–482.
14. Daniels N, Sabin J. Limits to health care: fair procedures, democratic deliberation, and the legitimacy problem for insurers. Philos Public Aff. 1997; 26 (4):303–350.
15. King D, Maynard A. Public opinion and rationing in the United Kingdom. Health Policy. 1999; 50 (1–2):39–53.
16. Halpern NA. Can the costs of critical care be controlled? Curr Opin Crit Care. 2009;15(6):591–596.

European countries), in which savings are reinvested in programs to improve the health of the population. Such rationing decisions are harder to justify in a for-profit health system with wasteful administrative mechanisms and in which most profits are passed on to employees and shareholders rather than invested in improving the quality of care for patients.

Levels and Transparency of Rationing

Rationing can occur at multiple levels. The clearest conceptual distinction exists between "macroallocation" and "microallocation" decisions.[17,18] Macroallocation occurs at the societal level and includes decisions about how to allocate funds across a range of public goods. For example, macroallocation decisions determine how a particular society's public funds are allocated across social goods, such as defense, education, infrastructure, public health, and health care. Microallocation decisions involve bedside decisions about whether an individual patient will or will not receive a scarce medical resource. Although conceptually distinct, macroallocation decisions and microallocation decisions are related. For example, restrictive macroallocation decisions regarding health-care funding will create more situations in which individual patients must be denied potentially beneficial treatments.

Perhaps the most straightforward examples of the rationing in medicine occur when there is an absolute scarcity of a medical resource, such as organs for transplantation. The United Network for Organ Sharing (UNOS) has developed policies to ration according to weighted organ-specific criteria, such as time on the waiting list, severity of illness, human leukocyte antigen matching, prognostic information, and other considerations.[19,20,21,22] These policies are examples of rationing at the micro level. UNOS explicitly acknowledges that many will die without receiving an organ because of the need to ration. Conceivably, more funding of initiatives to encourage organ donation at the macro level would decrease deaths of patients on transplant waiting lists but would likely come at the cost of funding other important social programs. Scarcity is unavoidable in the realm of social goods, and the need to ration is one consequence.

Rationing also occurs because of general fiscal scarcity rather than an absolute scarcity of a particular medical resource. For example, in the early 1990s, Oregon had to cope with escalating medical expenditures for Medicaid recipients in the face of budget deficits. The resulting Oregon Health Plan concurrently set a firm annual health-care budget and expanded the Medicaid eligibility criteria to include

17. Skowronski GA. Bed rationing and allocation in the intensive care unit. Curr Opin Crit Care. 2001; 7 (6):480–484.
18. Calabresi G, Bobbitt P. Tragic Choices: The Conflicts Society Confronts in the Allocation of Tragically Scarce Resources. New York, NY: W. W. Norton & Company; 1978.
19. Egan TM, Kotloff RM. Pro/Con debate: lung allocation should be based on medical urgency and transplant survival and not on waiting time. Chest. 2005;128(1):407–415.
20. Freeman RB Jr, Wiesner RH, Harper A, et al; UNOS/OPTN Liver Disease Severity Score, UNOS/OPTN Liver and Intestine, and UNOS/OPTN Pediatric Transplantation Committees. The new liver allocation system: moving toward evidence-based transplantation policy. Liver Transpl. 2002;8(9):851–858.
21. Renlund DG, Taylor DO, Kfoury AG, Shaddy RS; United Network for Organ Sharing. New UNOS rules: historical background and implications for transplantation management. J Heart Lung Transplant. 1999;18(11):1065–1070.
22. Childress J, Beauchamp T. Principles of Biomedical Ethics. New York, NY: Oxford University Press; 2009.

all below the federal poverty level.[2324] The initial macroallocation decision balanced state health-care spending against competing social goods, such as education, infrastructure, and prisons. The second macroallocation traded providing a larger range of health-care services to less than one-half the state's poor for providing a basic level of health care to all Oregonians living in poverty.[2526] Oregon covered services according to a published priority list until projected expenditures exhausted the budget; there was not publicly funded coverage for the remaining services. This entailed denying beneficial therapies to some patients (microallocation).

Both the UNOS strategy for organ allocation and the Oregon Health Plan are examples of explicit rationing; these rationing decisions arise from stated principles and rules. In contrast, implicit rationing occurs without formally stated rules or principles. The 46 million uninsured in the United States are an example of implicit rationing at the macro level.[2728] Intensivists' decisions about how much time to spend with each patient are also examples of implicit rationing because they are generally not based on publicly disclosed reasons. In general, implicit rationing raises more concerns about fairness than explicit rationing because the basis of the decisions is not disclosed and because unspoken and illegitimate biases may exert undue influence on the decisions.

Empiric Data on Rationing in ICUs

Empiric data from multiple countries document the rationing of medical services in ICUs. In. 10,000 ICU bed triage decisions across North America, Europe, Israel, and Hong Kong, at least 15% of patients were refused ICU admission, of which approximately 15% were attributed to lack of beds.[2930] Additionally, during times of ICU bed shortages, admitted patients were more ill at both ICU admission and discharge, average lengths of stay were shorter, and fewer patients were admitted for monitoring, which suggests that some patients are denied potentially beneficial treatment in times of ICU bed shortages. Some centers have attempted to reduce ICU use by making mechanical ventilation available on the wards. This also constitutes rationing

23. Hadorn D. The Oregon priority-setting exercise: quality of life and public policy. Hastings Cent Rep. 1991;21(3):11–16.
24. Kitzhaber J, Gibson M. The crisis in health care—The Oregon Health Plan as a strategy for change. Stanford Law & Policy Review. 1991;3:64–72.
25. Oberlander J, Marmor T, Jacobs L. Rationing medical care: rhetoric and reality in the Oregon Health Plan. CMAJ. 2001;164 (11):1583–1587.
26. Jacobs L, Marmor T, Oberlander J. The Oregon Health Plan and the political paradox of rationing: what advocates and critics have claimed and what Oregon did. J Health Polit Policy Law. 1999;24(1):161–180.
27. Feldman R. The cost of rationing medical care by insurance coverage and by waiting. Health Econ. 1994;3(6):361–372.
28. Kennedy J, Morgan S. Health care access in three nations: Canada, insured America, and uninsured America. Int J Health Serv. 2006;36(4):697–717.
29. Iapichino G, Corbella D, Minelli C, e t al. Reasons for refusal of admission to intensive care and impact on mortality. Intensive Care Med. 2010;36(10):1772–1779.
30. Reignier J, Dumont R, Katsahian S, et al. Patient-related factors and circumstances surrounding decisions to forego life-sustaining treatment, including intensive care unit admission refusal. Crit Care Med. 2008;36(7):2076–2083.

because ICU care is associated with lower rates of adverse events and mortality compared with providing mechanical ventilation outside ICUs.[31][32]

A survey of US intensivists suggests that many believe that they do not ration. These results may reflect a lack of understanding of what rationing is or may reflect a symbolic belief about what physicians should do. In either case, the lack of insight about the inevitability of rationing in ICUs is problematic, because it suggests that many intensivists are not well positioned to be informed participants in the social conversation about how best to make the difficult decisions regarding competing social goods.

What Principles Could Guide Rationing?

A substantial barrier to moving from implicit to explicit approaches to rationing health care is the failure to specify what principle(s) should guide allocation. Many principles could form the basis of rationing decisions in health care, each of which represents a different interpretation of distributive justice. For example, the following have been proposed as valid material principles of distributive justice: (1) to each person an equal share, (2) to each according to need, (3) to each according to effort, (4) to each according to free market conditions, (5) to each so as to maximize overall usefulness. A more comprehensive description of the principles—and how they might be combined into multiprinciple allocation strategies—can be found elsewhere.[33][34]

A foundational debate about distributive justice is how to navigate the conflicting impulses to maximize efficiency (making decisions so as to produce the most good with the least expenditure), equity (treating individuals equally), and prioritarian conceptions of justice (favoring the worst off). Therefore, we briefly discuss three approaches to allocating scarce resources grounded in these radically different philosophical notions of justice: utilitarianism, egalitarianism, and prioritarianism. We also introduce the "rule of rescue."

To Each to Maximize Overall Quality-Adjusted Life Years: Utilitarianism

In general terms, utilitarianism seeks to maximize overall benefits at the societal level. There are numerous approaches to quantifying benefits related to health care. Many health economists advocate use of the quality-adjusted life years (QALYs) as the best metric.[35] Rationing by QALYs involves two steps: selecting outcome measures that adjust life-years for quality, and then allocating so as to maximize QALYs. Use of QALYs allows comparisons regarding effectiveness across diseases and services that would otherwise be

31. Hersch M, Sonnenblick M, Karlic A, Einav S, Sprung CL, Izbicki G. Mechanical ventilation of patients hospitalized in medical wards vs the intensive care unit—an observational, comparative study. J Crit Care. 2007;22(1):13–17.
32. Lieberman D, Nachshon L, Miloslavsky O, et al. Elderly patients undergoing mechanical ventilation in and out of intensive care units: a comparative, prospective study of 579 ventilations. Crit Care. 2010;14(2):R48.
33. Persad G, Wertheimer A, Emanuel EJ. Principles for allocation of scarce medical interventions. Lancet. 2009;373(9661):423–431.
34. White DB, Katz MH, Luce JM, Lo B. Who should receive life support during a public health emergency? Using ethical principles to improve allocation decisions. Ann Intern Med. 2009;150(2):132–138.
35. Neumann PJ, Weinstein MC. Legislating against use of cost-effectiveness information. N Engl J Med. 2010;363(16):1495–1497.

difficult to compare. For example, ICU treatment of life-threatening drug intoxication costs approximately $620 per QALY, ICU treatment of acute renal failure costs approximately $30,625 per QALY, and drotrecogin a treatment of patients with systemic inflammatory response syndrome and APACHE (Acute Physiology and Chronic Health Evaluation) II scores, <25 costs > $400,000 per QALY.[363738]

Rationing by maximizing QALYs has limitations. First, there are important unanswered questions regarding the best methods to quantify quality of life. For example, a person who has over time adapted to using a wheelchair may rate her quality of life the same as someone who is ambulatory, whereas someone recently confined to a wheelchair might rate her quality of life lower. These differences would lead to substantially different cost per QALY calculations depending on the time point at which quality-of-life assessments were obtained.

Additionally, simple strategies to maximize QALYs fail to consider how the benefits are distributed. For example, saving 95 QALYs distributed among two people in a population of 10 with the disease is not necessarily superior to saving 94 QALYs that are equally distributed across all 10 patients (9.4 QALYs per patient),[39] because of egalitarian concerns about equal distribution of benefits among similarly situated patients. Discounting lower quality of life may also systematically disadvantage those with chronic illness compared with those with good health; such practice opposes a commonly held moral intuition that it is important to help the worst off, or at least not to enable their poor health to be a self-fulfilling prophesy.

Despite these limitations, the National Institute for Health and Clinical Excellence in the United Kingdom uses QALYs to guide coverage decisions.[40] For example, drug treatments costing >£20,000–30,000 per QALY are not considered cost-effective and often are not approved for funding. In the United States, public mistrust of policies incorporating cost considerations has made the use of QALYs and cost-effectiveness analysis a political quagmire.[41]

To Each an Equal Opportunity: Egalitarianism

Egalitarianism emphasizes the equal moral status of individuals by trying to provide equal opportunity to have the basic goods in life. A straightforward example of an egalitarian approach to rationing is a lottery to determine priority for receiving a scarce resource. Many citizens have strong moral intuitions toward egalitarian allocation strategies, even when they come at the expense of utility maximization.[42] For example, if there were an insufficient supply of ICU beds for the number of patients in need, an egalitarian

36. Woolf SH. Potential health and economic consequences of misplaced priorities. JAMA. 2007;297(5):523–526.
37. Sznajder M, Aegerter P, Launois R, Merliere Y, Guidet B, CubRea. A cost-effectiveness analysis of stays in intensive care units. Intensive Care Med. 2001;27(1):146–153.
38. Talmor D, Shapiro N, Greenberg D, Stone PW, Neumann PJ. When is critical care medicine cost-effective? A systematic review of the cost-effectiveness literature. Crit Care Med. 2006;34(11):2738–2747.
39. Kamm F. Morality, Mortality: Volume I: Death and Whom to Save from It. New York, NY: Oxford University Press; 1998.
40. Measuring effectiveness and cost effectiveness: the QALY. National Institute for Health and Clinical Excellence Web site. http://www.nice.org.uk/newsroom/features/measuringeffectivenessandcosteffectivenesstheqaly.jsp. Accessed January 25, 2011.
41. Neumann PJ, Rosen AB, Weinstein MC. Medicare and cost-effectiveness analysis. N Engl J Med. 2005;353(14):1516–1522.
42. Ubel PA, Baron J, Nash B, Asch DA. Are preferences for equity over efficiency in health care allocation "all or nothing"? Med Care. 2000;38(4):366–373.

might advocate for a lottery to randomly select which patients would be admitted. Lotteries require little knowledge about recipients, can occur rapidly, and resist corruption. On the other hand, lotteries—and egalitarian principles of justice in general—are insensitive to factors that are also intuitively important to many, such as patients' need and likelihood of deriving benefit from treatment.

First-come, first-served strategies to allocate scarce resources appear to be egalitarian, but often are not., Existing guidelines support allocating ICU beds in this way,[43,44] and prior to 2005 waiting time was the primary criterion for allocating lungs for transplantation. However, time on the wait list for organ transplantation is not "random" in two ways. First, it favors those with diseases who are well enough to wait the longest. Second, those with power, knowledge, and connections often have the social resources to more quickly secure a position in the queue compared with those who have poor health-care access.

To Each to Favor the Worst Off: Prioritarianism

In general terms, prioritarianism attempts to help those who are considered the worst off by giving them priority in situations in which all cannot receive a particular resource. For example, a prioritarian might preferentially allocate medical resources to the young over the old because the young have had the least chance to live through life's stages. This "life cycle principle"—which is one example of a prioritarian allocation strategy—has been advocated as a way to allocate scarce organs for transplantation and mechanical ventilators during an influenza pandemic.'[45] The justification for this principle does not rely on considerations of one's intrinsic worth or social usefulness. Rather, the goal is to give all individuals equal opportunity to live a normal life span. When used alone to guide allocation decisions, the life cycle principle ignores prognostic differences among individuals. This type of objection points to the possibility that multiprinciple allocation strategies may better account for the complex moral considerations at play in such decisions compared with single-principle allocation strategies.

The Rule of Rescue

The rule of rescue describes a powerful psychologic impulse to attempt to save those facing death, no matter how expensive or how small the chance of benefit. The philosopher Albert Jonsen coined the term and describes it as "the moral response to the imminence of death [which] demands that we rescue the doomed."[46] In many ways, the impulse underlying the rule of rescue is an admirable human response to suffering. However, it also can lead to decisions that confound priority setting meant to maximize population-level outcomes. When Oregon refused to cover a potentially lifesaving bone marrow transplantation for 7-year-old Coby Howard, there was tremendous public outrage and negative media coverage, which likely arose as a consequence of not satisfying the psychologic impulse to rescue

43. American Thoracic Society. Fair allocation of intensive care unit resources. Am J Respir Crit Care Med. 1997;156(4 pt 1):1282–1301.

44. Guidelines for intensive care unit admission, discharge, and triage. Task Force of the American College of Critical Care Medicine, Society of Critical Care Medicine. Crit Care Med. 1999;27(3):633–638.

45. Emanuel EJ, Wertheimer A. Public health. Who should get influenza vaccine when not all can? Science. 2006;312(5775):854–855.

46. Jonsen A R. Bentham in a box: technology assessment and health care allocation. Law Med Health Care. 1986;14(3–4):172–174.

identifiable persons facing death.[47] The emotional costs of rationing ICU care would likely be similarly high because it would lead to the loss of identifiable lives.

Conflicts Between Efficiency, Equity, and the Rule of Rescue

The deep moral tensions between efficiency, equity, and responding to those facing death should not be underestimated. In surveys of physicians, citizens, and economists about how to balance such trade-offs, people generally prioritize treatment that can be made available to everyone, but this view is tempered by impulses to maximize usefulness and to rescue those in need.[48,49,50,51,52] Finding an acceptable balance between these competing ethical goals remains a serious challenge for the development of explicit rationing policies.

Fair Processes of Rationing

In morally pluralistic societies, reasonable people may be unable to agree about which principles should guide rationing. When such conflicts arise concerning high-stakes outcomes, using fair processes to make decisions acquires special ethical importance.[53] Daniels and Sabin and Daniels have proposed four characteristics of fair processes related to allocation: oversight by a legitimate institution, transparent decision making, reasoning according to information and principles that all can accept as relevant, and procedures for appealing and revising individual decisions. A fifth aspect of procedural fairness is meaningful public engagement.[54] This step is important to identify unanticipated needs and values and to obtain public support.[55]

The approach used to develop the Oregon Health Plan priority lists had many elements of procedural fairness: The process was under the authority of the state government, which is a legitimate authority for

47. Egan T. Rebuffed by Oregon, patients take their life-or-death cases public. New York Times. May 1, 1988. http://www.nytimes.com/1988/05/01/us/rebuffed-by-oregon-patients-take-their-lifeor-death-cases-public.html?scp=1&sq=may%201%201988%20coby%20oregon&st=cse. Accessed November 6, 2010.

48. Ubel PA, DeKay ML, Baron J, Asch DA. Cost-effectiveness analysis in a setting of budget constraints—is it equitable? N Engl J Med. 1996;334(18):1174–1177.

49. Perneger TV, Martin DP, Bovier PA. Physicians' attitudes toward health care rationing. Med Decis Making. 2002;22(1):65–70.

50. Ubel PA, Loewenstein G, Scanlon D, Kamlet M. Individual utilities are inconsistent with rationing choices: A partial explanation of why Oregon's cost-effectiveness list failed. Med Decis Making. 1996;16(2):108–116.

51. Ubel PA, Loewenstein G. The efficacy and equity of retransplantation: an experimental survey of public attitudes. Health Policy. 1995;34(2):145–151.

52. Ubel PA. How stable are people's preferences for giving priority to severely ill patients? Soc Sci Med. 1999;49(7):895–903.

53. Daniels N. Accountability for reasonableness. BMJ. 2000;321(7272):1300–1301.

54. Baum NM, Jacobson PD, Goold SD. "Listen to the people": public deliberation about social distancing measures in a pandemic. Am J Bioeth. 2009;9(11):4–14.

55. Danis M, Ginsburg M, Goold S. Experience in the United States with public deliberation about health insurance benefits using the small group decision exercise, CHAT. J Ambul Care Manage. 2010;33(3):205–214.

such policies; there was extensive public engagement; priority setting was explicit and incorporated expert opinion; and mechanisms were created for review and refinement of the priority list.[56]

Recent work by Baum and colleagues and Danis and colleagues has demonstrated the feasibility of public engagement related to priority setting in health care. For example, focus groups with citizens about priority setting during a severe influenza outbreak revealed a strong sense of support for interventions focused on the well-being of the community at large. Citizens also raised other ethical, economic, religious, and social concerns that policy makers must consider to develop just policies that will garner compliance. Other research has focused on engaging community participants in setting priorities for health insurance plans. Similar exercises have been used for research and policy settings in nine states. Their use improved understanding of the need to limit benefits in order to limit health-care spending, increased community mindedness of group decisions, and allowed groups to set priorities that at least 85% of participants were willing to abide by.

Will Fair Processes Fail for Tragic Choices?

Although public engagement and transparency seem indispensable for ethical priority setting in medicine, critics have argued that the emotionally and morally difficult choices raised by the rationing of life-saving medical therapies may prove resistant to rational debate. In their book *Tragic Choices*, Calabresi and Bobbitt argue that society is unlikely to be able to produce a durable, acceptable solution to the issue of scarcity in medicine because the consequences of denying these treatments to individual patients are intolerable.

They argue that individuals collectively attempt to deny moral responsibility for their role in choices—no matter how ethical or necessary—that consign individuals to death. This denial involves creating the illusion that the suffering arises out of nature rather than from conscious choices. For example, the safety standards in the mining industry do not create the safest possible environment for coal miners; doing so would be prohibitively expensive and threaten the market competitiveness of mining companies. However, when there is a mine accident and identifiable miners are trapped, nothing is spared to save them. This response supports the illusion that the mining accident was not preventable and that all was done to safeguard the lives at stake, while ignoring the initial decision that allowed people to work in conditions with a certain level of risk.

Two repeating processes characterize tragic choices. First, society iteratively remakes macro-and microallocation decisions to make human suffering appear as infrequent and random as possible. Second, society chooses ostensibly noncontroversial values to justify rationing decisions until the inherent conflict with basic values is exposed. For example, when hemodialysis was first developed as a life-saving therapy for patients with renal failure, demand outstripped supply, and the Seattle Dialysis Committee was formed to determine who would receive dialysis.[57] This panel made decisions that entailed refusing treatment to

56. Daniels N. Is the Oregon rationing plan fair? JAMA. 1991;265(17):2232–2235.
57. Rescher N. The allocation of exotic medical lifesaving therapy. Ethics. 1969;79(3):173–186.

patients who died as a result. An exposé of the committee's decisions was published in *LIFE* magazine,[58] which generated a national public firestorm. The public's distaste for allowing identifiable patients to die partly led Congress to authorize universal coverage for hemodialysis. In doing so, society was able to better tolerate the (still unresolved) societal question of how to allocate scarce medical resources because the proposed solution minimized the number of identifiable lives lost. In the last decade, the debate has reemerged in a predictable way, now focused on controlling spending while ensuring a minimum acceptable level of basic care for all. It is not yet clear whether the next iteration of health care reform will produce substantive changes rather than changes that appease our consciences but leave unaddressed the inevitability of tragic choices.

Would Rationing ICU Care Near the End of Life Save Money?

ICU care is expensive and not always successful. In the United States, upward of 0.66% of the gross domestic product is spent on critical care services, and care for those who die in ICUs totals tens of billions of dollars a year.[59][60] It would seem then that the ICU might be an ideal location for rationing. In our experience, some physicians believe that healthcare costs should be substantially reduced by strategies that allow unilateral withdrawal of life support in ICUs when patients do not respond fully to a trial of intensive care. However, Luce and Rubenfeld's analysis of ICU cost structures reveals that the truth is less straightforward. Because > 80% of hospitals' budgets are independent of the volume of patients treated (ie, fixed—mortgage, maintenance, utilities, and essential personnel salaries), only 20% of costs are modifiable on a per-patient basis (ie, variable—medications, diagnostic and therapeutic equipment, or patient care supplies). The analysis suggests that authorizing unilateral withdrawal of life support when ICU care appears to be failing is unlikely to meaningfully reduce costs. Several empiric studies support this claim.[61][62] Limiting the number of ICU beds built—and closing existing ICU beds—presents much greater opportunities for cost savings because both fixed and variable costs would be reduced.

Nonetheless, it is certainly true that some cost savings could result from rationing ICU care for patients with relatively poor chances of benefit, especially if rules were developed that delineated situations in which palliative care rather than ICU care would be provided. However, these types of policies would likely be socially divisive and politically challenging, because they would violate the rule of rescue and result in the deaths of identifiable patients.[63] Because the modest savings achieved may be

58. Alexander S. They decide who lives, who dies. LIFE. November 19, 1962;53(19):102–125.
59. Luce JM, Rubenfeld GD. Can health care costs be reduced by limiting intensive care at the end of life? Am J Respir Crit Care Med. 2002;165(6):750–754.
60. Ward NS. Rationing critical care medicine: recent studies and current trends. Curr Opin Crit Care. 2005;11(6):629–632.
61. Halevy A, Neal RC, Brody BA. The low frequency of futility in an adult intensive care unit setting. Arch Intern Med. 1996;156(1):100–104.
62. Sachdeva RC, Jefferson LS, Coss-Bu J, Brody BA. Resource consumption and the extent of futile care among patients in a pediatric intensive care unit setting. J Pediatr. 1996;128(6):742–747.
63. Newman TB. The power of stories over statistics. BMJ. 2003;327(7429):1424–1427.

outweighed by the psychologic costs and social outrage, efforts to explicitly ration health care should likely begin with less controversial medical decisions.

Conclusions

Rationing of health care is necessary, unavoidable, and ethically complex. The levels at which health care is rationed, and the transparency of rationing, are important structural considerations in creating a sustainable and just health-care system. Ethical rationing requires deliberate choices guided by reasonably applied principles and fair procedures. How rationing occurs is important because it not only affects individual lives but also expresses what values are most important to society. We live in a world in which need is boundless but resources are not—and medicine is not immune to the consequences of this reality.

Principles for Allocation of Scarce Medical Interventions

Govind Persad, Alan Wertheimer, Ezekiel J. Emanuel

In health care, as elsewhere, scarcity is the mother of allocation.[1] Although the extent is debated,[23] the scarcity of many specific interventions—including beds in intensive care units,[4] organs, and vaccines during pandemic influenza[5]—is widely acknowledged. For some interventions, demand exceeds supply. For others, an increased supply would necessitate redirection of important resources, and allocation decisions would still be necessary.[6]

Allocation of scarce medical interventions is a perennial challenge. During the 1940s, an expert committee allocated—without public input—then-novel penicillin to American soldiers

1. Rawls J. A theory of justice. Oxford: Oxford University Press, 1999.

2. Harris J. QALYfying the value of life. *J Med Ethics* 1987; **13:** 117–23.

3. Caplan AL. Organ transplant rationing: a window to the future? *Health Prog* 1987; **68:** 40–45.

4. Truog RD, Brock DW, Cook DJ, et al. Rationing in the intensive care unit. *Crit Care Med* 2006; **34:** 958–63.

5. Emanuel EJ, Wertheimer A. Who should get influenza vaccine when not all can? *Science* 2006; **312:** 854–55.

6. Veatch RM. Disaster preparedness and triage. *Mount Sinai J Med* 2005; **72:** 236–41.

before civilians, using expected efficacy and speed of return to duty as criteria.[7] During the 1960s, committees in Seattle allocated scarce dialysis machines using prognosis, current health, social worth, and dependants as criteria. How can scarce medical interventions be allocated justly? This paper identifies and evaluates eight simple principles that have been suggested.[8,9,10,11,12] Although some are better than others, no single principle allocates interventions justly. Rather, morally relevant simple principles must be combined into multiprinciple allocation systems. We evaluate three existing systems and then recommend a new one: the complete lives system.

Simple Allocation Principles

Eight simple ethical principles for allocation can be classified into four categories, according to their core ethical values: treating people equally, favouring the worst-off, maximising total benefits, and promoting and rewarding social usefulness (table 3.8.1). We do not regard ability to pay as a plausible option for the scarce life-saving interventions we discuss.

Table 3.8.1   Simple principles and their core ethical values

	Advantages	Disadvantages	Examples of use	Recommendation
Treating people equally				
Lottery	Hard to corrupt; little information about recipients needed	Ignores other relevant principles	Military draft; schools; vaccination	Include
First-come, first-served	Protects existing doctor-patient relationships; little information about recipients needed	Favours wealthy, powerful, and well-connected; ignores other relevant principles	ICU beds; part of organ allocation	Exclude
Favouring the worst-off: prioritarianism				

7. McGough LJ, Reynolds SJ, Quinn TC, Zenilman JM. Which patients first? Setting priorities for antiretroviral therapy where resources are limited. *Am J Pub Health* 2005; **95:** 1173–80.

8. Kamm FM. Morality, mortality, volume 1: death and whom to save from it. New York: Oxford University Press, 1993.

9. Cookson R, Dolan P. Principles of justice in health care rationing. *J Med Ethics* 2000; **26:** 323–29.

10. Arras JD. Rationing vaccine during an avian influenza pandemic: why it won't be easy. *Yale J Biol Med* 2005; **78:** 287–300.

11. Rescher N. The allocation of exotic medical lifesaving therapy. *Ethics* 1969; **79:** 173–86.

12. Beauchamp T, Childress JF. Principles of biomedical ethics. New York: Oxford University Press, 2001.

Table 3.8.1 Simple principles and their core ethical values

Sickest first	Aids those who are suffering right now; appeals to "rule of rescue"; makes sense in temporary scarcity; proxy for being worst off overall	Surreptitious use of prognosis; ignores needs of those who will become sick in future; might falsely assume temporary scarcity; leads to people receiving interventions only after prognosis deteriorates; ignores other relevant principles	Emergency rooms; part of organ allocation	Exclude
Youngest first	Benefits those who have had least life; prudent planners have an interest in living to old age	Undesirable priority to infants over adolescents and young adults; ignores other relevant principles	New NVAC/ACIP pandemic flu vaccine proposal	Include
Maximising total benefits: utilitarianism				
Number of lives saved	Saves more lives, benefiting the greatest number; avoids need for comparative judgments about quality or other aspects of lives	Ignores other relevant principles	Past ACIP/NVAC pandemic flu vaccine policy; bioterrorism response policy; disaster triage	Include
Prognosis or life-years saved	Maximises life-years produced	Ignores other relevant principles, particularly distributive principles	Penicillin allocation; traditional military triage (prognosis) and disaster triage (life-years saved)	Include
Promoting and rewarding social usefulness				
Instrumental value	Helps promote other important values; future oriented	Vulnerable to abuse through choice of prioritised occupations or activities; can direct health resources away from health needs	Past and current NVAC/ACIP pandemic flu vaccine policy	Include but only in some public health emergencies
Reciprocity	Rewards those who implemented important values; past oriented	Vulnerable to abuse; can direct health resources away from health needs; intrusive assessment process	Some organ donation policies	Include only irreplaceable people who have suffered serious losses

Some people wrongly suggest that allocation can be based purely on scientific or clinical facts, often using the term "medical need".[13][14] There are no value-free medical criteria for allocation.[15][16] Although biomedical facts determine a person's post-transplant prognosis or the dose of vaccine that would confer immunity, responding to these facts requires ethical, value-based judgments. When evaluating principles, we need to distinguish between those that are insufficient and those that are flawed. Insufficient principles ignore some morally relevant considerations. Conversely, flawed principles recognise morally irrelevant considerations: inherently flawed principles necessarily recognise irrelevant considerations, whereas practically flawed principles allow irrelevant considerations to affect allocation. Principles that are individually insufficient could form part of an acceptable multiprinciple system, whereas systems that include flawed principles are untenable because they will always recognise irrelevant considerations.

Treating people equally

Many scarce medical interventions, such as organ transplants, are indivisible. For indivisible goods, benefiting people equally entails providing equal chances at the scarce intervention—equality of opportunity, rather than equal amounts of it. Two principles attempt to embody this value.

Lottery

Allocation by lottery has been used, sometimes with explicit judicial and legislative endorsement, in military conscription, immigration, education, and distribution of vaccines.[17][18]

Lotteries have several attractions. Equal moral status supports an equal claim to scarce resources.[19] Even among only roughly equal candidates, lotteries prevent small differences from drastically affecting outcome. Some people also support lottery allocation because "each person's desire to stay alive should be regarded as of the same importance and deserving the same respect as that of anyone else".[20] Practically, lottery allocation is quick and requires little knowledge about recipients. Finally, lotteries resist corruption.

The major disadvantage of lotteries is their blindness to many seemingly relevant factors.[21][22] Random decisions between someone who can gain 40 years and someone who can gain only 4 months, or

13. Langford MJ. Who should get the kidney machine? *J Med Ethics* 1992; **18:** 12–17.

14. Liss P-E. Hard choices in public health: the allocation of scarce resources. *Scand J Public Health* 2003; **31:** 156–57.

15. Hope T, Sprigings D, Crisp R. "Not clinically indicated": patients' interests or resource allocation? *BMJ* 1993; **306:** 379–81.

16. Brock DW. The misplaced role of urgency in allocation of persistently scarce life-saving organs. In: Gutmann T, Land W, Daar AS, Sells RA, eds. Ethical, legal, and social issues in organ transplantation. Lengerich, Germany: Pabst Science Publishers 2004: 41–48.

17. Silverman WA, Chalmers I. Casting and drawing lots: a time honoured way of dealing with uncertainty and ensuring fairness. *BMJ* 2001; **323:** 1467–68.

18. Broome J. Selecting people randomly. *Ethics* 1984; **95:** 38–55.

19. Ramsey P. The patient as person: exploration in medical ethics. New Haven, CT: Yale University Press, 2002.

20. Harris J. The value of life. London: Routledge & Kegan Paul, 1985.

21. Stein MS. The distribution of life-saving medical resources: equality, life expectancy, and choice behind the veil. *Soc Philos Policy* 2002; **19:** 212–45.

22. Elhauge E. Allocating health care morally. *Calif Law Rev* 1994; **82:** 1449–1544.

someone who has already lived for 80 years and someone who has lived only 20 years, are inappropriate. Treating people equally often fails to treat them as equals.[23] Ultimately, although allocation solely by lottery is insufficient, the lottery's simplicity and resistance to corruption suggests that it could be incorporated into a multiprinciple system.

First-come, first-served

Within health care, many people endorse a first-come, first-served distribution of beds in intensive care units[24] or organs for transplant.[25] The American Thoracic Society defends this principle as "a natural lottery—an egalitarian approach for fair [intensive care unit] resource allocation." Others believe it promotes fair equality of opportunity, and allows physicians to avoid discontinuing interventions, such as respirators, even when other criteria support moving those interventions to new arrivals.[26] Some people simply equate it to lottery allocation.

As with lottery allocation, first-come, first-served ignores relevant differences between people, but in practice fails even to treat people equally. It favours people who are well-off, who become informed, and travel more quickly, and can queue for interventions without competing for employment or child-care concerns.[27] Queues are also vulnerable to additional corruption. As New York State's pandemic influenza planners stated, "Those who could figuratively (and sometimes literally) push to the front of the line would be vaccinated and stand the best chance for survival".[28] First-come, first-served allows morally irrelevant qualities—such as wealth, power, and connections—to decide who receives scarce interventions, and is therefore practically flawed.

Favouring the worst-off: prioritarianism

Franklin Roosevelt argued that "the test of our progress is not whether we add more to the abundance of those who have much; it is whether we provide enough for those who have too little".[29] Philosophers call this preference for the worst-off prioritarianism.[30] Some define being worst-off as currently lacking valuable goods, whereas others define it as lacking valuable goods throughout one's entire life. Two principles embody these two interpretations.

23. Dworkin RM. Sovereign virtue: the theory and practice of equality. New York: Harvard University Press, 2002.

24. American Thoracic Society Bioethics Task Force. Fair allocation of intensive care unit resources. *Am J Respir Crit Care Med* 1997; **156:** 1282–1301.

25. Childress JF. Putting patients first in organ allocation: an ethical analysis of the US debate. *Camb Q Healthc Ethics* 2001; **10:** 365–76.

26. Lo B, White DB. Intensive care unit triage during an influenza pandemic: the need for specific clinical guidelines. Paper presented at: Ethical and legal considerations in mitigating pandemic disease. Washington, DC; 2007.

27. Daniels N. Fair process in patient selection for antiretroviral treatment in WHO's goal of 3 by 5. *Lancet* 2005; **366:** 169–71.

28. Billittier AJ. Who goes first? *J Public Health Manag Pract* 2005; **11:** 267–68.

29. Roosevelt FD. Second Inaugural Address, 1937; Washington, DC.

30. Parfit D. Equality and priority. *Ratio* 1997; **10:** 202–21.

Sickest first

Treating the sickest people first prioritises those with the worst future prospects if left untreated. The so-called rule of rescue, which claims that "our moral response to the imminence of death demands that we rescue the doomed", exemplifies this principle.[31] Transplantable livers and hearts, as well as emergency-room care, are allocated to the sickest individuals first.

Some people might argue that treating the sickest individuals first is intuitively obvious.[32] Others claim that the sickest people are also probably worst off overall, because healthier people might recover unaided or be saved later by new interventions.[33] Finally, sickest-first allocation appeals to prognosis if untreated—a criterion clinicians frequently consider.

On its own, sickest-first allocation ignores post-treatment prognosis: it applies even when only minor gains at high cost can be achieved. To circumvent this result, some misleadingly claim that sick people with a small but clear chance of benefit do not have a medical need. Sick recipients' prognoses are wrongly assumed to be normal, even though many interventions—such as liver transplants—are less effective for the sickest people.[34]

If the failure to take account of prognosis were its only problem, sickest-first allocation would merely be insufficient. However, it myopically bases allocation on how sick someone is at the current time—a morally arbitrary factor in genuine scarcity. Preferential allocation of a scarce liver to an acutely ill person unjustly ignores a currently healthier person with progressive liver disease, who might be worse off when he or she later suffers liver failure. Favouring those who are currently sickest seems to assume that resource scarcity is temporary: that we can save the person who is now sickest and then save the progressively ill person later. However, even temporary scarcity does not guarantee another chance to save the progressively ill person. Furthermore, when interventions are persistently scarce, saving the progressively ill person later will always involve depriving others. When we cannot save everyone, saving the sickest first is inherently flawed and inconsistent with the core idea of priority to the worst-off.

Youngest first

Although not always recognised as such, youngest-first allocation directs resources to those who have had less of something supremely valuable—life-years. Dialysis machines and scarce organs have been allocated to younger recipients fir st,[35] and proposals for allocation in pandemic influenza prioritise infants and children.[36] Daniel Callahan[37] has suggested strict age cut-offs for scarce life-saving interventions,

31. Jonsen AR. Bentham in a box: technology assessment and health care allocation. *Law Med Health Care* 1986; **14:** 172–74.
32. McKerlie D. Justice between the young and the old. *Philos Publ Aff* 2001; **30:** 152–77.
33. Veatch RM. Equity in liver allocation: Professor Veatch's reply. *Med Ethics* 2001: 7.
34. Howard DH. Hope versus efficiency in organ allocation. *Transplantation* 2001; **72:** 1169–73.
35. Rutecki GW, Kilner JF. Dialysis as a resource allocation paradigm: confronting tragic choices once again? *Semin Dial* 1999; **12:** 38–43.
36. Department of Health and Human Services. Draft guidance on allocating and targeting pandemic influenza vaccine. http://www.pandemicflu.gov/vaccine/prioritization.pdf (accessed Jan 19, 2009).
37. Callahan DD. Setting limits: medical goals in an aging society. Washington, DC: Georgetown University Press; 1995.

whereas Alan Williams[38] has suggested a system that allocates interventions based on individuals' distance from a normal life-span if left unaided.

Prioritising the youngest gives priority to the worst-off—those who would otherwise die having had the fewest life-years—and is thus fundamentally different from favouritism towards adults or people who are well-off. Also, allocating preferentially to the young has an appeal that favouring other worst-off individuals such as women, poor people, or minorities lacks: "Because [all people] age, treating people of different ages differently does not mean that we are treating persons unequally."[39] Prudent planners would allocate life-saving interventions to themselves earlier in life to improve their chances of living to old age. These justifications explain much of the public preference for allocating scarce life-saving interventions to younger people.[40][41]

Strict youngest-first allocation directs scarce resources predominantly to infants. This approach seems incorrect. The death of a 20-year-old young woman is intuitively worse than that of a 2-month-old girl, even though the baby has had less life. The 20-year-old has a much more developed personality than the infant, and has drawn upon the investment of others to begin as-yet-unfulfilled projects. Youngest-first allocation also ignores prognosis,[42] and categorically excludes older people. Thus, youngest-first allocation seems insufficient on its own, but it could be combined with prognosis and lottery principles in a multiprinciple allocation system.

Maximising Total Benefits: Utilitarianism

Maximising benefits is a utilitarian value, although principles differ about which benefits to maximise.

Save the Most Lives

One maximising strategy involves saving the most individual lives, and it has motivated policies on allocation of influenza vaccine and responses to bioterrorism.[43] Since each life is valuable, this principle seems to need no special justification. It also avoids comparing individual lives. Other things being equal, we should always save five lives rather than one.[44]

However, other things are rarely equal. Some lives have been shorter than others; 20-year-olds have lived less than 70-year-olds. Similarly, some lives can be extended longer than others. How to weigh these other relevant considerations against saving more lives—whether to save one 20-year-old, who might

38. Williams A. Inequalities in health and intergenerational equity. *Ethical Theory Moral Pract* 1999; **2:** 47–55.

39. Daniels N. Am I my parents' keeper? An essay on justice between the young and the old. Oxford University Press, 1988.

40. McKie J, Richardson J. Neglected equity issues in cost-effectiveness analysis, Part 1: severity of pre-treatment condition, realisation of potential for health, concentration and dispersion of health benefits, and age-related social preferences. Melbourne: Centre for Health Program Evaluation, 2005.

41. Tsuchiya A, Dolan P, Shaw R. Measuring people's preferences regarding ageism in health: some methodological issues and some fresh evidence. *Soc Sci Med* 2003; **57:** 687.

42. Brock DW. Children's rights to health care. *J Med Philos* 2001; **26:** 163–77.

43. Phillips S. Current status of surge research. *Acad Emerg Med* 2006; **13:** 1103–08.

44. Hsieh N-H, Strudler A, Wasserman D. The numbers problem. *Philos Publ Aff* 2006; **34:** 352–72.

live another 60 years if saved, or three 70-year-olds who could only live for 10 years each—is unclear.[45] Although insufficient on its own, saving more lives should be part of a multiprinciple allocation system.

Prognosis or Life-Years

Rather than saving the most lives, prognosis allocation aims to save the most life-years. This strategy has been used in disaster triage and penicillin allocation, and motivates the exclusion of people with poor prognoses from organ transplantation waiting lists.[46] Maximising life-years has intuitive appeal. Living more years is valuable, so saving more years also seems valuable.

However, even supporters of prognosis-based allocation acknowledge its inability to consider distribution as well as quantity. Making a well-off person slightly better off rather than slightly improving a worse-off person's life would be unjust; likewise, why give an extra year to a person who has lived for many when it could be given to someone who would otherwise die having had few?[47] Similarly, giving a few life-years to many differs from giving many life-years to a few. As with the principle of saving the most lives, prognosis is undeniably relevant but insufficient alone.

Promoting and Rewarding Social Usefulness

Unlike the previous values, social value cannot direct allocation on its own. Rather, social value allocation prioritises specific individuals to enable them to promote other important values, or rewards them for having promoted these values.

In view of the multiplicity of reasonable values in society and in view of what is at stake, social value allocation must not legislate socially conventional, mainstream values. When Seattle's dialysis policy favoured parents and church-goers, it was criticised: "The Pacific Northwest is no place for a Henry David Thoreau with kidney failure."[48] Allocators must also avoid directing interventions earmarked for health needs to those not relevant to the health problem at hand, which covertly exacerbates scarcity.[49] For instance, funeral directors might be essential to preserving health in an influenza pandemic, but not during a shortage of intensive-care beds.

Instrumental Value

Instrumental value allocation prioritises specific individuals to enable or encourage future usefulness. Guidelines that prioritise workers producing influenza vaccine exemplify instrumental value allocation to

45. Glover J. Causing death and saving lives. New York: Penguin, 1977.
46. Russell LB, Siegel JE, Daniels N, Gold MR, Luce BR, Mandelblatt JS. Cost-effectiveness analysis as a guide to resource allocation in health: roles and limitations. In: Gold MR, Siegel JE, Russell LB, Weinstein MC, eds. Cost-effectiveness in health and medicine. New York: Oxford University Press; 1996: 3–24.
47. Kappel K, Sandøe P. QALYs, age and fairness. *Bioethics* 1992; 6: 297–316.
48. Sanders D, Dukeminier J. Medical advance and legal lag: hemodialysis and kidney transplantation. *UCLA Law Rev* 1968; **15:** 357–419.
49. Brock DW. Separate spheres and indirect benefits. *Cost Eff Resour Alloc* 2003; **1:** 4.

save the most lives. Responsibility-based allocation—eg, allocation to people who agree to improve their health and thus use fewer resources—also represents instrumental value allocation.[50]

This approach is necessarily insufficient, because it derives its appeal from promoting other values, such as saving more lives: "all whose continued existence is clearly required so that others might live have a good claim to priority". Prioritising essential health-care staff does not treat them as counting for more in themselves, but rather prioritises them to benefit others. Instrumental value allocation thus arguably recognises the moral importance of each person, even those not instrumentally valuable.

Student military deferments have shown that instrumental value allocation can encourage abuse of the system.[51] People also disagree about usefulness: is saving all legislators necessary in an influenza pandemic? Decisions on usefulness can involve complicated and demeaning inquiries.[52] However, where a specific person is genuinely indispensable in promoting morally relevant principles, instrumental value allocation can be appropriate.

Reciprocity

Reciprocity allocation is backward-looking, rewarding past usefulness or sacrifice. As such, many describe this allocative principle as desert or rectificatory justice, rather than reciprocity. For important health-related values, reciprocity might involve preferential allocation to past organ donors, to participants in vaccine research who assumed risk for others' benefit,[53] or to people who made healthy lifestyle choices that reduced their need for resources. Priority to military veterans embodies reciprocity for promoting non-health values.[54]

Proponents claim that "justice as reciprocity calls for providing something in return for contributions that people have made". Reciprocity might also be relevant when people are conscripted into risky tasks. For instance, nurses required to care for contagious patients could deserve reciprocity, especially if they did not volunteer.

Reciprocity allocation, like instrumental value allocation, might potentially require time-consuming, intrusive, and demeaning inquiries, such as investigating whether a person adhered to a healthy lifestyle. Furthermore, unlike instrumental value, reciprocity does not have the future-directed appeal of promoting important health values. Ultimately, the appropriateness of allocation based on reciprocity seems to depend in a complex way on several factors, such as seriousness of sacrifice and irreplaceability. For instance, former organ donors seem to deserve reciprocity since they make a serious sacrifice and since there is no surplus of organ donors. By contrast, laboratory staff who serve as vaccine production workers do not incur serious risk nor are they irreplaceable, so reciprocity seems less appropriate for them.

50. Morreim EH. Lifestyles of the risky and infamous. From managed care to managed lives. *Hastings Center Report* 1995; **25:** 5–12.
51. Burgess EW. The effect of war on the American family. *Am J Sociol* 1942; **48:** 343–52.
52. Anderson ES. What is the point of equality? *Ethics* 1999; **109:** 287–337.
53. Macklin R. Ethics and equity in access to HIV treatment: 3 by 5 initiative. 2004.
54. Kass L. Session 5: Organ donation, procurement, allocation, and transplantation: policy options: The President's Council on Bioethics; 2006.

Assessing principles: allocation systems

Which principles best embody morally relevant values? First-come, first-served is flawed in practice because it unwittingly allows irrelevant considerations, such as wealth, to affect allocation decisions, whereas a lottery is insufficient but not flawed. Similarly, sickest-first allocation is inherently flawed, whereas the youngest-first principle, though insufficient, recognises the important value of priority to the worst-off. Both utilitarian principles—maximising lives saved and prognosis—are relevant but insufficient, and usefulness and reciprocity are relevant where irreplaceable individuals make serious sacrifices, such as those during public health emergencies.

Ultimately, no principle is sufficient on its own to recognise all morally relevant considerations. Combining principles into systems increases complexity and controversy, but is inevitable if allocations are to incorporate the complexity of our moral values (table 3.8.2). People disagree about which principles to include and how to balance them. Many allocation systems do not make their content explicit, nor do they justify their choices about inclusion, balancing, and specification. Elucidating, comparing, and evaluating allocation systems should be a research priority.

United Network for Organ Sharing (UNOS) points systems

The UNOS points systems are used for organ allocation (table 3.8.2). They combine three principles: sickest-first (current medical condition); first-come, first-served (waiting time); and prognosis (antigen, antibody, and blood type matching between recipient and donor). UNOS weights principles differently depending on the organ distributed. Kidney and pancreas allocation is mainly by waiting time, with some weight given to sickest-first and prognosis.[55] Conversely, heart allocation weights sickest-first principles heavily and waiting time less so. Lung and liver allocation takes into account waiting time, sickest-first, and prognosis. Historically, no UNOS system has emphasised prognosis, although UNOS's most recent policy discussions on lung allocation suggest such a change.[56]

Table 3.8.2 Four multiprinciple systems

	Principles included	Advantages	Objections
UNOS points systems for organ allocation in the USA	First-come, first-served; sickest-first; prognosis	Can combine all possible principles; flexible	Includes least justifiable principles: first-come, first-served and sickest-first; low priority given to prognosis; vulnerable to bias and manipulation, such as being listed on multiple transplantation lists and misrepresentation of health status; allows multiple organ transplants, thus saving fewer lives

55. United Network for Organ Sharing. Policies. http://www.unos.org/policiesandbylaws/policies.asp (accessed Sept 30, 2008).
56. Organ Procurement and Transplantation Network. Public Forum to Discuss Kidney Allocation Policy Development Synopsis, 2007; Dallas.

Table 3.8.2. Four multiprinciple systems

QALY allocation	Prognosis; excludes save the most lives	Maximises future benefits; considers quality of life; used in many existing, quantitatively sophisticated frameworks	Outcome measure disadvantages disabled people; incorrect conception of equality by focusing on equality of QALYs rather than equality of persons; does not incorporate many relevant principles
DALY allocation	Prognosis; instrumental value; excludes save the most lives	Maximises future benefits; includes instrumental value, saving people whose productivity is key to a flourishing society	Outcome measure disadvantages disabled people; age considered as modifying value of individual life-years, rather than from standpoint of distributive justice; definition of instrumental value is too focused on economic worth, and could justify bias towards heads of household and other "traditional" social positions; does not incorporate many relevant principles
Complete lives System	Youngest-first; prognosis; save the most lives; lottery; instrumental value, but only in public health emergency	Matches intuition that death of adolescents is worse than that of infants or elderly; everyone has an interest in living through all life stages; incorporates the largest number of relevant principles; resistant to corruption	Reduced chances for persons who have lived many years; life-years are not a relevant health care outcome; unable to deal with international differences in life expectancy; need lexical priority rather than balancing; complete lives system is not appropriate for general distribution of health care resources

UNOS=United Network for Organ Sharing. QALY=quality-adjusted life-years. DALY=disability-adjusted life-years.

The UNOS point systems are flexible: conceivably, they could include any simple principle by translating it into a points framework. The systems are easily revisable to weight one principle more heavily than others.

Current UNOS systems incorporate two flawed simple principles: first-come, first-served and sickest first. They are also vulnerable to additional exploitation. Taking advantage of the first-come, first-served principle, well-off patients place themselves on multiple waiting lists.[57] Exploiting the sickest-first element, some transplant centres have temporarily altered or misrepresented their patients' health state to get them scarce organs, making sickest-first both practically and inherently flawed.[58,59]

Furthermore, UNOS points systems do not appropriately consider the benefit-maximising principles, prognosis, and saving the most lives, nor do they include youngest-first allocation. Most dramatically, multiple-organ transplants to one individual are permitted, even when a heart-lung-liver combination could

57. Zink S, Wertlieb S, Catalano J, Marwin V. Examining the potential exploitation of UNOS policies. *Am J Bioethics* 2005; **5**: 6.

58. Murphy TF. Gaming the transplant system. *Am J Bioethics* 2004; **4**: W28.

59. Morreim EH. Another kind of end-run: status upgrades. *Am J Bioethics* 2005; **5**: 11.

save three lives if transplanted separately.[60] Similarly, policy revisions during the 1990s deemphasised organ-recipient matching even though poorer matching leads to fewer lives saved.[61]

Attempts to remedy these deficiencies have been covert and haphazard. In an effort to implement prognosis allocation tacitly, ill or old people have been excluded from supposedly first-come, first-served waiting lists.[62] Physicians can misdiagnose comorbidities as contra-indications, wrongly implying that transplants will harm recipients, rather than explicitly practising prognosis-based allocation.[63] Some have proposed so-called old-for-old policies that match donor organ age to recipient age—misrepresenting both youngest-first and prognosis-based allocation as biological fact.[64] Others have advocated local rather than national waiting lists to circumvent sickest-first allocation.[65] Explicit and public acknowledgment of allocation strategies would be preferable to this surreptitious and piecemeal approach.

Quality-adjusted life-years

Allocation systems based on quality-adjusted life-years (QALY) have two parts (table 3.8.2). One is an outcome measure that considers the quality of life-years. As an example, the quality-of-life measure used by the UK National Health Service rates moderate mobility impairment as 0.85 times perfect health.[66] QALY allocation therefore equates 8.5 years in perfect health to 10 years with moderately impaired mobility.[67] The other part of QALY allocation is a maximising assumption: that justice requires total QALYs to be maximised without consideration of their distribution.[68] QALY allocation initially constituted the basis for Oregon's Medicaid coverage initiative, and is currently used by the UK's National Institute for Health and Clinical Excellence (NICE).[6970] Both the ethics and efficacy of QALY allocation have been substantially discussed.

The QALY outcome measure has problems. Even if a life-year in which a person has impaired mobility is worse than a healthy life-year, someone adapted to wheelchair use might reasonably value an additional

60. Stein MS. The distribution of life-saving medical resources: equality, life expectancy, and choice behind the veil. *Soc Philos Policy* 2002: 19.
61. Mutinga N, Brennan DC, Schnitzler MA. Consequences of eliminating HLA-B in deceased donor kidney allocation to increase minority transplantation. *Am J Transplant* 2005; **5:** 1090.
62. Oniscu GC, Schalkwijk AAH, Johnson RJ, Brown H, Forsythe JLR. Equity of access to renal transplant waiting list and renal transplantation in Scotland: cohort study. *BMJ* 2003; **327:** 1261.
63. Miller LW. Listing criteria for cardiac transplantation: results of an American Society of Transplant Physicians-National Institutes of Health conference. *Transplantation* 1998; **66:** 947–51.
64. Arns W, Citterio F, Campistol JM. Old-for-old—new strategies for renal transplantation. *Nephrol Dial Transplant* 2007; **22:** 336–41.
65. Alexander GC, Werner RM, Ubel PA. The costs of denying scarcity. *Arch Intern Med* 2004; **164:** 593–96.
66. Kind P, Hardman G, Macran S, University of York Centre for Health E. UK Population Norms for EQ-5D: Centre for Health Economics, University of York; 1999.
67. National Institute for Clinical Excellence. Guide to the methods of technology appraisal. NICE: London; 2003.
68. McGregor M. Cost-utility analysis: Use QALYs only with great caution. *CMAJ* 2003; **168:** 433.
69. Rawlins MD, Culyer AJ. National Institute for Clinical Excellence and its value judgments. *BMJ* 2004; **329:** 224.
70. Hadorn DC. The Oregon priority-setting exercise: quality of life and public policy. *Hastings Center Report* 1991; **21:** S11–16.

life-year in a wheelchair as much as a non-disabled person would value an additional life-year without disability.[71] Allocators have struggled with this issue.[72]

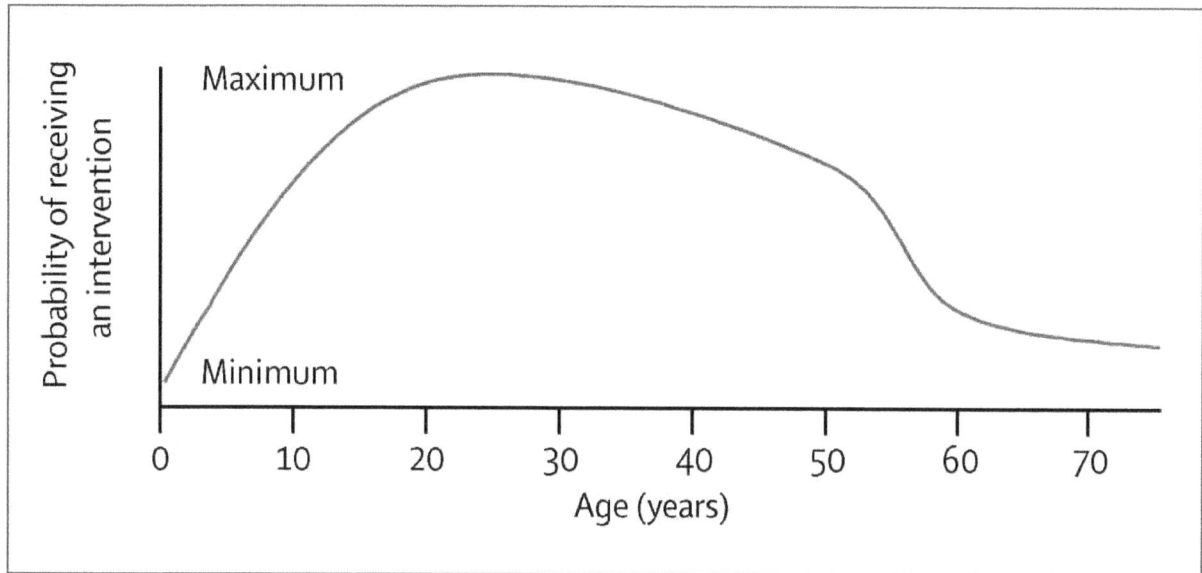

Figure 3.8.1   Age-based priority for receiving scarce medical interventions under the complete lives system

More importantly, maximising the number of QALYs is an insufficient basis for allocation. Although QALY advocates appeal to the idea that all QALYs are equal, people, not QALYs, deserve equal treatment.[73] Treatment of a serious disease such as appendicitis gives a few people many more QALYs, whereas treatment of a minor problem like uncapped teeth gives many people a few more QALYs. Even though the two strategies produce equal numbers of QALYs, they treat individuals very differently. Likewise, giving QALYs to someone who has had few life-years differs morally from giving them to someone who has already had many. Ultimately, QALY allocation systems do not recognise many morally relevant values—such as treating people equally, giving priority to the worst-off, and saving the most lives—and are therefore insufficient for just allocation.

Disability-adjusted life-years

WHO endorses the system of disability-adjusted life-year (DALY) allocation (table 2).[74] As with QALY allocation, DALY allocation does not consider interpersonal distribution. DALY systems also incorporate

71. Menzel P, Dolan P, Richardson J, Olsen JA. The role of adaptation to disability and disease in health state valuation: a preliminary normative analysis. *Soc Sci Med* 2002; **55:** 2149.

72. Ubel PA, Nord E, Gold M, Menzel P, Prades JL, Richardson J. Improving value measurement in cost-effectiveness analysis. *Med Care* 2000; **38:** 892.

73. Pronovost P, Angus DC. Economics of end-of-life care in the intensive care unit. *Crit Care Med* 2001; **29** (2 suppl): N46–N51.

74. Murray CJL, Acharya AK. Understanding DALYs. *J Health Econ* 1997; **16:** 703.

quality-of-life factors—for instance, they equate a life-year with blindness to roughly 0.6 healthy life-years. Additionally, DALY allocation ranks each life-year with the age of the person as a modifier: "The well-being of some age groups, we argue, is instrumental in making society flourish; therefore collectively we may be more concerned with improving health status for individuals in these age groups." This argument, although used to justify age-weighting, would equally justify counting the life-years of economically productive people and those caring for others for more.

DALY allocation wrongly incorporates age into the outcome measure, claiming that a year for a younger person is in itself more valuable. Priority for young people is better justified on grounds of distributive justice. Also, the use of instrumental value to justify DALY allocation resembles that used in Seattle's dialysis allocation, which inappropriately favoured wage earners and carers of dependants.

The Complete Lives System

Because none of the currently used systems satisfy all ethical requirements for just allocation, we propose an alternative: the complete lives system. This system incorporates five principles (table 2): youngest-first, prognosis, save the most lives, lottery, and instrumental value. As such, it prioritises younger people who have not yet lived a complete life and will be unlikely to do so without aid. Many thinkers have accepted complete lives as the appropriate focus of distributive justice: "individual human lives, rather than individual experiences, [are] the units over which any distributive principle should operate."[75][76] Although there are important differences between these thinkers, they share a core commitment to consider entire lives rather than events or episodes, which is also the defining feature of the complete lives system.

Consideration of the importance of complete lives also supports modifying the youngest-first principle by prioritising adolescents and young adults over infants (figure). Adolescents have received substantial education and parental care, investments that will be wasted without a complete life. Infants, by contrast, have not yet received these investments. Similarly, adolescence brings with it a developed personality capable of forming and valuing long-term plans whose fulfilment requires a complete life.[77] As the legal philosopher Ronald Dworkin argues, "It is terrible when an infant dies, but worse, most people think, when a three-year-old child dies and worse still when an adolescent does";[78] this argument is supported by empirical surveys.[79] Importantly, the prioritisation of adolescents and young adults considers the social and personal investment that people are morally entitled to have received at a particular age, rather than accepting the results of an unjust status quo. Consequently, poor adolescents should be treated the same as wealthy ones, even though they may have received less investment owing to social injustice.

The complete lives system also considers prognosis, since its aim is to achieve complete lives. A young person with a poor prognosis has had few life-years but lacks the potential to live a complete life. Considering prognosis forestalls the concern that disproportionately large amounts of resources will be

75. Nagel T. Mortal questions. New York: Cambridge University Press; 2000.
76. Aristotle. Nicomachean ethics. Cambridge University Press, 2000.
77. Shaffer DR, Kipp K. Developmental psychology: childhood and adolescence, 6th edn. London: Wadsworth, 2007.
78. Dworkin RM. Life's dominion. Knopf, 1993.
79. Richardson J. Age weighting and discounting: what are the ethical Issues? Melbourne: Centre for Health Program Evaluation; 1999.

directed to young people with poor prognoses. When the worst-off can benefit only slightly while better-off people could benefit greatly, allocating to the better-off is often justifiable. Some small benefits, such as a few weeks of life, might also be intrinsically insignificant when compared with large benefits.

Saving the most lives is also included in this system because enabling more people to live complete lives is better than enabling fewer. In a public health emergency, instrumental value could also be included to enable more people to live complete lives. Lotteries could be used when making choices between roughly equal recipients, and also potentially to ensure that no individual—irrespective of age or prognosis—is seen as beyond saving.[80] Thus, the complete lives system is complete in another way: it incorporates each morally relevant simple principle.

When implemented, the complete lives system produces a priority curve on which individuals aged between roughly 15 and 40 years get the most substantial chance, whereas the youngest and oldest people get chances that are attenuated (figure). It therefore superficially resembles the proposal made by DALY advocates; however, the complete lives system justifies preference to younger people because of priority to the worst-off rather than instrumental value. Additionally, the complete lives system assumes that, although life-years are equally valuable to all, justice requires the fair distribution of them. Conversely, DALY allocation treats life-years given to elderly or disabled people as objectively less valuable.

Finally, the complete lives system is least vulnerable to corruption. Age can be established quickly and accurately from identity documents. Prognosis allocation encourages physicians to improve patients' health, unlike the perverse incentives to sicken patients or misrepresent health that the sickest-first allocation creates.

Objections

We consider several important objections to the complete lives system.

The complete lives system discriminates against older people.[81,82] Age-based allocation is ageism. Unlike allocation by sex or race, allocation by age is not invidious discrimination; every person lives through different life stages rather than being a single age. Even if 25-year-olds receive priority over 65-year-olds, everyone who is 65 years now was previously 25 years. Treating 65-yearolds differently because of stereotypes or falsehoods would be ageist; treating them differently because they have already had more life-years is not.

Age, like income, is a "non-medical criterion" inappropriate for allocation of medical resources.[83] In

80. Schwappach DLB. Resource allocation, social values and the QALY: a review of the debate and empirical evidence. *Health Expectations* 2002; **5:** 210–22.
81. Jecker NS, Pearlman RA. Ethical constraints on rationing medical care by age. *J Am Geriatr Soc* 1989; **37:** 1067–75.
82. Rivlin MM. Protecting elderly people: flaws in ageist arguments. *BMJ* 1995; **310:** 1179–82.
83. American Medical Association. Allocation of limited medical resources. http://www.ama-assn.org/ama1/pub/upload/mm/Code_of_Med_Eth/opinion/opinion203.html (accessed Jan 19, 2009).

contrast to income, a complete life is a health outcome. Long-term survival and life expectancy at birth are key health-care outcome variables.[84] Delaying the age at onset of a disease is desirable.[8586]

The complete lives system is insensitive to international differences in typical lifespan. Although broad consensus favours adolescents over very young infants, and young adults over the very elderly people, implementation can reasonably differ between, even within, nation-states.[8788] Some people believe that a complete life is a universal limit founded in natural human capacities, which everyone should accept even without scarcity. By contrast, the complete lives system requires only that citizens see a complete life, however defined, as an important good, and accept that fairness gives those short of a complete life stronger claims to scarce life-saving resources.

Principles must be ordered lexically: less important principles should come into play only when more important ones are fulfilled. Rawls himself agreed that lexical priority was inappropriate when distributing specific resources in society, though appropriate for ordering the principles of basic social justice that shape the distribution of basic rights, opportunities, and income.As an alternative, balancing priority to the worst-off against maximising benefits has won wide support in discussions of allocative local justice. As Amartya Sen argues, justice "does not specify how much more is to be given to the deprived person, but merely that he should receive more".[89]

Accepting the complete lives system for health care as a whole would be premature. We must first reduce waste and increase spending.[90] The complete lives system explicitly rejects waste and corruption, such as multiple listing for transplantation. Although it may be applicable more generally, the complete lives system has been developed to justly allocate persistently scarce life-saving interventions. Hearts for transplant and influenza vaccines, unlike money, cannot be replaced or diverted to non-health goals; denying a heart to one person makes it available to another. Ultimately, the complete lives system does not create "classes of *Untermenschen* whose lives and well being are deemed not worth spending money on",[91] but rather empowers us to decide fairly whom to save when genuine scarcity makes saving everyone impossible.

Legitimacy

As well as recognising morally relevant values, an allocation system must be legitimate. Legitimacy requires that people see the allocation system as just and accept actual allocations as fair. Consequently, allocation

84. Mathers CD, Sadana R, Salomon JA, Murray CJL, Lopez AD. Healthy life expectancy in 191 countries, 1999. *Lancet* 2001; **357:** 1685.

85. Atkinson MA, Eisenbarth GS. Type 1 diabetes: new perspectives on disease pathogenesis and treatment. *Lancet* 2001; **358:** 221.

86. Tang M-X, Jacobs D, Stern Y, et al. Effect of oestrogen during menopause on risk and age at onset of Alzheimer's disease. *Lancet* 1996; **348:** 429.

87. Emanuel EJ. Finding new ethical conceptions through practical ethics: global justice and the "standard of care" debates. Paper presented at: University of Toronto Center for Ethics, Inaugural Conference: Is there progress in ethics? Toronto, Canada; 2006.

88. Rawls J. The Law of Peoples. Cambridge, MA: Harvard University Press, 2001.

89. Sen A. On economic inequality: Oxford University Press; 1973.

90. Lanken PN, Terry PB, Osborne ML. Ethics of allocating intensive care unit resources. Baltimore: New horizons, 1997: 5.

91. Evans JG. The rationing debate: Rationing health care by age: the case against. *BMJ* 1997; **314:** 822.

systems must be publicly understandable, accessible, and subject to public discussion and revision.[92] They must also resist corruption, since easy corruptibility undermines the public trust on which legitimacy depends. Some systems, like the UNOS points systems or QALY systems, may fail this test, because they are difficult to understand, easily corrupted, or closed to public revision. Systems that intentionally conceal their allocative principles to avoid public complaints might also fail the test.[93]

Although procedural fairness is necessary for legitimacy, it is unable to ensure the justice of allocation decisions on its own.[94][95] Although fair procedures are important, substantive, morally relevant values and principles are indispensable for just allocation.[96][97]

Conclusion

Ultimately, none of the eight simple principles recognise all morally relevant values, and some recognise irrelevant values. QALY and DALY multiprinciple systems neglect the importance of fair distribution. UNOS points systems attempt to address distributive justice, but recognise morally irrelevant values and are vulnerable to corruption. By contrast, the complete lives system combines four morally relevant principles: youngest-first, prognosis, lottery, and saving the most lives. In pandemic situations, it also allocates scarce interventions to people instrumental in realising these four principles. Importantly, it is not an algorithm, but a framework that expresses widely affirmed values: priority to the worst-off, maximising benefits, and treating people equally. To achieve a just allocation of scarce medical interventions, society must embrace the challenge of implementing a coherent multiprinciple framework rather than relying on simple principles or retreating to the status quo.

92. Daniels N. Accountability for reasonableness. *BMJ* 2000; **321:** 1300.
93. Calabresi G, Bobbitt P. Tragic choices: the conflicts society confronts in the allocation of tragically scarce resources. WW Norton and Company; 1978.
94. Daniels N. How to achieve fair distribution of ARTs in 3 by 5: fair process and legitimacy in patient selection. Geneva: World Health Organization, 2004.
95. Mielke J, Martin DK, Singer PA. Priority setting in a hospital critical care unit: qualitative case study. *Crit Care Med* 2003; **31:** 2764–68.
96. Hasman A, Holm S. Accountability for reasonableness: opening the black box of process. *Health Care Analysis* 2005; **13:** 261.
97. Friedman A. Beyond accountability for reasonableness. *Bioethics* 2008; **22:** 101–12.

Fair Allocation of Scarce Medical Resources in the Time of Covid-19

Ezekiel J. Emanuel, Govind Persad, Ross Upshur, Beatriz Thome, Michael Parker, Aaron Glickman, Cathy Zhang, Connor Boyle, Maxwell Smith, and James P. Phillips

Covid-19 is officially a pandemic. It is a novel infection with serious clinical manifestations, including death, and it has reached at least 124 countries and territories. Although the ultimate course and impact of Covid-19 are uncertain, it is not merely possible but likely that the disease will produce enough severe illness to overwhelm health care infrastructure. Emerging viral pandemics "can place extraordinary and sustained demands on public health and health systems and on providers of essential community services." Such demands will create the need to ration medical equipment and interventions.

Rationing is already here. In the United States, perhaps the earliest example was the near-immediate recognition that there were not enough high-filtration N-95 masks for health care workers, prompting contingency guidance on how to reuse masks designed for single use. Physicians in Italy have proposed directing crucial resources such as intensive care beds and ventilators to patients who can benefit most from treatment. Daegu, South Korea—home to most of that country's Covid-19 cases—faced a hospital bed shortage, with some patients dying at home while awaiting admission. In the United Kingdom, protective gear requirements for health workers have been downgraded, causing condemnation among providers. The rapidly growing imbalance between supply and demand for medical resources in many countries presents an inherently normative question: How can medical resources be allocated fairly during a Covid-19 pandemic?

Health Impacts of Moderate-to-Severe Pandemics

In 2005, the U.S. Department of Health and Human Services (HHS) developed a Pandemic Influenza Plan that modeled the potential health care impact of moderate and severe influenza pandemics. The plan was updated after the 2009 H1N1 outbreak and most recently in 2017. It suggests that a moderate pandemic will infect about 64 million Americans, with about 800,000 (1.25%) requiring hospitalization and 160,000 (0.25%) requiring beds in the intensive care unit (ICU) (Table 3.9.1). A severe pandemic would dramatically increase these demands (Table 3.9.1).

Modeling the Covid-19 pandemic is challenging. But there are data that can be used to project resource demands. Estimates of the reproductive number (R) of SARS-CoV-2 show that at the beginning of the epidemic, each infected person spreads the virus to at least two others, on average. A conservatively low estimate is that 5% of the population could become infected within 3 months. Preliminary data from China and Italy regarding the distribution of case severity and fatality vary widely. A recent large-scale analysis from China suggests that 80% of those infected either are asymptomatic or have mild symptoms, a finding that implies that demand for advanced medical services might apply to only 20% of the total infected. Of patients infected with Covid-19, about 15% have severe illness and 5% have critical illness. Overall mortality ranges from 0.25% to as high as 3.0%. Case fatality rates are much higher for vulnerable populations, such as persons over the age of 80 years (>14%) and those with coexisting conditions (10% for those with cardiovascular disease and 7% for those with diabetes). Overall, Covid-19 is substantially deadlier than seasonal influenza, which has mortality of roughly 0.1%.

The exact number of cases will depend on a number of factors that are unknowable at this time, including the effect of social distancing and other interventions. However, the estimate given above—that 5% of the population is infected—is low; new data are only likely to increase estimates of sickness and demand for health care infrastructure.

Table 3.9.1 Potential U.S. Health and Health Care Effects of Pandemic Covid-19 as Compared with Influenza.*

Category	Influenza		Covid-19[†]	
	Moderate	Severe	Moderate	Severe
Percentage of population infected (U.S. population, 320 million)	20	20	5	20
No. of ill persons	64,000,000	64,000,000	16,000,000	64,000,000
No. of outpatients	32,000,000	32,000,000	3,200,000	12,800,000
No. of hospitalized patients	800,000	3,800,000	1,280,000	5,120,000
No. of patients admitted to the ICU	160,000	1,200,000	960,000	3,840,000

No. of deaths	48,000	510,000	80,000	1,920,000

* Influenza numbers are based on the HHS Pandemic Influenza Plan. Moderate and severe cases differ with respect to case severity, not prevalence. Covid-19 infections and hospitalization estimates are based on references from China and Italy. ICU usage numbers are based on the Imperial College Covid-19 Response team predictions.

† The Covid-19 scenarios are much more conservative than the Imperial College Covid-19 Response team predictions that 81% of the population will be infected over the course of the epidemic without any action. The moderate and severe COVID-19 scenarios assume that public health measures such as social distancing reduce infection rates by roughly 95% and 75%, respectively. The moderate Covid-19 scenario is based on the following assumptions: 80% of infected patients are asymptomatic or have mild symptoms not requiring health care services; of the 20% requiring health care services, 40% (8% overall) need hospitalization; 6% of all infected patients—30% of those needing health care—need intensive care; and there is a death rate of 0.5%. The severe Covid-19 scenario is based on the following assumptions: 80% of infected patients are asymptomatic or have mild symptoms not requiring health care services; of the 20% requiring health care services, 40% (8% overall) need hospitalization; 6% of all infected patients—30% of those needing health care—need intensive care; and there is a death rate of 3.0%.

Health System Capacity

Even a conservative estimate shows that the health needs created by the coronavirus pandemic go well beyond the capacity of U.S. hospitals. According to the American Hospital Association, there were 5198 community hospitals and 209 federal hospitals in the United States in 2018. In the community hospitals, there were 792,417 beds, with 3532 emergency departments and 96,500 ICU beds, of which 23,000 were neonatal and 5100 pediatric, leaving just under 68,400 ICU beds of all types for the adult population. Other estimates of ICU bed capacity, which try to account for purported undercounting in the American Hospital Association data, show a total of 85,000 adult ICU beds of all types.

There are approximately 62,000 full-featured ventilators (the type needed to adequately treat the most severe complications of Covid-19) available in the United States. Approximately 10,000 to 20,000 more are estimated to be on call in our Strategic National Stockpile, and 98,000 ventilators that are not full-featured but can provide basic function in an emergency during crisis standards of care also exist. Supply limitations constrain the rapid production of more ventilators; manufacturers are unsure of how many they can make in the next year. However, in the Covid-19 pandemic, the limiting factor for ventilator use will most likely not be ventilators but healthy respiratory therapists and trained critical care staff to operate them safely over three shifts every day. In 2018, community hospitals employed about 76,000 full-time respiratory therapists, and there are about 512,000 critical care nurses—of which ICU nurses are a subset. California law requires one respiratory therapist for every four ventilated patients; thus, this number of respiratory therapists could care for a maximum of 100,000 patients daily (25,000 respiratory therapists per shift).

Given these numbers—and unless the epidemic curve of infected individuals is flattened over a very long period of time—the Covid-19 pandemic is likely to cause a shortage of hospital beds, ICU beds, and ventilators. It is also likely to affect the availability of the medical workforce, since doctors and nurses are already becoming ill or quarantined. Even in a moderate pandemic, hospital beds and ventilators are likely to be scarce in geographic areas with large outbreaks, such as Seattle, or in rural and smaller hospitals that have much less space, staff, and supplies than large academic medical centers.

Diagnostic, therapeutic, and preventive interventions will also be scarce. Pharmaceuticals like chloroquine, remdesivir, and favipiravir are currently undergoing clinical trials, and other experimental treatments are at earlier stages of study. Even if one of them proves effective, scaling up supply will take time. The use of convalescent serum, blood products from persons whose immune system has defeated Covid-19, is being contemplated as a possible treatment and preventive intervention. Likewise, if an effective vaccine is developed, it will take time to produce, distribute, and administer. Other critical medical supplies and equipment, such as personal protective equipment (PPE), are already scarce, presenting the danger that medical staff time will itself become scarce as physicians and nurses become infected. Technical and governmental failures in the United States have led to a persistent scarcity of tests. As more countries have been affected by Covid-19, worldwide demand for tests has begun to outstrip production, creating the need to prioritize patients.

Public health measures known to reduce viral spread, such as social distancing, cough etiquette, and hand hygiene, finally seem to be a U.S. national priority and may make resource shortages less severe by narrowing the gap between medical need and the available supply of treatments. But public health mitigation efforts do not obviate the need to adequately prepare for the allocation of scarce resources before it becomes necessary.

The choice to set limits on access to treatment is not a discretionary decision, but a necessary response to the overwhelming effects of a pandemic. The question is not whether to set priorities, but how to do so ethically and consistently, rather than basing decisions on individual institutions' approaches or a clinician's intuition in the heat of the moment.

Ethical Values for Rationing Health Resources in a Pandemic

Previous proposals for allocation of resources in pandemics and other settings of absolute scarcity, including our own prior research and analysis, converge on four fundamental values: maximizing the benefits produced by scarce resources, treating people equally, promoting and rewarding instrumental value, and giving priority to the worst off. Consensus exists that an individual person's wealth should not determine who lives or dies. Although medical treatment in the United States outside pandemic contexts is often restricted to those able to pay, no proposal endorses ability-to-pay allocation in a pandemic.

Each of these four values can be operationalized in various ways (Table 3.9.2). Maximization of benefits can be understood as saving the most individual lives or as saving the most life-years by giving priority to patients likely to survive longest after treatment. Treating people equally could be attempted by random selection, such as a lottery, or by a first-come, first-served allocation. Instrumental value could be promoted by giving priority to those who can save others, or rewarded by giving priority to those who have saved others in the past. And priority to the worst off could be understood as giving priority either to the sickest or to younger people who will have lived the shortest lives if they die untreated.

The proposals for allocation discussed above also recognize that all these ethical values and ways to operationalize them are compelling. No single value is sufficient alone to determine which patients should receive scarce resources. Hence, fair allocation requires a multivalue ethical framework that can be adapted, depending on the resource and context in question.

Who Gets Health Resources in a Covid-19 Pandemic?

These ethical values—maximizing benefits, treating equally, promoting and rewarding instrumental value, and giving priority to the worst off—yield six specific recommendations for allocating medical resources in the Covid-19 pandemic: maximize benefits; prioritize health workers; do not allocate on a first-come, first-served basis; be responsive to evidence; recognize research participation; and apply the same principles to all Covid-19 and non–Covid-19 patients.

Table 3.9.2. Ethical Values to Guide Rationing of Absolutely Scarce Health Care Resources in a Covid-19 Pandemic.

Ethical Values and Guiding Principles	Application to COVID-19 Pandemic
Maximize benefits	
Save the most lives Save the most life-years—maximize prognosis	Receives the highest priority Receives the highest priority
Treat people equally	
First-come, first-served Random selection	Should not be used Used for selecting among patients with similar prognosis
Promote and reward instrumental value (benefit to others)	
Retrospective—priority to those who have made relevant contributions Prospective—priority to those who are likely to make relevant contributions	Gives priority to research participants and health care workers when other factors such as maximizing benefits are equal Gives priority to health care workers
Give priority to the worst off	
Sickest first Youngest first	Used when it aligns with maximizing benefits Used when it aligns with maximizing benefits such as preventing spread of the virus

Recommendation 1: In the context of a pandemic, the value of maximizing benefits is most important. This value reflects the importance of responsible stewardship of resources: it is difficult to justify asking health care workers and the public to take risks and make sacrifices if the promise that their efforts will save and lengthen lives is illusory. Priority for limited resources should aim both at saving the most lives and at maximizing improvements in individuals' post-treatment length of life. Saving more lives and more years of life is a consensus value across expert reports. It is consistent both with utilitarian ethical perspectives that emphasize population outcomes and with nonutilitarian views that emphasize the paramount value of each human life. There are many reasonable ways of balancing saving more lives against saving more years of life; whatever balance between lives and life-years is chosen must be applied consistently.

Limited time and information in a Covid-19 pandemic make it justifiable to give priority to maximizing the number of patients that survive treatment with a reasonable life expectancy and to regard maximizing improvements in length of life as a subordinate aim. The latter becomes relevant only in comparing patients whose likelihood of survival is similar. Limited time and information during an emergency also counsel against incorporating patients' future quality of life, and quality-adjusted life-years, into benefit maximization. Doing so would require time-consuming collection of information and would present ethical and legal problems. However, encouraging all patients, especially those facing the prospect of intensive care, to document in an advance care directive what future quality of life they would regard as acceptable and when they would refuse ventilators or other life-sustaining interventions can be appropriate.

Operationalizing the value of maximizing benefits means that people who are sick but could recover if treated are given priority over those who are unlikely to recover even if treated and those who are likely to recover without treatment. Because young, severely ill patients will often comprise many of those who are sick but could recover with treatment, this operationalization also has the effect of giving priority to those who are worst off in the sense of being at risk of dying young and not having a full life.

Because maximizing benefits is paramount in a pandemic, we believe that removing a patient from a ventilator or an ICU bed to provide it to others in need is also justifiable and that patients should be made aware of this possibility at admission. Undoubtedly, withdrawing ventilators or ICU support from patients who arrived earlier to save those with better prognosis will be extremely psychologically traumatic for clinicians—and some clinicians might refuse to do so. However, many guidelines agree that the decision to withdraw a scarce resource to save others is not an act of killing and does not require the patient's consent. We agree with these guidelines that it is the ethical thing to do. Initially allocating beds and ventilators according to the value of maximizing benefits could help reduce the need for withdrawal.

Recommendation 2: Critical Covid-19 interventions—testing, PPE, ICU beds, ventilators, therapeutics, and vaccines—should go first to front-line health care workers and others who care for ill patients and who keep critical infrastructure operating, particularly workers who face a high risk of infection and whose training makes them difficult to replace. These workers should be given priority not because they are somehow more worthy, but because of their instrumental value: they are essential to pandemic response. If physicians and nurses are incapacitated, all patients—not just those with Covid-19—will suffer greater mortality and years of life lost. Whether health workers who need ventilators will be able to return to work is uncertain, but giving them priority for ventilators recognizes their assumption of the high-risk work of saving others, and it may also discourage absenteeism. Priority for critical workers must not be abused by prioritizing wealthy or famous persons or the politically powerful above first responders and medical staff—as has already happened for testing. Such abuses will undermine trust in the allocation framework.

Recommendation 3: For patients with similar prognoses, equality should be invoked and operationalized through random allocation, such as a lottery, rather than a first-come, first-served allocation process. First-come, first-served is used for such resources as transplantable kidneys, where scarcity is long-standing and patients can survive without the scarce resource. Conversely, treatments for coronavirus address urgent need, meaning that a first-come, first-served approach would unfairly benefit patients living nearer to health facilities. And first-come, first-served medication or vaccine distribution would encourage crowding and even violence during a period when social distancing is paramount. Finally, first-come, first-served approaches mean that people who happen to get sick later on, perhaps because of their strict adherence to recommended public health measures, are excluded from treatment, worsening outcomes without improving fairness. In the face of time pressure and limited information, random selection is also preferable to trying to make finer-grained prognostic judgments within a group of roughly similar patients.

Recommendation 4: Prioritization guidelines should differ by intervention and should respond to changing scientific evidence. For instance, younger patients should not be prioritized for Covid-19 vaccines, which prevent disease rather than cure it, or for experimental post- or preexposure prophylaxis. Covid-19 outcomes have been significantly worse in older persons and those with chronic conditions. Invoking the value of maximizing saving lives justifies giving older persons priority for vaccines immediately after health care workers and first responders. If the vaccine supply is insufficient for patients in the highest risk categories—those over 60 years of age or with coexisting conditions—then equality supports using random selection, such as a lottery, for vaccine allocation. Invoking instrumental value justifies prioritizing younger patients for vaccines only if epidemiologic modeling shows that this would be the best way to reduce viral spread and the risk to others.

Epidemiologic modeling is even more relevant in setting priorities for coronavirus testing. Federal guidance currently gives priority to health care workers and older patients, but reserving some tests for public health surveillance (as some states are doing) could improve knowledge about Covid-19 transmission and help researchers target other treatments to maximize benefits.

Conversely, ICU beds and ventilators are curative rather than preventive. Patients who need them face life-threatening conditions. Maximizing benefits requires consideration of prognosis—how long the patient is likely to live if treated—which may mean giving priority to younger patients and those with fewer coexisting conditions. This is consistent with the Italian guidelines that potentially assign a higher priority for intensive care access to younger patients with severe illness than to elderly patients. Determining the benefit-maximizing allocation of antivirals and other experimental treatments, which are likely to be most effective in patients who are seriously but not critically ill, will depend on scientific evidence. These treatments may produce the most benefit if preferentially allocated to patients who would fare badly on ventilation.

Recommendation 5: People who participate in research to prove the safety and effectiveness of vaccines and therapeutics should receive some priority for Covid-19 interventions. Their assumption of risk during their participation in research helps future patients, and they should be rewarded for that contribution. These rewards will also encourage other patients to participate in clinical trials. Research participation, however, should serve only as a tiebreaker among patients with similar prognoses.

Recommendation 6: There should be no difference in allocating scarce resources between patients with Covid-19 and those with other medical conditions. If the Covid-19 pandemic leads to absolute scarcity, that scarcity will affect all patients, including those with heart failure, cancer, and other serious and life-threatening conditions requiring prompt medical attention. Fair allocation of resources that prioritizes the value of maximizing benefits applies across all patients who need resources. For example, a doctor with an allergy who goes into anaphylactic shock and needs life-saving intubation and ventilator support should receive priority over Covid-19 patients who are not frontline health care workers.

Implementing Rationing Policies

The need to balance multiple ethical values for various interventions and in different circumstances is likely to lead to differing judgments about how much weight to give each value in particular cases. This highlights the need for fair and consistent allocation procedures that include the affected parties: clinicians, patients, public officials, and others. These procedures must be transparent to ensure public trust in their fairness.

The outcome of these fair allocation procedures, informed by the ethical values and recommendations delineated here, should be the development of prioritization guidelines that ensure that individual physicians are not faced with the terrible task of improvising decisions about whom to treat or making these decisions in isolation. Placing such burdens on individual physicians could exact an acute and life-long emotional toll. However, even well-designed guidelines can present challenging problems in real-time decision making and implementation. To help clinicians navigate these challenges, institutions may employ triage officers, physicians in roles outside direct patient care, or committees of experienced physicians and ethicists, to help apply guidelines, to assist with rationing decisions, or to make and implement choices outright—relieving the individual front-line clinicians of that burden. Institutions may also include appeals processes, but appeals should be limited to concerns about procedural mistakes, given time and resource constraints.

Conclusions

Governments and policy makers must do all they can to prevent the scarcity of medical resources. However, if resources do become scarce, we believe the six recommendations we delineate should be used to develop guidelines that can be applied fairly and consistently across cases. Such guidelines can ensure that individual doctors are never tasked with deciding unaided which patients receive life-saving care and which do not. Instead, we believe guidelines should be provided at a higher level of authority, both to alleviate physician burden and to ensure equal treatment. The described recommendations could shape the development of these guidelines.

Notes

1. Pandemic influenza plan: 2017 update. Washington, DC: Department of Health and Human Services, 2017 (https://www.cdc.gov/flu/pandemic-resources/pdf/pan-flu-report-2017v2.pdf).
2. Strategies for optimizing the supply of N95 respirators. Atlanta: Centers for Disease Control and Prevention, 2020 (https://www.cdc.gov/coronavirus/2019-ncov/hcp/respirators-strategy/index.html).
3. Vergano M, Bertolini G, Giannini A, et al. Clinical Ethics Recommendations for the Allocation of Intensive Care Treatments, in Exceptional, Resource-Limited Circumstances. Italian Society of

Anesthesia, Analgesia, Resuscitation, and Intensive Care (SIAARTI). March 16, 2020 (http://www.siaarti.it/SiteAssets/News/COVID19%20-%20documenti%20SIAARTI/SIAARTI%20-%20Covid-19%20-%20Clinical%20Ethics%20-Reccomendations.pdf).

4. Mounk Y. The extraordinary decisions facing Italian doctors. Atlantic. March 11, 2020 (https://www.theatlantic.com/ideas/archive/2020/03/who-gets-hospital-bed/607807/).

5. Kuhn A. How a South Korean city is changing tactics to tamp down its COVID-19 surge. NPR. March 10, 2020 (https://www.npr.org/sections/goatsandsoda/2020/03/10/812865169/how-a-south-korean-city-is-changing-tactics-to-tamp-down-its-covid-19-surge).

6. Campbell D, Busby M. 'Not fit for purpose': UK medics condemn Covid-19 protection. The Guardian. March 16, 2020 (https://www.theguardian.com/society/2020/mar/16/not-fit-for-purpose-uk-medics-condemn-covid-19—protection).

7. Livingston E, Bucher K. Coronavirus disease 2019 (COVID-19) in Italy. JAMA 2020 March 17 (Epub ahead of print).

8. Wu Z, McGoogan JM. Characteristics of and important lessons from the coronavirus disease 2019 (COVID-19) outbreak in China: summary of a report of 72 314 cases from the Chinese Center for Disease Control and Prevention. JAMA 2020 February 24 (Epub ahead of print).

9. Ferguson NM, Laydon D, Nedjati-Gilani G, et al. Impact of non-pharmaceutical interventions (NPIs) to reduce COVID-19 mortality and healthcare demand. London: Imperial College London, March 16, 2020 (https://www.imperial.ac.uk/media/imperial—college/medicine/sph/ide/gida-fellowships/Imperial-College-COVID19-NPI-modelling-16-03-2020.pdf).

10. Li Q, Guan X, Wu P, et al. Early transmission dynamics in Wuhan, China, of novel coronavirus–infected pneumonia. N Engl J Med 2020; 382:1199–207.

11. Wilson N, Kvalsvig A, Barnard LT, Baker MG. Case-fatality risk estimates for COVID-19 calculated by using a lag time for fatality. Emerging Infect Dis 2020 March 13 (Epub ahead of print).

12. AHA annual survey database. Chicago: American Hospital Association, 2018.

13. Sanger-Katz M, Kliff S, Parlapiano A. These places could run out of hospital beds as coronavirus spreads. New York Times. March 17, 2020 (https://www.nytimes.com/interactive/2020/03/17/upshot/hospital-bed-shortages-coronavirus.html).

14. Rubinson L, Vaughn F, Nelson S, et al. Mechanical ventilators in US acute care hospitals. Disaster Med Public Health Prep 2010;4: 199–206.

15. Jacobs A, Fink S. How prepared is the U.S. for a coronavirus outbreak? New York Times. February 29, 2020 (https://www.nytimes.com/2020/02/29/health/coronavirus-preparation-united-states.html).

16. Cohn J. How to get more ventilators and what to do if we can't. Huffington Post. March 17, 2020 (https://www.huffpost.com/entry/coronavirus-ventilators-supply-manufacture_n_5e6dc4f7c5b6747ef11e8134).

17. Critical care statistics. Mount Prospect, IL: Society of Critical Care Medicine (https://www.sccm.org/Communications/Critical-Care-Statistics).

18. Gold J. Surging health care worker quarantines raise concerns as coronavirus spreads. Kaiser Health News. March 9, 2020 (https://khn.org/news/surging-health-care-worker-quarantines-raise-concerns-as-coronavirus-spreads/).

19. Casadevall A, Pirofski LA. The convalescent sera option for containing COVID-19. J Clin Invest 2020 March 13 (Epub ahead of print).

20. Zimmer C. Hundreds of scientists scramble to find a coronavirus treatment. New York Times. March 17, 2020 (https://www.nytimes.com/2020/03/17/science/coronavirus-treatment.html).

21. Harrison C. Coronavirus puts drug repurposing on the fast track. Nat Biotechnol 2020 February 27 (Epub ahead of print).

22. Devlin H, Sample I. Hopes rise over experimental drug's effectiveness against coronavirus. The Guardian. March 10, 2020 (https://www.theguardian.com/world/2020/mar/10/hopes-rise-over-experimental-drugs-effectiveness-against-coronavirus).

23. Whoriskey P, Satija N. How U.S. coronavirus testing stalled: flawed tests, red tape and resistance to using the millions of tests produced by the WHO. Washington Post. March 16, 2020 (https://www.washingtonpost.com/business/2020/03/16/cdc-who-coronavirus-tests/).

24. Persad G, Wertheimer A, Emanuel EJ. Principles for allocation of scarce medical interventions. Lancet 2009; 373: 423–31.

25. Emanuel EJ, Wertheimer A. Public health: who should get influenza vaccine when not all can? Science 2006; 312: 854–5.

26. Biddison LD, Berkowitz KA, Courtney B, et al. Ethical considerations: care of the critically ill and injured during pandemics and disasters: CHEST consensus statement. Chest 2014; 146: 4 Suppl:e145S-e155S.

27. Interim updated planning guidance on allocating and targeting pandemic influenza vaccine during an influenza pandemic. Atlanta: Centers for Disease Control and Prevention, 2018 (https://www.cdc.gov/flu/pandemic—resources/national-strategy/planning—guidance/index.html).

28. Rosenbaum SJ, Bayer R, Bernheim RG, et al. Ethical considerations for decision making regarding allocation of mechanical ventilators during a severe influenza pandemic or other public health emergency. Atlanta: Centers for Disease Control and Prevention, 2011 (https://www.cdc.gov/od/science/integrity/phethics/docs/Vent_Document_Final_Version.pdf).

29. Zucker H, Adler K, Berens D, et al. Ventilator allocation guidelines. Albany: New York State Department of Health Task Force on Life and the Law, November 2015 (https://www.health.ny.gov/regulations/task_force/reports_publications/docs/ventilator_guidelines.pdf).

30. Christian MD, Sprung CL, King MA, et al. Triage: care of the critically ill and injured during pandemics and disasters: CHEST consensus statement. Chest 2014;146 4 Suppl:e61S-e74S.

31. Responding to pandemic influenza—the ethical framework for policy and planning. London: UK Department of Health, 2007 (https://webarchive.nationalarchives.gov.uk/20130105020420/http://www.dh.gov.uk/prod_consum_dh/groups/dh_digitalassets/@dh/@en/documents/digitalasset/dh_080729.pdf).

32. Toner E, Waldhorn R. What US hospitals should do now to prepare for a COVID-19 pandemic. Baltimore: Johns Hopkins University Center for Health Security, 2020 (http://www.centerforhealthsecurity.org/cbn/2020/cbnreport-02272020.html).

33. Influenza pandemic—providing critical care. North Sydney, Australia: Ministry of Health, NSW, 2010 (https://www1.health.nsw.gov.au/pds/ActivePDSDocuments/PD2010_028.pdf).

34. Kerstein SJ. Dignity, disability, and lifespan. J Appl Philos 2017;34:635–50.

35. Hick JL, Hanfling D, Wynia MK, Pavia AT. Duty to plan: health care, crisis standards of care, and novel coronavirus SARS-CoV-2. NAM Perspectives. March 5, 2020 (https://nam.edu/duty-o-plan-health-care-crisis-standards-of-care-and-novel-coronavirus-sars-cov-2/).

36. Irvin CB, Cindrich L, Patterson W, Southall A. Survey of hospital healthcare personnel response during a potential avian influenza pandemic: will they come to work? Prehosp Disaster Med 2008;23:328–35.

37. Biesecker M, Smith MR, Reynolds T. Celebrities get virus tests, raising concerns of inequality. Associated Press. March 19, 2020 (https://apnews.com/b8dcd1b369001d5a70eccdb1f75ea4bd).

38. Updated guidance on evaluating and testing persons for coronavirus disease 2019 (COVID-19). Atlanta: Centers for Disease Control and Prevention, March 8, 2020 (https://emergency.cdc.gov/han/2020/han00429.asp).

39. COVID-19 sentinel surveillance. Honolulu: State of Hawaii Department of Health, 2020 (https://health.hawaii.gov/docd/covid-19-sentinel-surveillance/).

Ethics and Euthanasia in Ethics

Clive Seale

Summary

Public support for laws that allow medical practitioners to end life by active measures has risen in recent years, but the medical profession in the UK has been reluctant to endorse this development. The obvious benefits to a few people who experience extremes of suffering towards the end of life need to be balanced against the interests of those who might feel pressurised to opt for death in a society where euthanasia becomes an acceptable and well-known solution to the problems of old age. Additionally, the effect on practitioners (usually doctors) who are called on to administer lethal treatments requires consideration. This chapter reports surveys of the relatives and friends of people who have died, as well as surveys of medical practitioners, to provide empirical evidence that deepens understanding of how moral and ethical dilemmas play themselves out in practice.

Introduction

End of life decision making requires consideration of numerous potential harms and benefits that may arise from particular decisions. Some of these consequences may be immediate, obvious and personal. For example, there are obvious benefits in relieving an individual's suffering and in avoiding inappropriate life-sustaining therapies. Other harms and benefits are less obvious and often unintended. For example, potential harm may be done to efforts to establish good palliative care services if the option of legal euthanasia is available. There may be harms involved in allowing a system that places pressure on vulnerable people to opt for euthanasia. On the other hand it may be argued that in a system that permits medical actions to end life there are beneficial effects of open disclosure that allows scrutiny of these actions.

For the general public of media-saturated countries like the UK, the more obvious consequences are more easily appreciated. Mass media therefore often focus on these outcomes, providing a diet of personalised stories of end of life care that generally demonstrate the benefits of relieving individual suffering through acts of euthanasia (McInerney, 2000; Hausmann, 2004). Coupled with a general decline in religious attachment and the rise in rationalist and consumerist ideologies, the overall effect, in recent years, has been to raise levels of public support for legal measures that allow medical practitioners to end life by active measures (Seale, 1997). It is harder and apparently less appealing to most consumers of mass media to explain the less obvious and often harmful consequences of such policies, or to describe the negative impact that such actions may have on those given the task of carrying them out.

Capacities to make decisions and follow them through with actions are frequently constrained, by physical or mental capacity for example, or by legal and professional proscriptions. Cultural and ideological factors, such as the degree of attachment to religious as against rationalist belief systems, or changing patterns of family obligations, also play a part in influencing the wishes of individuals. In this complex and changing climate a number of important types of end of life decision have emerged in ethical debates that include:

1. The active termination of life by another person at the request of the individual who dies (made either contemporaneously, or at some point in the past by means of a 'living will'). This is often called 'active euthanasia'.
2. The active termination of life by another person without such an explicit request (although carers may judge this situation to be the course that the person who died might have chosen had they been able to do so).
3. Physician-assisted suicide, where a medical practitioner provides an individual with the means to end their own life.
4. The provision of treatment intended to relieve suffering in the knowledge that the treatment will also shorten life (an action involving 'double effect').
5. The withdrawal or withholding of life-sustaining treatment.

In this [reading] ethical issues are explored by reference to research studies undertaken by myself and other colleagues over the past 15 years. These studies, firstly, have described the views of lay people reporting on the situations and preferences of their recently deceased relatives. Secondly, and more recently, my intention has been to discover the experiences of medical practitioners in this area of practice, as well as to compare UK doctors with those in other countries, some of which have more permissive legal systems, where comparable research has been done.

In choosing this focus, of course, a great deal about this subject is missed. Doctors are not the only ones involved in taking these actions; relatives, nurses and other carers are also sometimes involved.

The views of relatives and their reports of deceased persons' wishes while alive may not be an adequate substitute for direct access to the views of people who approach the end of life, or indeed for the many opinion polls of general public views that have been done over the years. There is a vast literature that describes these other matters that would not be feasible to review here. It will become evident too that this is not, primarily, a discussion of the general ethical or philosophical principles that lie behind end of life decisions. I am not a philosopher or an ethicist, but a sociologist and therefore bring an empirical element to bear on this subject that is often not present in discussions that seek to elaborate underlying principles. At the same time I hope that it will be seen that these empirical investigations have numerous points of relevance for philosophical and ethical debates.

Views of Bereaved Relatives and People Approaching Death

In collaboration with other researchers I was involved in organising and analysing a survey to investigate the views and experiences of relatives, friends and others who had known a sample of 3,696 people dying in 1990 in 20 areas of the UK. Our aim was to find out their views about the quality of care experienced by both the person who had died and by themselves, where relevant. The survey is, to date, the largest survey of this sort and provides the best evidence currently available for the preferences of a UK-based population of individuals facing death and caring for dying people concerning end of life decision making. The sampling covered all causes of death and enabled comparison between cancer and other illnesses that cause death, being to all intents and purposes a random and representative sample of deaths in the UK.

As well as a series of questions enquiring about the quality of care, the incidence of distressing symptoms and bodily restrictions and other matters, we took the opportunity of this survey to ask some questions about what we called 'euthanasia'. To be precise, these two questions were added to the survey:

- 'Looking back now, and taking (the deceased's) illness into account, do you think s/he died at the best time—or would it have been better if s/he had died earlier or later?'
- 'What about (the deceased)? Did s/he ever say that they wanted to die sooner?' and '(If yes) did s/he ever say that s/he wanted euthanasia?'

The study was published as four papers (Seale and Addington-Hall, 1994, 1995a, 1995b; Seale et al, 1997). What follows is based on a summary of these reports.

The study established for the first time the prevalence of requests for 'euthanasia' (based on what respondents understood by this term) and the relative role played in this context by pain as against dependency. The study also provided evidence that the 'slippery slope' argument against the legalisation of voluntary euthanasia may hold true for certain very elderly individuals vulnerable to subtle pressures to opt for death when they perceive themselves to be a burden on others. Evidence was also provided that contradicted the common argument that good quality health and social care, particularly that associated with hospice and palliative care, is associated with reductions in the incidence of euthanasia requests. Here are the details.

We showed that 28% of respondents and 24% of the deceased were said to have expressed the view that an earlier death would be, or would have been, preferable (Seale and Addington-Hall, 1994). In addition, 3.6% of the people who died were said to have asked for euthanasia at some point in the last year of life. We also examined factors that might have been causally related to the incidence of such requests and sentiments. We found that although much of the public debate about euthanasia concentrates on the role of pain, the experience of dependency was also a significant factor behind the request. We also found that this was a particularly important consideration for people dying with conditions that were not included under hospice and palliative care services, which largely provide for people with cancer. Additionally, although much of the public debate about the legalisation of euthanasia is influenced by religious considerations, religious faith was found to be largely insignificant in influencing the views of people actually facing their, or their relatives', deaths. This finding has important implications for the interpretation of opinion polls, since these are usually conducted on samples of healthy people who may be more willing to be influenced by ideology. By contrast we concluded:

> When nearing one's own death ... it appears that religious considerations and cultural influences fade into insignificance in the face of the overwhelming physical and emotional experience of suffering. (Seale and Addington-Hall, 1994, p 653)

'Slippery Slope' Argument

We then turned to an analysis that was to relate to the 'slippery slope' argument that is often used to oppose the legalisation of assisted dying. The argument is that such legislation would eventually fail to protect the interests of vulnerable elderly people who may experience subtle and not so subtle pressures to opt for euthanasia. In the light of demographic trends that leave more elderly people—particularly elderly women—living on their own or in institutional care towards the end of life than was once the case (see Seale, 2000), this issue is a serious consideration.

To address this argument, then, we examined some of the factors that influenced our respondents to say that an earlier death would have been desirable (Seale and Addington-Hall, 1995a). In particular, we were interested in comparing respondents who were spouses with other kinds of respondent, such as the (adult) children of the deceased. We found various indicators to suggest that spouses were more attached to the deceased person than any other group of respondents. Spouses were more likely than others, for example, to say they missed the deceased person, or that looking after the person had not been a burden even when spouses reported quite considerable labours of care. Spouses were less likely than others to feel that it would have been better if the person had died earlier and this held true even when we manipulated the statistics to control for differential levels of reported pain, distress, dependency and age in the deceased. Non-spouses (children and other relatives of the deceased, friends, neighbours and a few officials), on the other hand, were more likely than spouses to say an earlier death would have been better.

While this might be as one would expect (and of course it is equally possible that spouses' own judgements about the desirability of an earlier death were coloured by their own needs for companionship), this finding has some quite disturbing and systematic consequences for the very old. These people are more likely to be women because women live longer than men and tend to marry men somewhat older than themselves. Because of these underlying demographic trends older people were more likely to be cared for by people who, in retrospect, felt that it would have been better if the old person had died earlier. We found, too, that older people and women in particular, were more likely to be reported as having felt they themselves wanted to die earlier, even where they shared similar levels of symptom distress and dependency with others. This is consistent with the view that such people felt themselves to be a burden, or to have lives not worth living (although an alternative argument suggests that the sentiment is an expression of altruism towards those who feel obliged to care for them). It is not difficult to see the implications of this for the 'slippery slope' argument against the legalisation of voluntary euthanasia, which suggests a movement towards an involuntary state whereby a 'right' to die becomes a 'duty' to die.

Role of Hospice and Palliative Care

Finally, we turned (Seale and Addington-Hall, 1995b) to another argument commonly put forward by those who advocate the provision of hospice and palliative care services in place of the legalisation of euthanasia: that such good quality care can help people feel that their lives are worth living to their natural end, without recourse to euthanasia. Our findings suggest that the picture is in fact more complex. We found, even when we controlled for differences in reported levels of symptom distress and dependency levels, that people who received hospice care were, if anything, more likely to have respondents who felt that it would have been better if the people had died earlier. Investigation of the reported wishes of dying people suggested a similar picture, although here it was not possible to establish the time order of events, so it is possible that the reported wish had occurred before the episode of hospice care. In general, however, when we looked for associations between reports of good quality care (from whatever source) and the wish to die earlier, we found nothing to support the view that good care led to a reduced incidence.

Planning for Death

Finally, in the last paper in the series (Seale et al, 1997) we drew out the implications of a key difference on which people facing death differed: the degree to which they wished to plan for their deaths. People with cancer who wanted to plan in this way were more likely than others both to encounter hospice and palliative care services and be reported as having made requests for euthanasia. Hospice and palliative care appears to attract the kind of people who are also interested in considering euthanasia because such individuals are more able than others to accept and plan for their own deaths. It remains the case, of course, that such care may help people feel that euthanasia is not the best solution, but the argument for this view as yet remains unproven. We ended up questioning the contribution made by hospice and palliative care services to a reduction in the incidence of requests for assisted dying, even suggesting the opposite conclusion that such institutions foster a climate that actually encourages such a planned approach to death.

Subsequent research in Oregon, US, where physician-assisted suicide has been legal since 1998, has provided further evidence to support this view (Ganzini, 2004). Initially, there were concerns that physician-assisted suicide would be opted for disproportionately by poorer people in Oregon, by African Americans and by the uninsured without access to palliative care. In fact, the opposite is the case: in the first five years of legalisation no African Americans opted for physician-assisted suicide. It was largely chosen by people with higher levels of income and education, the vast majority of whom were enrolled on hospice and palliative care programmes.

Our findings then both established, for the first time, the incidence of requests of euthanasia in a random, representative sample of people at the end of life and demonstrated some of the factors that led to this request. On the way, we were able to shed light on some important ethical and policy debates that concern the legalisation of euthanasia. These debates included the claim that legalisation might lead to a slippery slope of obligation to die, as well as providing a deeper understanding of the relation between palliative care (largely restricted to cancer patients) and sentiments about the desirability of a hastened death.

Medical Practice

Although countries differ as to whether their legal systems allow for the practice of active euthanasia, or of physician-assisted suicide, these practices are known to occur in most countries. Either laws are not applied vigorously, or prosecutions fail to stick once public sympathy is recruited to support a doctor who has actively ended the life of his or her patient, or penalties for those convicted are mild, again reflecting a degree of sympathy for the professional dilemmas that can face doctors attending patients with terminal or otherwise debilitating illness. The discovery that some doctors are quite often willing to end patients' lives with active measures in spite of laws that prohibit this practice has, in Australia and Belgium, resulted in relaxations of the law in recent years (although in Australia this was confined to the Northern Territories only; and the law has since been nullified by actions taken by the national government). Here, the argument has been that if doctors are ending their patients' lives anyway, a wiser course would be to make the actions legal so that they can be exposed to a greater degree of public scrutiny. Thus surveys that seek to document medical actions in this area can have potentially important effects on arguments for legalisation. Although medical practices have been described in a number of countries, researchers have until recently been slow to investigate UK medical practice in this area. An exception is Ward and Tate (1994), who surveyed 273 general practitioners (GPs) and hospital consultants in one area of England, of whom 38 (14%) indicated that they had at one time or another 'taken active steps to bring about the death of a patient who asked them to do so'.

While this seems a high rate at which doctors appear to have been willing to contravene UK law, the figure is somewhat deceptive. It is well known that the wording of questions can influence the rates at which particular actions or opinions are expressed. In this case, all depends on what respondents thought the term 'active steps' actually meant. Clearly, the authors of the survey believed this to mean that the doctor had taken an action that was something like decisions 1 and 3 above ('active euthanasia' or 'physician-assisted suicide'). It is quite feasible, however, that decisions involving the withdrawal or withholding of life-sustaining treatment, or 'double effect' actions, were understood by respondents to be 'active steps'. Indeed, it is quite possible that no neutral question can be designed to elucidate the actual incidence of particular actions because of enduring problems with the variability of meaning in fixed choice questions, inherent in the process of questionnaire design. In these circumstances, it is much more illuminative to use such questionnaire devices to conduct *comparative* work, using the same questions across different groups of respondents—either people at different points in time, or practising in different parts of the world. Survey data of this sort then needs to be understood as providing estimates of *relative* rates at which decisions are taken, rather than absolute rates.

Additionally, surveys of doctors are an inadequate substitute for surveys of deaths. Different types of doctors deal with different types of patients. Ward and Tate (1994) found that GPs were more willing to contemplate active euthanasia, but such doctors see far fewer dying patients than do certain kinds of hospital consultant. A survey that adjusts for these differences between doctors is the most likely to give an adequate account of the proportion of deaths where various kinds of end of life decision are taken.

International Comparisons

In the Netherlands, where active euthanasia is legally permitted as long as certain safeguards are followed, surveys of this sort have been reported for a number of years, starting with a report by Maas et al (1991) published in *The Lancet*, which was based on interviews and mailed questionnaires to physicians who had attended people selected from a random sample of death certificates. This initial survey found that the most common forms of end of life decision to be carried out were those involving the withholding or withdrawal of life-sustaining treatment, or the provision of 'double effect' therapies, both of which accounted for 17.5% of Dutch deaths. A further 1.8% involved the administering of lethal drugs at the patients' request; 0.3% involved assisted suicide; and 0.8% involved 'life-terminating acts without explicit and persistent request', which, elsewhere in their report, the authors (unfortunately) translated as 'involuntary' euthanasia. The authors did not mean to imply by this term that these patients had been euthanised *against* their will, indeed the report states that "In more than half of these cases the decision had been discussed with the patient, or the patient had expressed in a previous phase of the disease a wish for euthanasia if his/her suffering became unbearable" (Maas et al, 1991, p 671). Nevertheless, critics have often pointed to these 'involuntary' cases in the Netherlands as evidence of a policy that contravenes the wishes of dying people.

It is instructive to examine the rates at which Dutch doctors reported 'ever' having practised euthanasia or assisted in a suicide: 54% reported having taken this action and GPs were particularly likely to say they had done (62%). This puts the finding of Ward and Tate (1994), reported above, into perspective since these authors found only 14% of UK doctors saying they had 'taken active steps' to end a patient's life. Although 14% may seem like a 'lot', the Dutch example shows that very large numbers of doctors (much more than in the UK) may report this, while the actual rate of euthanasia remains quite small when expressed as a proportion of deaths. If one were to use the Dutch proportions to extrapolate from Ward and Tate's (1994) figure to make an estimate of the proportion of UK deaths receiving such 'active steps', the estimate would be very small indeed.

The survey undertaken by the Dutch investigators involved a standardised questionnaire that has been translated into several languages, including English, and has been used by various teams of investigators to survey medical practice over time in the Netherlands (for example, Onwuteaka-Philipsen et al, 2003), in five other European countries (Deliens et al, 2000; van der Heide et al, 2003) as well as Australia (Kuhse et al, 1997) and New Zealand (Mitchell and Owens, 2003). The most recent of these surveys was done in the UK in late 2004 (Seale, 2006), providing for the first time an estimate of the extent of the main end of life decisions taken in UK medical practice that is comparable with a number of other European and other countries.

On the whole the survey (Seale, 2006) reveals that UK doctors report fewer decisions than doctors in other countries that involve the active termination of life (for example, active euthanasia at a patient's request where 0.16% of deaths were estimated to have involved such an action, or physician-assisted suicide where no cases were reported). Decisions to withhold or withdraw treatment, on the other hand, were more common than in a number of other European countries. Very few doctors (4.6% of 857 doctors) felt that UK law had inhibited or interfered with their preferred management of the patient on whom they reported. A culture of decision making informed by a palliative care philosophy (which prioritises comfort care and avoids taking active steps to end life) is therefore evident in UK medical practice. This emphasis is consistent with the UK having been centrally involved in the origination and development of palliative care as a medical and nursing specialty in the latter half of the 20th century.

Conclusion and Contemporary Challenges

In many countries with advanced economies and highly developed systems of health care, there is periodic interest in the possibility of changes to laws that prohibit doctors from becoming involved in actively hastening patients' deaths. Such ethical and legal debates appear not to occur very much in poorer countries where, it may be guessed, medical care is less widely available and professional–client relations are less subject to public debate. In only a few countries though—and the Netherlands is the most well known example—is euthanasia more or less legal.

In the UK there has long been an active lobby to legalise euthanasia and there are periodic upsurges of public interest and parliamentary debate about this matter. At the time of writing, it appears that the issue is once again on the parliamentary agenda, this time because of a House of Lords proposed Bill to legalise physician-assisted suicide, which was accompanied by an inquiry report into the matter (House of Lords, 2005). Support for this kind of medical action is easier to gain than is support for active euthanasia (where a doctor, for example, administers a lethal injection). This is because the responsibility of the doctor is at one remove: the doctor's role is simply to provide the means for death without personally administering a lethal substance, a matter that is left to the patient themselves. Thus medical objections to involvement are somewhat reduced. Significantly, the British Medical Association dropped its long-standing objection to such a relaxation of the law in June 2005 (Sommerville, 2005). However, in adopting a neutral policy, rather than one that would involve campaigning for a relaxation of the law, the British Medical Association reflected some enduring concerns of its membership, all of which have been touched on in this chapter. These concerns are worth setting out below at the chapter's conclusion (adapted from Sommerville, 2005), as they provide a good indication of the key moral and practical issues involved:

- patients should be competent, informed and unpressured, able to change their mind at any stage;
- alternatives, such as good palliative care, ought to be available;
- doctors must have the right to object to involvement in such acts, without any prejudice to their careers;

- doctors who engage in such acts need special training that would focus, among other things, on dealing with the emotional consequences of such involvement.

These concerns draw attention to the continuing importance of avoidance of harms, while trying to ensure that a system is created that will not deny benefits to a small proportion of people who would otherwise endure intolerable levels of suffering. Given the range of ethical, moral and practical issues involved in any proposed legislation for physician-assisted suicide, both support and opposition are potential outcomes. Contemporary challenges are therefore likely to play a key part in any future developments.

References

Deliens, L., Mortier, F., Bilsen, J., Cosyns, M., van der Stichele, R., Vanoverloop, J. and Ingels, K. (2000) 'End-of-life decisions in medical practice in Flanders, Belgium: a nationwide survey', *The Lancet*, vol 356, pp 1806–11.

Ganzini, L. (2004) 'The Oregon experience', in T. Quill and M. Battin (eds) *Physician-assisted dying: The case for palliative care and patient choice*, Baltimore, MD: Johns Hopkins University Press, pp 165–83.

Hausmann, E. (2004) 'How press discourse justifies euthanasia', *Mortality*, vol 9, no 3, pp 206–22.

House of Lords Select Committee on the Assisted Dying for the Terminally Ill Bill (2005), *Assisted Dying for the Terminally Ill Bill: First report*, London: The Stationery Office.

Kuhse, H., Singer, P., Baume, P., Clark, M. and Rickard, M. (1997) 'End-of-life decisions in Australian medical practice', *Medical Journal of Australia*, vol 166, pp 191–6.

Maas, P., Delden, J., Pijnenborg, L. and Looman, C. (1991) 'Euthanasia and other medical decisions concerning the end of life', *The Lancet*, vol 338, pp 669–74.

McInerney, F. (2000) '"Requested death": a new social movement', *Social Science and Medicine*, vol 50, pp 137–54.

Mitchell, K. and Owens, G. (2002) 'National survey of medical decisions at end of life made by New Zealand general practitioners', *British Medical Journal*, vol 327, pp 202–3.

Onwuteaka-Philipsen, B., van der Heide, A., Koper, D., KeijDeerenberg, I., Rietjens, J., Rurup, M., Vrakking, A., Georges, J., Muller, M., van der Wal, G. and van der Maas, P. (2003) 'Euthanasia and other end-of-life decisions in the Netherlands in 1990, 1995, and 2001', *The Lancet*, vol 362, pp 395–9.

Seale, C. (1997) 'Social and ethical aspects of euthanasia: a review', *Progress in Palliative Care*, vol 5, no 4, pp 141–6.

Seale, C. (2000) 'Changing patterns of death and dying', *Social Science and Medicine*, vol 51, pp 917–30.

Seale, C. (2006) 'End of life decision making in UK medical practice', *Palliative Medicine*, vol 20, no 1, pp 1–8.

Seale, C. and Addington-Hall, J. (1994) 'Euthanasia: why people want to die earlier', *Social Science and Medicine*, vol 39, no 5, pp 647–54.

Seale, C. and Addington-Hall, J. (1995a) 'Dying at the best time', *Social Science and Medicine*, vol 40, no 5, pp 589–95.

Seale, C. and Addington-Hall, J. (1995b) 'Euthanasia: the role of good care', *Social Science and Medicine*, vol 40, no 5, pp 581–7.

Seale, C., Addington-Hall, J. and McCarthy, M. (1997) 'Awareness of dying: prevalence, causes and consequences', *Social Science and Medicine*, vol 45, no 3, pp 477–84.

Sommerville, A. (2005) 'Changes in the BMA policy on assisted dying', *British Medical Journal*, vol 331, pp 686–8.

van der Heide, A., Deliens, L., Faisst, K., Nilstun, T., Norup, M., Paci, E., van der Wal, G. and van der Maas, P. (2003) 'End-of-life decision-making in six European countries: descriptive study', *The Lancet*, vol 362, pp 345–50.

Ward, B. and Tate, P. (1994) 'Attitudes among NHS doctors to requests for euthanasia', *British Medical Journal*, vol 308, pp 1332–4.

Physician-Assisted Suicide

Safe, Legal, Rare?

Margaret P. Battin

Margaret P. Battin, "Physician-Assisted Suicide: Safe, Legal, Rare?," *Physician Assisted Suicide: Expanding the Debate*, ed. Rosamond Rhodes and Anita Silvers, pp. 63-72. Copyright © 1998 by Taylor & Francis Group. Reprinted with permission.

D espite the vigor of the debate over physician-assisted suicide, both proponents and opponents of legalization appear to agree that if adequate pain control were available, requests for physician-assisted suicide would and should be rare, a last resort in those few cases in which pain control proves inadequate after all. This ubiquitous view treats concern with physician-assisted suicide as a "phenomenon of discrepant development," a symptom of the disparity between our capacities to prolong life and to control pain. However, interest in physician-assisted suicide can also be viewed as a symptom of far more substantial cultural, religious, and epidemiological changes, involving a shift towards self-directed dying: Death is no longer seen as "something that happens to you," but "something you do." In this essay I explore what might motivate such a shift, and how changes in a decisional perspective from an "enmeshed" to a distanced but still personal perspective may make physician-assisted suicide a societally preferred alternative.

The Way It Looks Now

Observe the current debate over physician-assisted suicide: On the one side, supporters of legalization appeal to the principle of autonomy, or self-determination, to insist that terminally ill patients have the right to extricate themselves from pain and suffering and to control as much as possible the ends of their lives. On the other, opponents resolutely insist on various religious, principled, or slippery-slope grounds that physician-assisted suicide cannot be allowed, whether because it is sacrilegious, immoral, or poses risks of abuse. As vociferous and politicized as these two sides of the debate have become, however, proponents and opponents (tacitly) agree on a core issue: that the patient may choose to avoid suffering and pain. They disagree, it seems, largely about the means the patient and his or her physician may use to do so.

They also disagree about the actualities of pain control. Proponents of legalization insist that currently available forms of pain and symptom control are grossly inadequate and unsatisfactory. Citing such data as the SUPPORT study, they point to high rates of reported pain among terminally ill patients, inadequately developed pain-control therapies, physicians' lack of training in pain-control techniques, and obstacles and limitations to delivery of pain-control treatment, including restrictions on narcotic and other drugs.[1] Pain and the suffering associated with other symptoms just aren't adequately controlled, proponents of legalization insist, so the patient is surely entitled to avoid them—if he or she so chooses—by turning to earlier, humanely assisted dying.

Opponents of legalization, on the other hand, insist that these claims are uninformed. Effective methods of pain control include timely withholding and withdrawal of treatment, sufficient use of morphine or other drugs for pain (even at the risk of foreseen, through unintended, shortening of life), and the discontinuation of artificial nutrition and hydration. When all other measures to control pain and suffering fail, there is always the possibility of terminal sedation: the induction of coma with concomitant withholding of nutrition and hydration, which, though it results in death, is not to be seen as killing.

Proponents laugh at this claim. Terminal sedation, they retort, like the overuse of morphine, is functionally equivalent to *causing* death.

Despite these continuing disagreements about the effectiveness, availability, and significance of current pain control, both proponents and opponents in the debate appear to agree that *if* adequate pain control were available, there would be far less call for physician-assisted suicide. This claim is both predictive and normative. *If* adequate pain control were available, both sides argue, then physician-assisted suicide would be and should be quite infrequent—a "last resort," as Timothy Quill puts it, to be used only in exceptionally difficult cases when pain control really does fail. Borrowing an expression used by President Clinton to describe his view of abortion, proponents insist that physician-assisted suicide should be "safe, legal, and rare." Opponents do not believe that it should be legal, but they also think that if it cannot be suppressed altogether or if a few very difficult cases remain, it should be very, very rare. The only real disagreement between opponents and proponents concerns those cases in which adequate pain control cannot be achieved.

What accounts for the opposing sides' underlying agreement that physician-assisted suicide should be rare is, I think, an unexamined assumption they share. This assumption is the view that the call for physician-assisted suicide is what might be called a *phenomenon of discrepant development:* a symptom

---

1. According to the SUPPORT study, about 50 percent of dying hospitalized patients were reported to have experienced moderate to severe pain at least 50 percent of the time in their last three days of life. The Support Principal Investigators, "A Controlled Trial to Improve Care for Seriously Ill Hospitalized Patients," *Journal of the American Medical Association* 274 (20) (1995): 1951–98.

of the disparity in development between two distinct capacities of modern medicine, the capacity to extend or prolong life and the capacity to control pain. Research, development, and delivery of technologies for the prolongation of life have raced far ahead; those for control of pain lagged far behind. It is this situation of discrepant development that has triggered the current concern with physician-assisted suicide and the volatile public debate over whether to legalize it or not.

The opposing sides both also hold in common the view that what would lead to the resolution of the problem is whatever set of mechanisms would tend to equalize the degree of development of medicine's capacities to prolong life and to control pain. To achieve this equalization, two simultaneous strategies are recommended: cutting back on overzealous prolongation of life (as Dan Callahan, for example, has long recommended), and at the same time (as Hospice and others have been insisting) accelerating the development of technologies, modes of delivery, and physician training for more effective methods of pain control.[2] As life prolongation is held back a bit, pain control can catch up, and the current situation of discrepant development between the two can be alleviated. Thus calls for physician-assisted suicide can be expected to become rarer and rarer, and as medicine's capacities for pain control are finally equalized with its capacities for life prolongation, finally virtually to disappear. Almost no one imagines that there will not still be a few difficult situations in which life is prolonged beyond the point at which pain can be effectively controlled, but these will be increasingly infrequent, it is assumed, and in general, as the disparity between our capacities for life prolongation and for pain control shrinks, interest in and need for physician-assisted suicide will decrease and all but disappear.

Fortunately, this view continues, the public debate over physician-assisted suicide now so intense will not have been a waste, since it has both warned against the potential cruelty of overzealous prolongation of life and at the same time stimulated greater attention to imperatives of pain control. The current debate serves as social pressure for bringing equalization of the disparity about. Yet as useful as this debate is, this view holds, it will soon subside and disappear; we're just currently caught in a turbulent—but fleeting—little maelstrom.

The Longer View

That's how things look now. But I think we can also see our current concern with physician-assisted suicide in a longer-term, historically informed view. Consider just three of the many profound changes that affect matters of how we die. First, there has been a shift, beginning in the middle of the last century, in the ways in which human beings characteristically die. Termed the "epidemiological transition," this change involves a shift away from death due to parasitic and infectious disease (ubiquitous among humans in all parts of the globe prior to about 1850) to death in later life of degenerative disease—especially cancer and heart disease, which together account for almost two-thirds of deaths in the developed countries.[3] This means

2. See, e.g., Daniel Callahan, *Setting Limits: Medical Goals in an Aging Society* (New York: Simon and Schuster, 1987), *What Kind of Life? The Limits of Medical Progress* (New York: Simon and Schuster, 1990), and *Tile Troubled Dream of Life: Living with Mortality* (New York: Simon and Schuster, 1993). On acceleration of pain-control development, see especially the work of Kathleen Foley, "Pain, physician-assisted suicide, and euthanasia," *Pain Forum* 4 (3) (1995) and other works.
3. The term originates with A. R. Omran, "The Epidemiologic Transition: A Theory of the Epidemiology of Population Change," *Milbank*

dramatically extended lifespans and also deaths from diseases with characteristically extended downhill terminal courses. Second, there have been changes in religious attitudes about death: People are less likely to see death as divine punishment for sin, or to see suffering as a prerequisite for the afterlife, or to see suicide as a highly stigmatized and serious sin rather than the product of mental illness or depression. Third among the major shifts in cultural attitudes that affect the way we die is the increasing emphasis on the notion of individual rights of self-determination, reinforced in the latter part of this century by the civil rights movement's attention to individuals in vulnerable groups. This shift has affected self-perceptions and attitudes towards the terminally ill, and patients, including dying patients, are now recognized to have a wide array of rights previously eclipsed by the paternalistic practices of medicine.

These three transitions, along with many other concomitant cultural changes, invite us to see our current concern with physician-assisted suicide in a quite different way—not just as a phenomenon resulting from the currently disparate development of life-prolonging and pain-controlling technologies, a temporary anomaly, but as a precursor, an early symptom of a much more substantial sea change in attitudes about death. We might call this shift in attitudes a shift towards "directed dying" or "self-directed dying," in which the individual who is dying plays a far more prominent, directive role than in earlier eras in determining how and when his or her death shall occur. In this changed view, dying is no longer *something that happens to you* but *something you do*.

To be sure, this shift—if it is one—can be seen as already well under way. Taking its legally visible start with the California Natural Death Act of 1976, terminally ill patients have already gained dramatically enlarged rights of self-determination in matters of guiding and controlling their own deaths, including rights to refuse treatment, discontinue treatment, stipulate treatment to be withheld at a later date, designate decisionmakers, and to negotiate with their physicians, or have their surrogates do so, such matters as DNR orders, withholding and withdrawal of ventilators, surgical procedures, nutrition and hydration, the use of opioids, and even terminal sedation. Some patients also negotiate, or attempt to negotiate, physician-assisted suicide or physician-performed euthanasia with their physicians. In all of this, we already see the patient playing a far more prominent role in determining the course of his or her dying process and its character and timing, and far more willingness on the part of physicians, family members, the law, and other parties to respect the patient's preferences and choices in these matters.

But this may be just the tip of a looming iceberg. for we may ask whether, much as we human beings have made dramatic gains in control over our own reproduction (particularly rapidly in very recent times—the birth control pill was introduced just thirty years ago), we human beings are beginning to make dramatic gains in control over our own dying, particularly rapidly in the last several decades. We cannot keep from dying altogether, of course. But by using directly caused death, as in physician-assisted suicide, it is possible to control many of dying's features: its timing in the downhill course of a terminal disease, its place, the exact agents which cause it, its observers, and so on. Indeed, as Robert Kastenbaum has argued,

Memorial Fund Quarterly 49 (4): 509–38 (1971); and the theory is augmented in A. Jay Olshansky and A. Brian Ault, "The Fourth Stage of the Epidemiologic Transition: The Age of Delayed Degenerative Disease," in Timothy M. Smeeding et al., eds., *Should Medical Care Be Rationed By Age?* (Totowa, NJ: Rowman and Littlefield, 1987, pp. 11–43.

because it makes it possible to control the time, place, manner and people present at one's death, assisted suicide will become the *preferred* manner of dying.[4]

But this conjecture doesn't yet show what could actually motivate such substantial social change, away from a culture which sees dying primarily as *something that happens to you,* to a culture which sees it as *something you do*—a deliberate, planned activity, one's final and culminative activity. What might do this, I think, is a conceptual change, or, more exactly, a shift in decisional perspective in choice-making about pain, suffering, and other elements of dying. It is the kind of shift in decisional perspective that evolves on a society-wide scale as a populace gains understanding of and control over a matter, a shift in choice-making perspective from a stance we might describe as immediately involved or "enmeshed," to one that is distanced and reflective. (I'll use two Latin names for these stances later.) This shift can occur for many features of human experience—it has already largely occurred in the developed world with respect to reproduction—but it has not yet occurred with respect to death and dying. It has not yet occurred—or rather, perhaps, it has just begun.

Take a patient, an average man. This particular man is so average that he just happens to have contracted that disease which is the usual diagnosis (as we know from the Netherlands) in cases of physician-assisted suicide—cancer—and he is also so average that this disease will kill him at just the average life-expectancy for males in the United States, 72.8 years.[5] Furthermore, he is also so average that if he does turn to physician-assisted suicide, he will choose to forgo just about the same amount of life that, on average, Dutch patients receiving euthanasia or physician-assisted suicide do, less than 3.3 weeks.[6] He has been considering physician-assisted suicide since his illness was first diagnosed (since he is an average man, this was about 29.6 months ago), but now, as his condition deteriorates, he thinks more seriously about it. His motivation includes both preemptive elements, the desire to avoid some of the very worst things that terminal cancer might bring him, and reactive elements, the desire to relieve some of the symptoms and other suffering that he is already experiencing. *It's bad enough now,* he tells his doctor, *and it will probably get worse.* He asks his doctor for the pills. He is perfectly aware of what he may miss—a number of weeks of continued life, the possibility of an unexpected cure, the chance, even if it is a longshot, of spontaneous regression or remission, and—not to be overlooked—the possibility that that the worst is over, so to speak, and that the remainder of his down-hill course in terminal cancer won't be so bad. He is also well aware that even a bad agonal phase may nevertheless include moments of great intimacy and importance with his family or friends. But he makes what he sees as a rational choice, seeking to balance the risks and possible benefits of easy death now, versus a little more continuing life

4. Robert Kastenbaum, "Suicide as the Preferred Way of Death," in Edwin S. Shneidman, ed. *Suicidology: Contemporary Developments* (New York: Grune and Stratton, 1976), pp. 425–41.

5. Data on physician-assisted suicide and euthanasia in the Netherlands is provided by what is called the "Remmelink Commission Report." Paul J. van der Maas, Johannes J. M. van Delden, and Loes Pijnenborg, "Euthanasia and Other Medical Decisions Concerning the End of Life," published in full in English as a special issue of *Health Policy* 22, nos. 1 and 2 (1992); and, with Caspar W. M. Looman, in summary in *The Lancet* 338 (Sept. 14, 1991): 669–74; and the five-year update in Paul J. van der Maas, et al., "Euthanasia, Physician-Assisted Suicide, and Other Medical Practices involving the End of Life in the Netherlands, 1990–1995," *New England Journal of Medicine* 335 (22): 1699–1705 (1996).

6. See Ezekiel J. Emanuel and Margaret P. Battin, "The Economics of Euthanasia: What are the Potential Cost Savings from Legalizing Physician-Assisted Suicide?" MSS in progress, citing data from the Netherlands.

with a greater possibility of a hard death. He is making his choice *in medias res,* in the middle of things, as the physical, social, and emotional realities of terminal illness engulf him. He is enmeshed in his situation, caught in it, trapped between what seem like two bad alternatives—suffering, or suicide.

But, of course, he might have done his deciding about how his life shall end and whether to elect physician-assisted suicide in preference to the final stages of terminal illness from a quite different, more distanced perspective, a secular version of the view *sub specie aeternitatis.* This is not just an objective, depersonalized view—anybody's view—but his own, distinctively personal view not confined to a specific timepoint.[7] Rather than assessing his prospects from the point of view he has at the time at which he would continue or discontinue his life-that point late in the course of his illness when things have already become "bad enough" and are likely to get worse-he might have done his deciding, albeit rather more hypothetically, from the perspective of a more generalized view of his life.

From this alternative perspective, what he would have seen is the overall shape of his life, and it is with respect to this that he would have made his choices about how it shall end. Of course, he could not know in advance whether he will contract cancer, or succumb to heart disease, or be hit by a bus—though he does know that he will die sometime or other. Consequently, his choices are necessarily conditional in form: "*If* I get cancer, I'll refuse aggressive treatment and use hospice care"; "*If* I get AIDS, I'll ask for physician-assisted suicide"; "If I get Alzheimer's, I'll commit suicide on my own, since no physician besides Jack Kevorkian would help me," and so on. Although conditional in form and predicated on circumstances that may not occur, these may be real choices nonetheless, and, particularly because they are reiterated and repeated over the course of a lifetime, have real motive force.

The difference, then, between these two views is substantial. In the first, our average man with an average terminal cancer, doing his deciding *in medias res,* is deciding whether or not to take the pills his physician has given him now. It is his last possible couple of weeks or a month (on average, 3.3 weeks) that he is deciding about. Even if continuing life threatens pain and other suffering, it is still all he has left, and while it may be difficult to live this life—all he has left—it may also be very difficult to relinquish it.

In contrast, if our average man were doing his deciding *sub specie aeternitatis,* from a distanced though still personal viewpoint not tied to a specific moment in his life, he would have been deciding all along between two different conceptions of his own demise, between two possible lives for himself. One of his possible lives would, on average, be 72.8 years long, the average lifespan for a male in the United States, with the possibility of substantial suffering at the end—on average, as the SUPPORT study finds, a 50 percent chance of moderate to severe pain at least 50 percent of the time during the last three days before his death. The other of his possible lives would be about 72.7 years long, foreshortened on average 3.3 weeks by physician-assisted suicide, but with a markedly reduced possibility of substantial suffering at the end. (This shortening of the lifespan is not age-based but time-to-death based, planned for, on average, 3.3 weeks before an unassisted death would have occurred; it occurs in this example at age 72.7 just because our man is so average.) This latter, shortened life also offers our man the opportunity to control

---

7. The distinction I am drawing here between personal views *in medias res* and *sub specie aeternitatis* is thus not quite the same as that drawn by Thomas Nagel between subjective and objective views, though it has much in common with Nagel's distinction in contexts concerning death. See Nagel, *The View from Nowhere* (New York: Oxford University Press, 1986), especially chapter XI, section 3, on death.

the timing, the place, the manner, and other features of his death in the way he likes. Viewed *sub specie aeternitatis,* at any or many earlier points in one's life or from a vantage point standing outside life, so to speak, the difference between 72.8 and 72.7 seems negligible: These are both lives of average length not interrupted by grossly premature death. Why not choose the one in which the risk of agonal pain—as high as 50/50, according to the SUPPORT study—is far, far less great, and the possibility of conscious, culminative experience, surrounded by family members, trusted friends, and permitting final prayers and goodbyes, is far, far greater?

It may seem difficult to distinguish these two choices in practice. This is because we typically make our decisions about death and dying *in medias res,* not *sub specie aeternitatis,* and our medical practices, our bioethics discussions, and our background culture strongly encourage this. The call for assisted dying, like other patient pleas, is seen as a reaction to the circumstances of dying, not a settled, longer term, preemptive preference.[8] True, some independently minded individuals consider these issues in a kind of background, hypothetical way throughout their lives, but this is certainly not the practical norm. We can only really understand this view as involving a substantial cultural shift from our current perspective.

But if this shift occurs, a slightly abbreviated lifespan in which there is dramatically reduced risk of pain and suffering will not only seem to be preferable to one which is negligibly longer but carries substantial risk of pain and suffering in its agonal phase, it will also be seen as rational and normal to plan for this abbreviated lifespan and to plan the means of bringing it about. The way to ensure it, of course, is to plan for direct termination of life. After all, one cannot count on being able to discontinue some life-prolonging treatment or other—refusing antibiotics, disconnecting a respirator—to hasten death and thus avoid what might be the worst weeks at the end. This most likely means planning for physician-assisted suicide. From this distanced perspective, a 72.7-year life with a virtually assured good end looks much, much better than a 72.8-year life that has an even chance of coming to a bad end. Arguably, it would be rational for any individual, except those for whom religious commitments or other scruples rule out suicide altogether, to plan to ensure this. But if it looks this way to one individual, it will look this way to many; and it is thus plausible to imagine that physician-assisted suicide would not be rare but rather a choice viewed as rational and preemptively prudent by many or most members of the culture. Thus it can come to be seen as a normal course of action, not a rarity or a "last resort." To be sure, there are other ways of abbreviating a lifespan to avoid terminal suffering—withdrawing or withholding treatment, overusing of morphine or other pain-relieving drugs, discontinuing artificial nutrition and hydration, and terminal sedation—but these cannot be used unless the patient's condition has already worsened and is thus likely to involve that pain or suffering the person might choose to avoid. Thus these other modalities function primarily reactively; it is assisted suicide that can function preemptively.

But, as soon as planning for a normal, slight abbreviation in the lifespan by means of assisted suicide becomes conceptually possible not just for our average man but for actual persons in general, it also becomes possible to imagine a wide range of context-specific cultural practices which might emerge surrounding physician-assisted suicide. After all, that a person understands and expects his life-span to be one which will end in an assisted death a few weeks before he might otherwise have died, while he is still

8. See C. G. Prado, *The Last Choice: Preemptive Suicide in Advanced Age* (Westport, Conn.: Greenwood Press, 1990).

conscious, alert, and capable of deciding what location he wants it to take place in, what family members, caregivers, clergy, or others he wants to have present, what ceremonies, religious or symbolic, he wants conducted, etc., suggests that more general social practices would grow up around these possibilities. After all, our average man sees his life this way; but it is possible for him to do this partly because the others in his society see their lives this way as well. Attitudes about death are heavily socially conditioned, and so are the perspectives from which choice-making about death is seen.

This is the precondition for the development of a whole range of social practices supporting such choices. These might include various kinds of practical supports, such as legal, insurance, and other policies that treat assisted dying as acceptable and normal; various sorts of cultural and religious practices that similarly treat assisted dying as acceptable and normal (for instance by developing rituals and rites concerning the forthcoming death); familial supports within the family, including family gatherings, preparing for the death, and sharing reminiscences and goodbyes; pre-death dispositions of wills and life insurance (we already recognize viaticums, pre-death payoffs of life insurance for terminally ill patients); and even such now-inconceivable practices as pre-death funerals, understood as ceremonies of leavetaking and farewell, expressions of both celebration of a life complete and grief at its loss. In turn, such social practices come to function as positive reasons for choosing a somewhat earlier, elective death—formerly and rudely called "physician-assisted suicide," even when pain control is no longer the issue at all—and the new social pattern, so different from our current one-reinforces itself. This has nothing to do with a *Soylent Green* sort of view, in which people are forced into choices they do not genuinely make (this film can be understood only from our current, *in medias res* view); but a world in which their normal choices have genuinely changed, and changed for reasons which seem to them good.

Furthermore, if the culture-wide view of choice making about death and dying were more fully held *sub specie aeternitatis* in this distanced, less enmeshed and less merely reactive way, in which earlier, elective death becomes the norm, we could also expect the more frequent practice of "setting a date," as people who have contracted predictably terminal illnesses carry out the plans they had been developing all along for their own demises. Setting a date for one's own death—presumably, a couple of weeks or so before the date it might naturally have been, revisable of course in the light of any changes in the diagnosis or prognosis—would still be both preemptive and reactive in character, but far more preemptive than choices made *in medias res,* where choices will be highly reactive to the then current circumstances the patient finds himself or herself in. The timing of such choices might always be revised in consultation with the physician; but what would be culturally reinforced would be the general commitment to advance planning for one's own death as well as a commitment to assuming a comparatively autonomist, directive role in it. Self-directed dying would be the norm, though of course different people would direct their deaths in quite different ways.

If profound changes affecting matters of how we die are already underway—the epidemiological transition, shifting from parasitic and infectious disease deaths to deaths of predictably degenerative disease; the changes in religious conceptions of suicide so that it is not understood primarily as sin; and the steadily increasing attention to patients' and terminally ill patients' rights of self-determination—it is an open conjecture whether this is where we may be going. Are we in fact experiencing just a temporary aberration in our basic cultural patterns of death and dying, an aberration which is a function of the discrepant development of technologies for life prolongation and for pain control? Or are we seeing the first breaking waves of a sea-change from one perspective on death and dying to another, a far more autonomist and directive one much as we have seen changes in reproduction?

Obviously, I can't say. But I can say that if this is what is happening, the assumption that physician-assisted suicide would or should be rare, an assumption still held by both sides in the current debate, will collapse. We would have no reason to assume that assisted dying should be rare, whatever the relationship between capacities for life prolongation and pain control. Of course, such a picture is very difficult to envision, since we do not think that way about death and dying now. But if we can at least see what is different about viewing personal choices about one's own death *sub specie aeternitatis* and in our current way, *in medias res*, enmeshed in particular circumstances, we can understand why it might occur.

Would it be a good thing, or a bad thing? I can hardly answer that question here, but let me close with a story I heard somewhere in the Netherlands several years ago. I do not remember the exact source of the story nor the specific dates or names, and it is certainly not representative of current practice in Holland. But it was told to me as a true story, and it went something like this:

> Two friends, old sailing buddies, are planning a sailing trip in the North Sea in the summer. It is late February now, and they are discussing possible dates.
>
> "How about July 21?" says Willem. "The North Sea will be calm, the moon bright, and there's a music festival on the southern coast of Denmark we could visit."
>
> "Sounds great," answers Joost. "I'd love to get to the music festival. But I can't be gone then; the twenty-first is the date of my father's death."
>
> "Oh, I'm so sorry, Joost," Willem replies. "I knew your father was ill. Very ill, with cancer. But I didn't realize he had died."
>
> "He hasn't," Joost replies. "That's the day he will be dying. He's picked a date and made up his mind, and we all want to be there with him."

Such a story seems just that, a story, a fiction, somehow horrifying and also somehow liberating, but in any case virtually inconceivable to us. But it was not told to me as a fiction, but as a true story. I've tried to explore the conceptual assumptions that might lie behind such a story, and to consider whether in the future such stories might become more and more the norm. I have not tried to say whether this would be good or bad, but only that this might well be where we are going. In fact, I think it would be good—just as I think increasing personal control over reproduction is good—but I haven't argued for that view here.

In this respect, what the Supreme Court has done in its 1997 *Washington* v. *Glucksberg* and *Vacco* v. *Quill* decision may make a substantial difference. To ban physician-assisted suicide altogether would have been to reinforce the conception that physician-assisted suicide, if it occurs at all, should be rare; to recognize it as a constitutionally based right would have been to begin to create the psychological and legal space within which individuals could reflect in a longer term way about their own future choices when they come to dying, perhaps making physician-assisted suicide an eventual part of their plans, and indeed planning whatever family gatherings, ceremonies, and religious observances they might wish—not as a desperate last resort or reactive escape from bad circumstances, but as a preemptively prudent, significant, culminative experience. To leave the matter with the states, as the Supreme Court in fact did, will be somewhere in between, depending on whether most individual states respond by reinforcing prohibitions or permitting legalization; here, only time will tell.

www.ingramcontent.com/pod-product-compliance
Lightning Source LLC
Chambersburg PA
CBHW061349210326
41598CB00035B/5936